AN INTRODUCTION

TO HEALTH POLICY

AN INTRODUCTION
TO HEALTH POLICY

TOBA BRYANT

Canadian Scholars' Press Inc.
Toronto

An Introduction to Health Policy
by Toba Bryant

First published in 2009 by
Canadian Scholars' Press Inc.
180 Bloor Street West, Suite 801
Toronto, Ontario
M5S 2V6

www.cspi.org

Canadian Scholars' Press Inc. gratefully acknowledges financial support for our publishing activities from the Government of Canada through the Book Publishing Industry Development Program (BPIDP) and the Government of Ontario through the Ontario Book Publishing Tax Credit Program.

Library and Archives Canada Cataloguing in Publication

Bryant, Toba
    An introduction to health policy / Toba Bryant.

Includes bibliographical references and index.
ISBN 978-1-55130-349-9

    1. Medical policy—Canada. 2. Medical policy. I. Title.

RA395.C3B793 2009   362.10971   C2008-906678-2

Interior design and composition: Brad Horning and Stewart Moracen
Cover design: John Kicksee/KIX BY DESIGN
Cover art: "Operation room," © istookphoto.com/Gizmo

09 10 11 12 13   5 4 3 2 1

Printed and bound in Canada by Marquis Book Printing Inc.

Canada

For Alexander and Dennis

TABLE OF CONTENTS

PREFACE

There are many books on health policy and public policy that have been designed for the policy specialist. This book was developed with the intent of making health policy accessible to students and practitioners in a range of health sectors. These include health professionals such as nurses, physicians, social workers, and other allied health care professionals who are on the front lines of health care delivery. The second audience is post-secondary students in these same areas, as well as those studying health policy and public policy.

This book is not a compendium of every health policy or health policy initiative undertaken in Canada. Rather, the book explores some of the key developments in health policy in Canada and elsewhere. It does not regard health policy as a process that simply requires management of facilities and human resources. It is a public policy area that is driven and influenced by social, political, and economic forces.

The book draws upon the approach taken by Gill Walt in her excellent book, *Health Policy: An Introduction to Process and Power*. In that 1994 book, Walt presented a framework of health policy focused on process and power. She was specifically interested in the political, economic, and social forces that shape how policy is developed and implemented. While it is a highly readable text, Walt focused largely on health policy in the United Kingdom.

I wanted to write a book that considered health policy in Canada and did so within the context of recent international developments in economic and public policy, including economic globalization and free trade agreements. Therefore, an important theme in this volume is the impact of economic globalization on health policy and health care in Canada, and the impact of the market on health policy, not only in terms of health care provision, but also on the health-related public policy that shapes the health of the population.

While it is true that the major health problems in the world today are found in developing nations, this volume focuses on health policy among developed economies such as Canada, the United States, the United Kingdom, and others.

Much of the existing health policy literature in Canada focuses on health care policy to the exclusion of public policy that shapes a jurisdiction's population health. Public policy that influences population health through the provision of economic, political, and social resources is also health policy. This recognition— that what are now termed the social determinants of health strongly influence health outcomes—appeared during the 19th-century writings of Rudolph Virchow and Friedrich Engels. The implications of this knowledge have been integrated into health policy in Europe, but less so in Canada. This book therefore considers the political, economic, and social forces that shape both health care policy and health-related public policy in Canada. By doing so, it aims to make understandable the processes and means of producing health policy in the service of health.

The first few chapters of this book serve as a road map to this inquiry. It first lays out the theoretical terrain that underpins health policy by examining key public policy frameworks and various paradigms of health and paradigms of knowledge. It outlines four health lenses: (1) the biomedical; (2) lifestyle; (3) socio-environmental; and (4) critical/structural. It also discusses how the dominant theoretical approaches in the social sciences—positivism, interpretive/hermeneutics, and the critical social science perspective—help explain how health policy comes about. The paradigms have different assumptions about the world and how it can be understood and studied with clear implications for understanding how health policy is made.

The book then discusses how health care delivery is organized in Canada by examining federal legislation on health care financing and administration from 1958 to the present day. It details how health care reform has dominated health policy discussions since 2000, and some of the emerging themes in health policy are examined. These include issues of public versus private financing and delivery of health care services, the impact of economic globalization on health policy, and how various sectors come to shape health policy. How these developments shape health-related public policy related to income, housing, and other social determinants of health is also examined.

Each chapter contains boxed inserts that illustrate the key concepts discussed. Tables and figures further clarify the concepts examined in each chapter. In addition, each chapter concludes with critical thinking questions, URLs for resources available on the Internet, and recommended further readings. These resources are intended to help extend discussion on the issues and enhance students' conceptual understanding of health policy concepts and issues.

Understanding health policy and how it is developed and implemented are essentials skills for those concerned about health care and health in Canada. I hope that those reading this book come away with a better understanding of these processes and how they can be influenced in the service of health.

■ ACKNOWLEDGEMENTS

Few books are written without the support of many people. I would like to thank Megan Mueller, editorial director at Canadian Scholars' Press Inc., who encouraged this project from the prospectus. Megan is thoroughly professional, warm, and always encouraging. As well, I would like to thank the reviewers—David Coburn, Suzanne Jackson, Duncan Sinclair, and Paula Goering—for their insights and constructive comments. All helped to strengthen the prose and the content of the book.

The beginnings of this book are found in my doctoral thesis on health and social policy change. The supervision and constructive contributions and insights of David Hulchanski, my thesis supervisor, and my diligent committee members— Ron Manzer, Sheila Neysmith, and Irv Rootman—also helped to shape this volume.

Finally, I would also like to thank Dennis Raphael, my husband and scholar, who provided support during the writing. Also, a special thank-you to Alexander, my son. For a seven-and-a-half-year-old, he is a very perceptive little boy who coped well while Mother worked doggedly to complete this project.

Toba Bryant
Toronto, July 2008

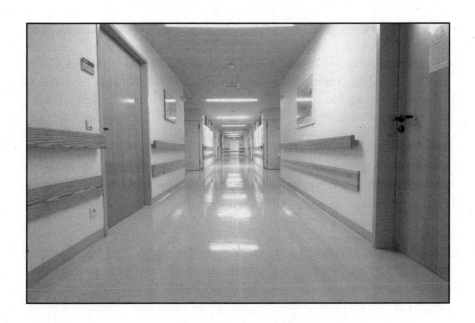

Chapter 1
INTRODUCING HEALTH POLICY
AND POLICY STUDIES

■ INTRODUCTION: WHAT IS HEALTH POLICY?

Policy refers to plans and procedures developed and implemented by governments, agencies, organizations, and associations to achieve desired goals. *Public* policy refers to a course of action or inaction chosen by *public* authorities to address a given problem or interrelated set of problems (Pal, 2006). Health policy is a subset of public policy and is concerned with addressing various health-related issues. The focus of this book is on health policy and how it is developed by governments and implemented by health authorities.

Since health policy is a subset of public policy, it is important to understand what public policy is. Public policy is a course of action that is anchored in a set of values regarding appropriate public goals and a set of beliefs about the best way to achieve those goals. The idea of public policy is that an issue is not a private affair, but one that needs to be addressed by the larger society in the public domain (Pal, 2006).

At another level, health policy is also about politics, power, and process (Walt, 1994). In other words, who has power and who does not have power to influence health policy outcomes? Who benefits and who does not benefit from health policy changes? What is the nature of the political or policy change process? For example, in Canada, the medical doctor or physician is usually the gatekeeper to many aspects of the health care system, including being seen by medical specialists, physiotherapists, and other health care providers. The dominance of the medical profession creates particular dynamics that affect the delivery of care and the ability of other health professionals such as nurses, pharmacists, and physiotherapists to influence health policy.

Medical dominance also influences the public's ability to influence health policy by having governments either address or neglect certain issues. Many health policy issues are of special importance to the medical profession, and their dominance shapes whether and how governments address them. This dynamic also influences the nature of health policy itself and leads to an emphasis on health care organization and delivery as opposed to development and implementation of other public policies that shape health. Various groups all attempt to influence health policy debates and outcomes, but clearly all do not participate on a level playing field. Therefore, politics—in all its meanings—permeates the study of health policy (see Box 1.1).

Box 1.1: What Is Politics?

Politics is multidimensional.

- *Politics as government:* Politics is primarily associated with the art of government and the activities of the state.
- *Politics as public life:* Politics is primarily concerned with the conduct and management of community affairs.
- *Politics as conflict resolution:* Politics is concerned with the expression and resolution of conflicts through compromise, conciliation, negotiation, and other strategies.
- *Politics as power:* Politics is the process through which desired outcomes are achieved in the production, distribution, and use of scarce resources in all areas of social existence.

Source: Bambra, C., Fox, D. & Scott-Samuel, A. (2005). Towards a politics of health. *Health Promotion International, 20,* 187–193.

■ THE SCOPE OF HEALTH POLICY

Health policy encompasses both health care and other health-related public policies. The state, represented by the government of the day, determines the organization of health care and resource allocations for the delivery of health care services to the population. In countries that have public health care systems such as Canada, the state has a very direct role in this. In other words, Canada has a publicly financed system of public health care insurance. But the state also affects health policy in nations where the private sector plays a significant part even if that governmental role is one of allowing the private sector to dominate policymaking. For example, the United States' public policy is dominated by market-driven approaches so that its health care system consists primarily of a wide range of private health insurance plans (Navarro, 1994). Many employers in the US provide health benefits to their employees, but 47 million Americans have no health insurance coverage. There, the only populations who receive health benefits from the government as a matter of right are seniors and people identified as destitute or close to being destitute. But even then, health care is dominated by a for-profit model provided by a multitude of health care institutions.

Health policy has a broad scope and is concerned not only with health care but also with improving and maintaining population health (Canadian Population Health Initiative, 2004). In North America, this broader approach to promoting health is not as developed as it is in other nations. In Canada, consideration of health-related public policy beyond the purview of the health care system is rare. As an example, Canada's concern with health status indicators is usually focused on the effects of health care access and delivery (Canadian Institute for Health Information & Statistics Canada, 2002). Even though Canadian policy documents have argued that there are many factors that lie outside the health care sector—the social determinants of health or people's living conditions—that influence these indicators and hence the health of a population, there has been little policy action in support of these arguments (Raphael, 2007).

In contrast, in many European nations, health policy has a much broader meaning than the delivery of health care services (Mackenbach & Bakker, 2002). In many European nations, health policy is also concerned with addressing the broader policy issues associated with various determinants of health such as income, housing, and education (European Policy Health Impact Assessment Project, 2004). This concern is grounded in frameworks that consider the provision of income, housing, and food security as ensuring that people are provided the resources necessary for health. As a result, there is particular attention given to how the provision of citizen security plays out in health status indicators (such as infant and adult mortality rates) and the incidence and mortality from a range of diseases (such as cardiovascular disease, diabetes, and other chronic diseases) (Mackenbach & Bakker, 2003).

In these jurisdictions governments are seen as having an important role in promoting the health and well-being of its citizens not only through the provision of health care, but also by addressing these social determinants of health. In this volume, the broader definition of health policy is applied. Health policy is concerned with a range of issues that affect health and well-being in addition to its obvious concern with health care organization and provision.

■ THE EVOLUTION OF HEALTH POLICY

The provision of health care as an entitlement in many industrialized nations began in earnest at the end of the Second World War (Teeple, 2000). By the mid-1970s, virtually all these industrialized nations, with the exception of the United States, developed public health care systems as part of the postwar welfare state. In terms of health-related public policies—which are normally defined as encompassing the welfare state such as those providing income, employment, and other forms of security—the postwar period was also a time of expansion. This was especially the case in nations such as Canada, the US, and the UK. Interestingly, the seeds of the welfare state were planted much earlier in many European nations, especially in the Scandinavian nations (Einhorn & Logue, 2003).

The driving value in health care developments was on the provision of health services on the basis of need rather than the ability to pay. (This principle eventually became enshrined in Canadian health policy statements.) The creation of a public health care system, similar to developments in other public policy areas such as public education, was an expression of societal will to share the cost of health care across the population. This sharing would ensure universal access to health care services for all citizens regardless of the ability to pay or the place of residence. Relating back to the definition of public policy provided earlier, health care in Canada had become a public issue to be provided by the state on the basis of need. The guiding value was universality, whereby all Canadians were entitled to receive health services without user fees.

Prior to the development of medicare, many people did without health care or, in some cases, lost their homes in order to pay medical costs. At that time, health care was considered a responsibility to be borne by the individual or family. Despite the creation of Canada's health care system during a period of economic prosperity, some argue that Canadian medicare was developed as a response to poverty, not affluence (Yalnizyan, 2006). The experience of the Depression (1929–1939) convinced the Canadian public—with politicians coming on board rather later— that a health care system based on universality provided the preferred solution to

. meeting the health care needs of the population. In addition, returning veterans who had fought in the Second World War wanted something in return for their sacrifices overseas. The initial establishment of a medicare system in Saskatchewan by Premier Tommy Douglas reflected these influences.

Box 1.2: Tommy Douglas: The Greatest Canadian

My friends, watch out for the little fellow with an idea.
—Tommy Douglas, 1961

For more than 50 years, his staunch devotion to social causes, rousing powers of speech, and pugnacious charm made Tommy C. Douglas an unstoppable political force. From his first foray into public office politics in 1934 to his post-retirement years in the 1970s, Canada's "father of medicare" stayed true to his socialist beliefs—often at the cost of his own political fortune—and earned himself the respect of millions of Canadians in the process.

The child of Scottish immigrants, Douglas spent his formative years in Winnipeg, Manitoba, in a home where politics, philosophy, and religion were side dishes at the dinner table. His father, a veteran of two wars, worked part-time in an iron foundry. When money was tight, Douglas and his two sisters had to drop in and out of school as they worked occasional jobs to help pay the bills.

His family's socialist leanings were solidified after Douglas was hospitalized at the age of 10. Due to a bone infection suffered four years earlier, Douglas's knee required several operations, none of which were successful.

Without the money to pay for a specialist, his parents were told that the only option was to amputate their son's leg before the infection spread to the rest of his body. But before that could happen, a visiting surgeon offered to operate on Douglas for free, as long as his students were allowed to attend. The surgery saved Douglas's leg—quite possibly his life—and would serve as his inspiration for his dream of universally accessible medical care.

Not long after this, Douglas would witness first-hand the violent end of Canada's first general strike on a day known as "Bloody Saturday." In the summer of 1919, a teenaged Douglas watched from a rooftop as officers fired on participants in the Winnipeg General Strike and killed two men. The forceful and violent end of the strike further mobilized his dedication to the working man.

During his youth, he tried many different occupations: amateur actor, boxer, and apprentice printer. Douglas found his true calling in 1924 when he enrolled in a liberal arts college run by the Baptist church. It was here that he refined his notion of the "social gospel," a vision of religion-in-action that he would carry through his life. Following several post-graduation years working as a minister in Depression-era Saskatchewan, Douglas made the move to politics in 1935 when he was elected as an MP in the Co-operative Commonwealth Federation, or CCF.

After nine years in the House of Commons polishing his fiery public-speaking talent, Douglas was elected the leader of the provincial CCF in Saskatchewan. With interest in socialism peaking in postwar Canada, the party won a landslide victory in 1944 and Douglas found himself an instant celebrity as the head of North America's first-ever socialist government.

Amid widespread skepticism, Premier Douglas mobilized aggressively, passing more than 100 bills during his first term. He introduced paved roads, sewage systems, and power to most farmers and managed to reduce the provincial debt by $20 million. Over the next 18 years he weathered communist fear campaigns and a province-wide doctors' strike. Elected to five terms, he introduced Saskatchewan residents to car insurance, labour reforms, and his long-standing dream of universal medicare.

But the years spent reforming his home province worked against him when he made his transition to national politics. By the time he was elected to the leadership of the newly formed national New Democratic Party in 1961, many provincial governments had already adopted many of his ideas, diluting his progressive lustre. That, combined with a fervent anti-medicare campaign by Saskatchewan's medical professionals, helped to deal him his first significant defeat in the 1961 federal election. The NDP won only 19 seats, and Douglas lost his cherished seat in Regina.

Douglas continued to promote his socialist policy through the 1960s, but never managed to secure the highest office in the land. The adoption of national medicare and a pension plan by Lester B. Pearson's Liberals gave him hope.

He took his final and most controversial stand during the October Crisis of 1970, when he voted against the implementation of the War Measures Act in Quebec. The move was devastating to his popularity at the time, but he would be heralded years later for sticking by his principles of civil liberty.

He stepped down as leader in 1971, but he stayed on with the party. In 1979, he resigned his seat in Parliament and retired to a house in the Gatineau Hills, just outside Ottawa, where he devoted himself to reforesting his land. He continued to make appearances at NDP functions where he gave his trademark speeches. Douglas died of cancer in 1986.

Tommy Douglas's legacy as a social policy innovator lives on. Social welfare, universal medicare, old age pensions, and mothers' allowances— Douglas helped keep these ideas, and many more, watching as more established political parties eventually came to accept these once-radical ideas as their own.

Source: http://www.cbc.ca/greatest/top_ten/nominee/douglas-tommy.html

The form that public health care takes in Canada reflects a particular policy approach that is grounded in particular principles and values. The public provision of health care is financed through taxation rather than fees for services. Since wealthier people generally pay more taxes and the less wealthy require greater health services, public financing of a universally accessible health care system effectively serves as a form of redistribution of resources from high- to low-income groups (Teeple, 2006). Despite the potential of this transfer serving as a source of conflict among the Canadian public, surveys consistently find medicare to be Canada's most prized social program (Yalnizyan, 2006).

Box 1.3: The Two Phases of Medicare

"When we began to plan medicare (35 years previously), we pointed out that it would be in two phases. The first phase would be to remove the financial barrier between those giving the service and those receiving it. The second phase would be to reorganize and revamp the delivery system—and of course, that's the big item. It's the big thing we haven't done yet."

—Tommy Douglas

Source: Tommy Douglas, from the 1982 film *Folks Call Me Tommy*, as quoted in Saskatchewan Health, *A Saskatchewan vision for health: A framework for change* (Regina: Saskatchewan Health, 1992).

■ THE ROLES OF FEDERAL AND PROVINCIAL GOVERNMENTS IN HEALTH CARE

Canadian federalism is a key institutional concept necessary for understanding the development of medicare. Federalism refers to the division of legislative authority between a central or national government and regional governments. In Canada, these regional governments are the provincial and territorial governments.

In Canada, the federal and provincial governments share responsibility for health care. Section 91 of the Canadian Constitution Act enumerates the powers of the federal government with emphasis on its spending power (Government of Canada, 1867/1982). Thus, the federal government pays some of the costs of provincial health care programs, sets some of the rules for health service provision by the provinces and territories, and provides health care services to some groups such as Aboriginal Canadians on reserves and to members of the military (Brooks & Miljan, 2003).

Section 92, subsection 7 of the Constitution, specifies the powers of the provincial governments and, most notably, invests responsibility for the administration and delivery of health care in these provincial governments. The specific wording of Section 92, subsection 7, assigns provincial legislatures exclusive power to make laws concerning "The Establishment, Maintenance, and Management of Hospitals, Asylums, Charities and Eleemosynary Institutions in and for the Province, other than Marine Hospitals" (Government of Canada, 1867/1982). The wording reflects the state of health care in 1867 when governments played a minimal role in financing, regulating, and funding health care (Brooks & Miljan, 2003). Private organizations and charities built hospitals, which derived revenues from fees paid by patients for the services they received. Hospitals for those with mental illness received a small sum from the provincial governments. In addition, doctors billed patients directly for their services.

Public health issues, such as epidemics and sanitary conditions that adversely affected health, eventually led to the development of public health boards at the local or municipal level. The position of minister of health at the provincial level of government did not emerge until the 1880s. Provincial boards of health were also created at this time. At the federal level the Dominion Department of Health was created in 1919. The much larger state presence in health care did not occur until the middle of the 20th century.

Together, sections 91 and 92 determine that federal influence upon health care occurs through its control of revenue transfers to the provinces. These transfers support provincial health care programs. In turn, the provincial health care plans must comply with the five principles of medicare articulated in the Canada Health Act (1984).

Consistent with this analysis and the structure of the Canadian welfare state, the federal government has attempted to use its spending powers to enforce national standards of medicare and other social programs that have been shown to influence health. These powers and their associated attempts to influence public policy have been a source of ongoing conflict between the federal and provincial governments.

In the past, this power provided means to maintain national standards for both health and social programs. From the 1960s to the 1980s, the federal government played a significant role in financing health care services. The 1980s, however, saw the federal government reducing its health transfers—that is, financial resources, as well as other related transfers—to the provinces while attempting to maintain control over health care. Control of resources for Canadian health care and health-related public policy is a key theme explored in this book.

■ THEORIES OF PUBLIC POLICY

In order to understand the various dimensions of Canadian health policy, it is necessary to lay out various theoretical approaches that attempt to explain how health policy, a subset of public policy, is made and implemented. As an introductory overview, most theories of public policy—and this is especially the case with regard to health policy—fall within one of two camps: consensus or conflict/critical approaches (Walt, 1994). Consensus approaches are concerned with how various groups compete to influence public policy, including health policy, debates. These theories of public policy assume that policy is made based on a rational consideration of various alternative courses of action with choices based on a cost and benefit analysis.

Consistent with this approach, many applied models of policy development and change are built on assumptions drawn from the physical and natural sciences but adapted for consideration of public policy issues. This was an attempt by early public policy theorists to make the world of policy analysis and politics more like science (Albaek, 1995; Brunner, 1991). The intention was to improve the quality of policy decisions by applying scientific principles of rationality and objectivity. In essence, Lasswell, credited as the founder of the policy sciences, attempted to remove consideration of values from public policy inquiry (Lasswell, 1970).

These consensus models tend to concentrate on technical issues such as the day-to-day organization and delivery of health care and analysis of the various roles that various groups and professions play in delivering care and influencing policy development (Walt, 1994). They say little about the economic, political, and social forces that shape the overall organization and delivery of health care services and other public policies that shape health.

Consensus models are important as there are always significant activities that attempt to provide incremental improvements to existing services and other policies that shape health (Walt, 1994). But how useful are they for dealing with broad issues of how health care is organized and delivered? How useful are they for understanding whether there is adequate provision of income, housing, and food security, which are known to be the primary determinants of the health of the population? Can rational cost-benefit type of analyses explain how the broad strokes of health care and health-related public policy come about?

In response to these concerns, some see consensus models as sorely neglecting the important role that political ideology, values, and power play in shaping complex issues such as public policy in general and health policy in particular (Teeple, 2000). Political ideology is a system of ideas about how problems should be addressed, and include issues such as whether government has a responsibility for social provision to the population and whether such provision should be carried out by the public or private sector.

Values are beliefs that come to influence political ideology and come with a significant emotional investment to add to its ideas component. Since it is apparent that ideology and values play important roles in shaping policy, it makes sense that conflict should exist among various competing constituencies who are interested in shaping public policy.

Why would we expect that large for-profit health care corporations and working-class financially insecure Canadians would share the same ideology and values with regard to the provision of health care? And why would we assume that these two groups would have equal ability to influence the development of health policy? Conflict models consider the role that ideology and power and their different manifestations among differing groups play in shaping health policy.

Conflict models, therefore, usually consider broader macro issues in the organization and development of health care policy in particular and health-related public policy in general (Armstrong, Armstrong & Coburn, 2001). There is particular emphasis on the extent to which health policy debates are influenced by social class politics and inequalities in influence and power. Differences in power associated with gender, race, social class, disability, or sexual orientation, among others, not only have implications for the ability to influence policy development (Grabb, 2002), they also have implications for who will be affected—for better or worse—by public policy decisions.

Canadians with less power—working-class Canadians, women, people with low income, those of colour, among others—not only have less influence upon policy development, but are more likely to lack access to health care, as well as resources such as income and employment that support health. As one example, the organization of health care is especially important for populations with health conditions such as HIV/AIDS, yet these groups have less power and influence in society. How would these differences in power and influence affect their ability to influence health policy? And how do these differences influence their health outcomes?

Each model has its place in explaining the development and implementation of health policy, but it may be that some issues may best be understood by drawing on one model rather than another. I argue throughout this volume that health policy issues in particular are driven by strong ideological convictions—shaped by political, economic, and social forces—about how health should be maintained.

■ INDIVIDUALISM IN HEALTH

Another key issue in understanding policy development is that of individualism as an explanatory discourse on health. Individualism is the belief that the focus of attention with regard to health care and health policy should be on the person rather than on environments and societal institutions or structures (Hofrichter, 2003). With respect to health care, it provides a narrow lens focused on treatments and remedies. It may also focus on individual screening for biomedical indicators, and identifying individual risk factors such as poor diet, lack of exercise, and alcohol and tobacco consumption (Nettleton, 1997). Within this approach, concern with broader aspects of the health care system and the political, economic, and social forces that shape health care services and delivery and other health-related public policies tend to be neglected.

Similarly, with regard to health-related public policies concerned with health maintenance or promotion, the focus is again upon individual characteristics and individual behaviours (Hofrichter, 2003). Attention is given to public policies that may influence biomedical indicators such as cholesterol, glucose levels, or weight. Policy actions that shape incidence of risk behaviours such as poor diet, lack of activity, or tobacco and alcohol use also dominate attention. Health policy comes to be narrowly conceived as a means of changing such behaviours. The end result of individualist approaches is a narrow health care focus on individual treatment plans and remedies and ways of shaping individual health-related behaviours.

Individualism can lead to victim-blaming whereby poor health outcomes are attributed to individual "lifestyle choices" rather than the environments and societal institutions that are known to have primary influence upon health outcomes. In Box 1.4, Hofrichter succinctly states the problem with such an approach for both health care policy in particular and health policy broadly conceived.

Box 1.4: Individualism in Health

With exceptions, few decision makers examine the relationship of inequalities in health status to racism or social, political, and economic inequality. None suggest the need for major political and economic transformations to eliminate health inequities. Many analysts and policymakers instead focus on symptoms and treatments, microanalysis of individual risk factors, and changing people's behavior and lifestyles, not conditions or places. They present options primarily through a biomedical model and remedial solutions, mostly associated with health care, rarely stressing social transformation.

Individualism, a powerful philosophy and practice in North America, limits the public space for social movement activism. By transforming public issues into private matters of lifestyle, self-empowerment, and assertiveness, individualism precludes organized efforts to spur social change. It fits perfectly with a declining welfare state and also influences responses to health inequities. From this perspective, each person is self-interested and possessed of a fixed, competitive human nature. Everyone has choice and the potential for upward mobility through hard work—ignoring how we develop through the process of living in society (Tesh, 1988). Individualism presumes that individuals exist in parallel with society instead of being formed by society.

Source: Hofrichter, R. (2003). The politics of health inequities: Contested terrain. In R. Hofrichter (Ed.) *Health and social justice: A reader on ideology, and inequity in the distribution of disease* (pp. 25, 28). San Francisco: Jossey Bass.

Consistent with Hofrichter's analysis, individualist approaches to health dominate policy activity in Canada. Broad questions about health policy give way to the management of health systems and concerns with wait times. Rather than consider the provision of a program to provide prescription drugs to all citizens as a matter of entitlement, focus is upon whether to provide one drug or another to patients undergoing chemotherapy for cancer or heart patients undergoing life-prolonging surgeries.

In the health-related policy arena, governments promulgate messages that promote individual responsibility for reducing the risk of developing chronic diseases, such as heart disease and diabetes, through proper diet and exercise. There is less attention to health-related public policy issues such as income, housing, and food security and how these issues increase the risk of developing these chronic diseases (Raphael, Anstice & Raine, 2003; Raphael & Farrell, 2002). Some argue that governments foster these approaches to justify less government involvement in the provision of social and health services (Raphael, 2007).

Narrow views of health policy also neglect the conflicts and politics endemic to policy discussion. I therefore highlight the idea that health policy is not exclusively about health care and its provision to the larger population. It is about politics, values, and conflict among groups in society and arguments about what contributes to health and well-being. Consistent with Rudolph Virchow's famous dictum "Medicine is social science and politics is medicine on a larger scale," full attention is provided on these issues throughout this volume.

■ EMERGING ISSUES IN HEALTH CARE POLICY IN CANADA

As noted, Canadian federalism has shaped the organization and delivery of health care in Canada. It also shapes the distribution of responsibilities for health care between the two levels of government. It helps explain the continuing debates between them in the health care policy arena. Much has been written about Canadian federalism and its implications for health care. These key issues characterize health care and health-related policy and must be considered in any analysis of health policy.

For example, *the vertical fiscal imbalance* is considered to lie at the heart of the current debate on the future of health care in Canada and has been "the main irritant in intergovernmental relations" for many years (St-Hilaire & Lazar, 2003, p. 60). The imbalance refers to the division of powers for health care and the different revenue-generating capacities of each level of government. In other words, the federal government has the revenue capacity (i.e., the ability to raise money through tax collection) and the provinces and territories have the responsibility to respond to health care needs. The Constitution has thus created a situation in which the taxing powers of the two levels of government do not always match their responsibilities for service provision to the population.

The greater revenue-generating—and funding—power of the federal government has enabled it to exert control over the provinces by dictating in part how the provinces and territories should deliver health care services. In short, at the heart of vertical fiscal imbalance is the capacity of each level of government to generate its own revenues to finance its own expenditures (St-Hilaire & Lazar, 2003). Some observers see advantages to this arrangement. For example, having more taxation occurring at the federal level of government promotes tax harmonization and reduces economic inequalities among provinces and territories.

However, the downside is continuing intergovernmental wrangling over the financing of health care and increasing concern about the future of medicare. Such wrangling and the resultant perception that governments are unable to respond to pressing policy needs may prompt calls to remove health care from the realm of government responsibility and allow a parallel private system of health care to develop.

■ THE CHANGING ROLE OF GOVERNMENT IN HEALTH CARE

Recent funding changes have altered the role of the state in health care and health-related policy. During the 1980s and 1990s federal spending declined, and the provinces and territories had to pick up the slack (Teeple, 2000). While this trend began to reverse with greater federal contributions, there has been growing interest in creating a third level of governmental responsibility in health care by devolving responsibility for health care and other health-related matters to municipal governments. All provinces have devolved health care services to regional bodies (Church & Barker, 1998).

Regionalization is an organizational arrangement that sees development of more locally based administrative and governance structures (Church & Barker,

1998). This structure is authorized to perform functions or exercise authority that was previously the responsibility of provincial or local governments, such as cities. For example, regionalization could involve the transfer of responsibility for public health activities such as sanitation and prenatal care from local health boards to a regional agency. At the same time it could devolve health care authority from a central governing agency such as a provincial government to these same regional bodies.

Regionalization activity stems from a belief within governments that a regional health care system runs more effectively and can be more responsive to local health needs (Church & Barker, 1998). Church and Barker suggest that advocates of regionalization believe that regionalized health care systems deal better with many of the problems currently associated with health care by promoting better service coordination and realizing economies of scale. Greater equity in service delivery containment of health care expenditures may occur.

On the downside, the organization and management of regionalization may fail to involve citizens in health care decision making and reduce accountability even more than may have been the case previously (Church & Barker, 1998; Sutcliffe, Deber & Pasut, 1997). This transfer of power to these regional authorities is an important trend in health care in Canada. What are the implications of these kinds of transfers of power for access to health care and the quality of health care provision?

▇ HEALTH CARE REFORM

Most Canadians agree that medicare can be improved. Several commissions on health care reform have gathered much attention. The predominant reports on health care reform were *A Framework for Reform*, prepared by former federal Minister of Finance Don Mazankowski for the Alberta government, Senator Michael Kirby's *The Health of Canadians: The Federal Role*, and former Saskatchewan Premier Roy Romanow's *Building on Values: The Future of Medicare*, prepared for the federal Liberal government of Prime Minister Jean Chrétien (Kirby, 2002; Mazankowski, 2001; Romanow, 2002). Mazankowski and Kirby favour user fees and private sector involvement in health care delivery and consider health care to represent a "rich commercial opportunity" (Grieshaber-Otto & Sinclair, 2004, p. 9).

Romanow, in contrast, calls for renewal of medicare around the key principles of public financing and not-for-profit delivery. He rejects an increased role for the private sector in health care itself, yet is open to an expanded private sector role in the delivery of ancillary health services such as food services, cleaning services, maintenance services, and other services that are critical to the health care system (Armstrong et al., 2002; Grieshaber-Otto & Sinclair, 2004).

One outcome of all of these activities and commissions has been the federal, provincial, and territorial governments agreeing to focus their efforts on reducing wait times for various medical procedures and devising a health care guarantee (Government of Canada, 2007). Indeed, such a guarantee was recommended by the Mazankowski and Kirby reports (Grieshaber-Otto & Sinclair, 2004; Kirby, 2002; Mazankowski, 2001). This guarantee and its implications suggest another important theme informing Canadian health policy: that of public versus private financing and delivery of health care.

■ HEALTH CARE REFORM AND THE PUBLIC VERSUS PRIVATE HEALTH CARE DEBATE

As noted, the 1980s and 1990s saw—ostensibly to assure the sustainability of medicare—Canadian governments reducing the role of the state in health care by reducing their financial commitments to the provinces. This reduction has been associated with increasing private sector involvement in the financing and delivery of health services. Indeed, Canada now has one of the largest proportion of such private sector involvement in health care among developed nations (Organisation for Economic Co-operation and Development, 2005).

Interacting with these cutbacks, the outlining of health care treatment guarantees has influenced debate regarding public versus private financing and delivery of services. These health care guarantees involve establishing a maximum wait time for each type of major procedure or treatment. When the maximum time has been reached, the insurer (government) would be required to pay for the patient to receive the procedure in another jurisdiction.

It has been suggested that this arrangement could lead to more locally managed and delivered private care if the publicly financed and managed systems become unable to meet these guarantees and the private sector becomes mandated to step in (Rachlis, 2005). Privatization can assume many different forms such as establishing public-private partnerships to build a new hospital, allowing private specialized clinics to provide cataract surgery or hip replacements, or allowing private insurance schemes to support a new tier of health services thereby substituting for the publicly managed system.

Supporters of private health care argue that it is more efficient and has shorter wait times for care. However, studies show that the quality of private care is poorer and has been associated with worse outcomes, in some cases even higher mortality rates (Woolhandler, Campbell & Himmelstein, 2003). Part of this may be related to lack of sufficient staff to provide quality care.

In reality, claims that allowing a parallel private health care system would relieve wait times in the public system are not accurate. Only people of wealth

---

Box 1.5: The Chaoulli Decision and Private Health Care in Canada

The decision by the Supreme Court that struck down a Quebec ban on private health insurance has fuelled calls for a parallel private system (Rachlis, 2005). Many medicare supporters view this decision as a nail in the coffin of medicare. If banning private health insurance to protect the public health care system is seen as violating the Charter of Rights and Freedoms, how can medicare be preserved and protected? What are the key costs and benefits associated with public versus private health care? Is increasing privatization going to create more problems than currently exist?

Source: Rachlis, M. (2005). *Public solutions to health care wait lists.* Ottawa: Canadian Centre for Policy Alternatives.

---

who can afford to pay will jump the queue by seeking private care, while others will remain in the public system (Rachlis, 2004). But since these private clinics will draw physicians from the public system by enticing them with higher salaries and other incentives, waiting lists would increase, not decline. These issues are taken up in later chapters of this book.

There is much evidence to support the view that the public health care system could be improved in some ways. Many of the problems with the system can be attributed to under-resourcing by governments (Armstrong & Armstrong, 2003). However, there is also a need for an emphasis within the public system on preventative care consistent with the vision of Tommy Douglas, the father of medicare. Use of the broader definition of health policy as including other health-related public policies in this book would assure consideration of these broader issues and their implications for the future of the health care system.

■ ECONOMIC GLOBALIZATION AND TRADE TREATIES

Another important theme that informs health policy is that of economic globalization, which is the economic integration of national economies into the global economy (Banting, Hoberg & Simeon, 1997). Canadian governments have justified reduced health and social spending as necessary to maintain medicare and to ensure Canada's competitiveness in the global economy. Economic globalization—with its associated increase in the influence and power of multinational corporations—has contributed to the growing responsiveness of governments to allow private financing and for-profit delivery of health care (Teeple, 2000). While the provided reason is that of increasing Canada's competitiveness in the new global economy, it is important to consider how increasing influence of the private sector in a wide range of policy debates is contributing to such governmental responsiveness.

In addition, Canada is signatory to the North American Free Trade Agreement (NAFTA) and the General Agreement on Trade in Services (GATS). The terms of these trade agreements have implications for Canadian health care and population health as they could lock in privatization and market-driven health care reforms (Grieshaber-Otto & Sinclair, 2004). Some critics argue that economic globalization threatens national sovereignty and the capacity of national governments to set domestic policy (Teeple, 2000). These issues are explored in later chapters of this book.

■ POLIS VERSUS THE MARKET

One way to consider how issues such as economic globalization and increasing privatization of health care can be understood is presented by Deborah Stone's dimension of the polis versus the market in public policymaking. This dimension runs through many themes discussed in this chapter. The distinction also lies at the heart of many debates in the Canadian health policy field.

In *Policy Paradox and Political Reason*, Deborah Stone defines two models of political society: the polis and the market (Stone, 1988). *Polis* is the Greek word for city-state and the term that Stone applies to a model of political society whose primary objective is to act in the interests or welfare of the collective. The polis operates with the community as the level of organization rather than the individual. Political activities are organized around providing for the common good. Such activities may create conflicts among various sectors and groups, but communal, rather than individual, interest is always seen as paramount (see Box 1.6).

In contrast, the *market* is defined as a social system in which individuals engage in various activities, usually economic, to enhance their welfare. They do so by exchanging goods and services with the expectation that such trades will be beneficial to both sides. It works as follows. Participants in the market compete with each other for scarce resources. Each individual attempts to obtain goods and services at the lowest possible cost and to transform raw materials into more valuable items to be sold at the highest possible price.

In the market model then, individuals engage in activities for the sole purpose of maximizing self-interest, defined in whatever ways they wish for themselves. In this context, self-interest can also include acting to protect the welfare of family and friends. Stone argues, however, that the market as a social system can profoundly distort political life by neglecting the role that ideology, politics, and values may play in shaping the organization of society.

Box 1.6: Concepts of Society

	Market Model	Polis Model
1. Unit of analysis	individual	community
2. Motivations	self-interest	public interest (as well as self-interest)
3. Chief conflict	self-interest vs. self-interest	self-interest vs. public interest (commons problems)
4. Source of people's ideas and preferences	self-generation within the individual	influences from outside
5. Nature of collective activity	competition	co-operation and competition
6. Criteria for individual decision making	maximizing self-interest, minimizing cost	loyalty (to people, places, organizations, products), maximize self-interest, promote public interest
7. Building blocks of social action	individuals	groups and organizations
8. Nature of information	accurate, complete, fully available	ambiguous, interpretive, incomplete, strategically manipulated
9. How things work	laws of matter (e.g., material resources are finite and diminish with use)	laws of passion (e.g., human resources are renewable and expand with use)
10. Sources of change	material exchange, quest to maximize	ideas, persuasion, alliances, pursuit of power, pursuit of the public interest

Source: Stone, D. (1988). *Policy paradox and political reason*. Glenview: Scott, Foresman.

Stone notes the launch of what she terms "the rationality project," which is dominated by the market as the model of society (Stone, 1988). She sees the fields of political science, public administration, law, and policy analysis adopting a common mission to save public policy "from the irrationalities and indignities of politics" in order to imbue public policy with rational, analytical, and scientific methods.

In essence, the rationality project depoliticizes inherently political activities such as policymaking by removing values and conflict from consideration. Society is conceived as a "collection of autonomous, rational decision-makers who have no community life" (Stone, 1997, p. 9). As defined above, individuals maximize self-interest through rational calculation of the options before them, whether it is buying a car, a house, or health care.

There is evidence that the increasing emphasis on the market has shaped Canadian policymaking in Canada. The rise of neo-liberalism—the belief that the marketplace should be the arbiter of the creation and distribution of various resources—has driven this development (Coburn, 2001). At a broad governmental level, powerful interests have urged governments to consider health services as an area for investment and trade opportunities. What does this mean for the development of health care policy and the survival of the health care system in Canada? The distorting nature of public policymaking under such a market view is considered in later chapters.

Box 1.7: Neo-liberalism, Public Policy, and Population Health

Neo-liberalism has also influenced health policy as more broadly conceived. One aspect of neo-liberalism is a withdrawal of the state from involvement in the delivery of health services. It has also led to significant reduction in government support of important social determinants of health such as income, housing, and food security, among others. To what extent has the resurgence of neo-liberal ideology associated with governmental withdrawal of resources affected the health status of Canadians? What are the implications of neo-liberal ideology for developing and implementing health care policies and health-related public policies that maintain health?

While all of these health care issues are critical in the study of health policy, they are not the only health-related policy issues that need to be to be considered. Governments also set health-related policies that have differing impacts on the health of different populations. These include issues that impact the incidence of poverty and social exclusion.

Indeed, it is increasingly evident that the way a society organizes the production and distribution of economic and social resources within it influences health outcomes (Marmot & Wilkinson, 2006; Raphael, 2008). These processes can lead to social and economic marginalization, which has been associated with adverse health outcomes. Interestingly, the economic, political, and social forces that affect health care policy are frequently the same that influence health policy as broadly conceived here. It is the intention of this book to define and explain how these forces influence health care policy, health-related policy, and the health of a population as a whole.

■ HEALTH POLICY AND PUBLIC POLICY

Health policy is often separated from public policy theory, and this has limited understanding of how health policy is made. By linking health policy to the broader public policy literature, it becomes possible to articulate the influences and differential impacts on health policy by different societal groups. Such an analysis illustrates how health policy reflects ideological commitments—and action in support of such ideologies—of governments and various interests, sectors, and society (see Box 1.8).

Box 1.8: Unfinished Health-Care Revolution

By Carol Goar
Toronto Star

Twelve years ago, the Ontario Hospital Association set up a health policy think-tank called The Change Foundation. It gave the new organization a generous endowment and set it free to tackle the big questions that no one—not politicians, not bureaucrats, not hospital administrators, not doctors or nurses or drug makers—wanted to touch.

Last week, the foundation invited the country's top health care thinkers to Toronto to grapple with a simple but sensitive question: Has the multi-billion-dollar decentralization of medicare worked?

Every province in the country has divided its health care system into regional units over the last 35 years. Quebec was first, Ontario last. Patients were promised better care. Communities were promised the chance to set their own priorities. Taxpayers were promised a seamless system in which all the players worked together.

Were these promises kept? Did some jurisdictions do better than others? Can Ontario, whose Local Health Integration Networks are still in the formative stages, learn from provinces with more experience?

It was a closed-door symposium. The 40 participants were encouraged to speak freely on the understanding that they would be guaranteed anonymity. But the two lead-off speakers, Ken Fyke, who led Saskatchewan's

Commission on Medicare in 2000, and Steven Lewis, research director of The Change Foundation, agreed that their remarks could be reported. They had plenty to say, little of it complimentary.

Fyke's basic contention was that regionalization was a good idea, badly implemented. "I know of no province that has totally succeeded," he said. "Too many governments have made the structure an end in itself. Until health is the core business, regionalization will fail."

He pointed to four recurring mistakes:

- Political leaders told the public they were decentralizing health care to bring decision making closer to home. But, in most cases, they were trying to insulate themselves from the fallout of closing hospital beds, firing highly paid administrators and reining in spending.
- No one wanted to take on the medical profession, so doctors remained outside the system, operating their private practices on a fee-for-service basis.
- Major chunks of the health-care system—mental health and chronic care—were overlooked, leaving patients without access to a full range of services.
- No clear lines of accountability were set. Governments and regional health boards blamed each other whenever an unpopular decision was made. Patients couldn't figure out who was in charge. Taxpayers didn't know where their money was going.

"All too often, it (regionalization) has been a structure without a mission," Fyke concluded.

Lewis offered an even harsher indictment. He thinks the provinces blew an historic opportunity.

They had a chance to transform Canada's fragmented illness treatment system into an intelligently designed network of health services. Instead, they created another level of administration to shore up the old system.

"It's certainly not the ambitious model we hoped it would be."

Most policy-makers knew, when they embarked on regionalization, that more high-tech equipment, more drugs, and more doctors wouldn't make people healthier. But they took the path of least resistance, Lewis said.

It wasn't entirely a case of political cowardice. Just as regionalization got rolling, the economy stumbled. "In a sense, it was born under a bad sign."

With limited resources, governments focused on hot-button issues: doctor shortages, surgical wait times, emergency-room backups. They mandated regional health boards to do likewise.

For the next 15 years, those priorities prevailed. Ontario, which decentralized its health-care system in the friendlier economic climate of 2006, could have carved out a bolder path, but didn't.

No one at the 1 1/2-day meeting wanted to turn back the clock. But none of the participants could say with assurance that regionalization has improved health, enhanced teamwork, or strengthened medicare.

The good news is that the people in the system have a vision of patient-centred health care.

The bad news is that their political bosses either don't share it or don't have the courage to follow their convictions.

Source: The Toronto Star (May 26, 2008), AA6.

■ CONCLUSION

Health policy is frequently narrowly conceived as being concerned with health care, but should be conceived more broadly. Health policy is a vehicle for governments to respond to health care needs and provide means of supporting a population's health through the development and implementation of health-related public policies. An important issue is the extent to which these activities are best carried out by the public sector or turned over to the private sector as a source of investment and profit.

The understanding of health policy can be advanced by placing it within the broader domain of public policy. Various models for considering public policy are available and these can be designated as consisting of consensus and conflict models. Conflict models consider the role that political ideology, values, and power play in shaping the development and implementation of health policy in particular and public policy in general. These frameworks help to make sense of some of the emerging issues in health policy in Canada: funding and financing, organization and delivery of services, and emphasis upon public versus private organization and delivery of health care. These models also illuminate how public policy in the service of maintaining health is created as well.

■ REFERENCES

Albaek, E. (1995). Between knowledge and power: Utilization of social science in public policy-making. *Policy Sciences, 28*(1)', 79–100.

Armstrong, H. & Armstrong, P. (2003). *Wasting away: The undermining of Canadian health care.* Toronto: Oxford University Press.

Armstrong, P., Armstrong, H. & Coburn, D. (Eds.). (2001). *Unhealthy times: The political economy of health and care in Canada.* Toronto: Oxford University Press.

Armstrong, P., Boscoe, M., Clow, B., Grant, K., Pederson, A. & Willson, K. (2002). *Reading Romanow.* Ottawa: Canadian Women's Health Network.

Banting, K., Hoberg, G. & Simeon, R. (Eds.). (1997). *Degrees of freedom: Canada and the United States in a changing world.* Montreal & Kingston: McGill-Queen's University Press.

Brooks, S. & Miljan, L. (2003). *Public policy in Canada: An introduction.* Toronto: Oxford University Press.

Brunner, R.D. (1991). The policy movement as a policy problem. *Policy Sciences, 24*(1), 65–98.

Canadian Institute for Health Information & Statistics Canada. (2002). *Health care in Canada 2002.* Retrieved from http://secure.cihi.ca/cihiweb/products/HR2002eng. pdf

Canadian Population Health Initiative. (2004). *Improving the health of Canadians.* Ottawa: Canadian Population Health Initiative.

Church, J. & Barker, P. (1998). Regionalization of health services in Canada: A critical perspective. *International Journal of Health Services, 28*(3), 467–486.

Coburn, D. (2001). Health, health care, and neo-liberalism. In P. Armstrong, H. Armstrong & D. Coburn (Eds.), *Unhealthy times: The political economy of health and care in Canada,* 45-65. Toronto: Oxford University Press.

Einhorn, E.S. & Logue, J. (2003). *Modern welfare states: Scandinavian politics and policy in the global age.* Westport: Praeger.

European Policy Health Impact Assessment Project. (2004). *European policy health impact assessment: A guide.* Geneva: European Policy Health Impact Assessment Project.

Government of Canada. (1867/1982). *Canadian Constitution.* Retrieved from http://laws. justice.gc.ca/en/const/c1867_e.html

Government of Canada. (2007). *Canada's new government announces patient wait times guarantees.* Retrieved from http://pm.gc.ca/eng/media.asp?id=1611

Grabb, E. (2002). *Theories of social inequality.* Toronto: Harcourt Canada.

Grieshaber-Otto, J. & Sinclair, S. (2004). *Bad medicine: Trade treaties, privatization, and health care reform in Canada.* Ottawa: Canadian Centre for Policy Alternatives.

Hofrichter, R. (2003). The politics of health inequities: Contested terrain. In R. Hofrichter (Ed.), *Health and social justice: A reader on ideology, and inequity in the distribution of disease,* 1–56. San Francisco: Jossey Bass.

Kirby, M.J. (2002). *The health of Canadians: The federal role.* Ottawa: Standing Senate Committee on Social Affairs, Science, and Technology.

Lasswell, H. (1970). The emerging conception of the policy sciences. *Policy Sciences, 1*(1), 3–14.

Mackenbach, J. & Bakker, M. (Eds.). (2002). *Reducing inequalities in health: A European perspective.* London: Routledge.

Mackenbach, J. & Bakker, M. (2003). Tackling socioeconomic inequalities in health: Analysis of European experiences. *Lancet, 362,* 1409–1414.

Marmot, M. & Wilkinson, R. (2006). *Social determinants of health* (2nd ed.). Oxford: Oxford University Press.

Mazankowski, D. (2001). *A framework for reform: Report of the Premier's Advisory Council on Health.* Edmonton: Government of Alberta.

Navarro, V. (1994). *The politics of health policy: The US reforms 1980–1994.* Cambridge: Blackwell Publishers.

Nettleton, S. (1997). Surveillance, health promotion, and the formation of a risk identity. In M. Sidell, L. Jones, J. Katz & A. Peberdy (Eds.), *Debates and dilemmas in promoting health,* 314–324. London: Open University Press.

Organisation for Economic Co-operation and Development. (2005). *Health at a glance: OECD indicators 2005.* Paris: Organisation for Economic Co-operation and Development.

Pal, L. (2006). *Beyond policy analysis: Public issue management in turbulent times.* Toronto: Nelson.

Rachlis, M. (2004). *Prescription for excellence: How innovation is saving Canada's health care system.* Toronto: HarperCollins.

Rachlis, M. (2005). *Public solutions to health care wait lists.* Ottawa: Canadian Centre for Policy Alternatives.

Raphael, D. (2007). The future of the Canadian welfare state. In D. Raphael (Ed.), *Poverty and policy in Canada: Implications for health and quality of life,* 365–398. Toronto: Canadian Scholars' Press Inc.

Raphael, D. (Ed.). (2008). *Social determinants of health: Canadian perspectives* (2nd ed.). Toronto: Canadian Scholars' Press Inc.

Raphael, D., Anstice, S. & Raine, K. (2003). The social determinants of the incidence and management of type 2 diabetes mellitus: Are we prepared to rethink our questions and redirect our research activities? *Leadership in Health Services, 16,* 10–20.

Raphael, D. & Farrell, E.S. (2002). Beyond medicine and lifestyle: Addressing the societal determinants of cardiovascular disease in North America. *Leadership in Health Services, 15,* 1–5.

Romanow, R.J. (2002). *Building on values: The future of health care in Canada.* Saskatoon: Commission on the Future of Health Care in Canada.

St-Hilaire, F. & Lazar, H. (2003). He said, she said: The debate on vertical fiscal imbalance and federal health-care funding. *Policy Options* (February), 60–67.

Stone, D. (1988). *Policy paradox and political reason.* Glenview: Scott, Foresman.

Sutcliffe, P., Deber, R. & Pasut, G. (1997). Public health in Canada: A comparative study of six provinces. *Canadian Journal of Public Health, 88*(4), 246–249.

Teeple, G. (2000). *Globalization and the decline of social reform: Into the twenty-first century.* Aurora: Garamond Press.

Teeple, G. (2006). Foreword. In D. Raphael, T. Bryant & M. Rioux (Eds.), *Staying alive: Critical perspectives on health, illness, and health care,* 1–4. Toronto: Canadian Scholars' Press Inc.

Walt, G. (1994). *Health policy: An introduction to process and power.* London: Zed Books.

Woolhandler, S., Campbell, T. & Himmelstein, D.U. (2003). Costs of health care administration in the United States and Canada. *New England Journal of Medicine, 349*(8), 768–775.

Yalnizyan, A. (2006). *Controlling vosts: Canada's single-payer system is costly—but least expensive.* Ottawa: Canadian Centre for Policy Alternatives.

CRITICAL THINKING QUESTIONS

1. What does the term "health policy" mean to you? What has informed your understanding of health policy?
2. How does the media report health policy issues? What issues do they highlight? What is missing from these reports?
3. In your other courses, how is health policy defined? What issues have been highlighted?

4. How has what you have read in this chapter about health policy and health care in Canada been consistent or inconsistent with your understandings prior to reading this chapter?

5. If you consider recent federal and provincial election campaigns, how have health issues been presented? Which political party or parties have discussed health policy in broad terms?

FURTHER READINGS

Brunner, R. (1991) The policy movement as a policy problem. *Policy Sciences 24*(1), 65–98.

The author examines the problem of applying a technical definition to complex policy problems. While it is not focused on health policy specifically, it is an interesting assessment of the focus on the rational model and its weaknesses as an analytic tool.

Hofrichter, R. (2003). *Health and social justice: A reader on ideology, and inequity in the distribution of disease.* San Francisco: Jossey Bass.

This volume brings together the recent literature on key aspects of health policy, particularly inequalities in health. Each essay examines particular aspects of health inequalities and shows how inequalities are rooted in public policy.

Pal, L.A. (2006). *Beyond policy analysis: Public issue management in turbulent times.* Toronto: Nelson.

This book is a useful guide to public policy analysis. It defines key concepts and explains the stages of policy formulation, design, implementation, and evaluation. The author factors in the changing political and social environment while focusing on the analytic tools of policy analysis and conceptual dimension of public policy.

Stone, D. (1988). *Policy paradox and political reason.* Glenview: Scott, Foresman.

This text examines the paradox of the polis versus the market. Stone discusses the origins of the current focus on the market and how it depoliticizes politics. Although this is an analysis of American politics, the trends identified pertain to Canadian politics and health policy.

Walt, G. (1994). *Health policy: An introduction to process and power.* London: Zed Books.

This volume is a good basic text on health policy. It is concerned with health policy as process and power. Examples are drawn from health policy in the United Kingdom and Europe.

RELEVANT WEBSITES

Canadian Policy Research Networks
www.cprn.org

The Canadian Policy Research Networks is a non-profit, charitable, policy research think tank. Its health policy network produces research reports on current health policy and health care issues. Their reports and other resources are available on the website.

Centre for Health Services and Policy Research
www.chspr.ubc.ca

The Centre for Health Services and Policy Research is based at the University of British Columbia. This website provides useful information and reports on health care and health policy.

European Community Health Policy
tinyurl.com/2s83r9

The European Community addresses a full scope of health policy, including living conditions and health care. The website identifies health policy priorities for the European Union and links to health policy resources.

Government of Sweden Health Policy
www.sweden.gov.se/sb/d/2942

This is the website of the government of Sweden, a world leader in the social determinants of health and exemplar in developing healthy public policy. This website outlines its priorities in public health and provides access to several resources that discuss Swedish health policy.

International Health Impact Assessment Consortium
www.ihia.org.uk/about.html

Based at the University of Liverpool in the United Kingdom, this excellent website provides a wide range of information and resources on the impact of policies and programs on the health of a population. It provides access to articles, research, and case studies on health policy issues.

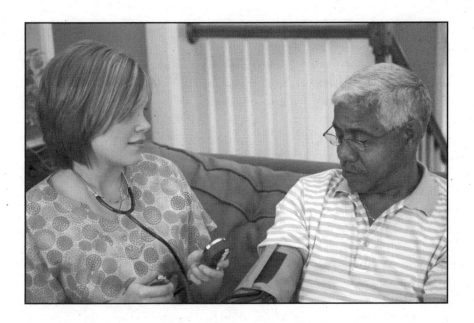

Chapter 2
WAYS OF KNOWING: HEALTH POLICY AND HEALTH STUDIES

■ INTRODUCTION: THE SCOPE OF HEALTH STUDIES AND HEALTH POLICY

The scope of health studies and health policy has traditionally been narrowly focused on clinical health care interventions provided by health care professions such as medicine, nursing, physiotherapy, and occupational therapy. In the early to mid-20th century, the focus of health studies was on treatments carried out by physicians and other health professionals and their effects on the health of individuals. In health policy, the emphasis was on the organization and delivery of clinical health care services. Much of these health study activities examined what took place in hospital settings.

But there is also a tradition of studying health and health care issues in the social sciences that has existed alongside that of the health sciences (Teeple, 2000, 2006). In the mid-19th century, Chadwick, Virchow, and Engels began to connect the health of populations to living conditions. Sociology of health, illness, and medicine grew out of this tradition, and this is now a standard undergraduate course offered in most sociology programs across Canada. In this approach, social scientists have applied broader concepts to illuminate the organization and delivery of medical services and their impact on health. This broader scope has also been concerned with understanding the determinants of health that exist outside of the clinical or hospital setting.

Social scientists have identified critical questions about health concerned with understanding how economic, political, and social forces influence the organization of the health care system as well as the health of the population (Raphael, Bryant & Rioux, 2006). They have also linked structures and political ideology to explain the organization of health care and health outcomes. The role that societal institutions play in perpetuating political, economic, and social inequalities in power and influence has also been an area of study (Grabb, 2002).

As a result of these social science influences, the study of health is no longer limited to strict experimental studies of how one or more factors predict the incidence of a disease and/or its treatment and outcome. The scope of health studies now includes the determinants of health, the meaning of health held by individuals, and identifying public policy approaches by which health can be maintained.

As one such example of social science analysis, Figure 2.1 identifies the societal structures that underlie social inequality (Grabb, 2002). Grabb states: "Social inequality can refer to any of the differences between people (or the socially defined positions they occupy) that are consequential for the lives they lead, more particularly, for the right or opportunities they exercise and the rewards or privileges they enjoy" (p. 2). The model suggests that the economic structure of a society whose components are the market (i.e., the systems of production, finance, and exchange), the political structure of the state (i.e., governments and the civil service), and associated ideological structures (comprised of religious beliefs, the mass media, educational systems, and others) play important roles in shaping the distribution of resources within a society.

These structures are of such importance in the organization and operation of society that it would also be expected that these societal structures would shape the organization of the health care system and related public policy domains that influence health, i.e., health policy, and this indeed appears to be the case. The analysis of how these societal structures—the market and other economic forces, governments, and ideological concepts—influence health policy is a primary goal of this book.

Figure 2.1: The Major Means of Power, Structures of Domination, and Bases for Social Inequality

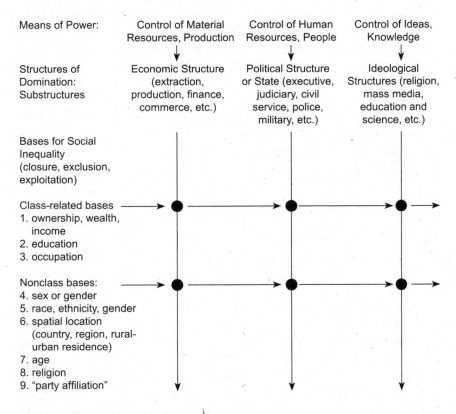

Source: Grabb, E. (2002). *Theories of social inequality* (p. 224). Toronto: Harcourt Canada.

■ REDEFINING HEALTH

Since the 1970s, growing evidence has supported the belief that health—and its maintenance—is more complex than examining physical health and treating disease (World Health Organization, 1986). Moreover, the evidence suggests that health can best be seen as a multidimensional concept that is influenced by a range of factors that fall outside the traditional sphere of clinical health care (Epp, 1986; Evans, Barer & Marmor, 1994; Lalonde, 1974). The social sciences contributed to this concept of health as a multidimensional concept and have offered critical insights into the organization and delivery of health care services and the factors that promote health (Teeple, 2006).

The proliferation of undergraduate and graduate health studies programs at Canadian universities in recent years is testament to the growing interest in health. Some of these programs attempt to link traditional health science studies with social science theory in order to raise critical questions about the impact of societal institutions and forces that shape public policies, thereby influencing the health of populations.

The social science disciplines, in particular sociology and political science, have contributed the greatest insights to the discipline of health studies (Armstrong, Armstrong & Coburn, 2001). They have done so by identifying and investigating critical questions about the different meanings of health, the influence of public policy upon the organization and delivery of health care services, and upon the other factors that affect health.

In particular, the political economy perspective has been concerned with identifying the economic, political, and social structures (that is, societal institutions and forces) that influence health (Coburn, 2006). These analyses take two forms. The first focuses on the organization of the health care system. What role does the economic system, the state, and societal ideologies play in shaping the form of the health care system?

Second, how does the organization of society in general influence the non-health care determinants of health of populations? A political economy analysis of health is very helpful in answering this question. These social determinants include living conditions such as income, housing availability and quality, access to education, nutritious food, and health care, the influence of gender, among others (Raphael, 2008).

A political economy perspective therefore directs attention to a broad range of health issues that include how the production and distribution of economic, political, and social resources shape the health care system as well as the broader determinants of health. These analyses also help explain how individuals make certain assumptions about their society and their own health, and their expectations of what health care services and health supporting public policies should be in place (Coburn, 2006).

■ WAYS OF THINKING ABOUT HEALTH

Both the traditional health sciences and the social sciences have developed various ways of thinking about health. These paradigms range from identifying individual biomedical and behavioural risk factors for specific health conditions, such as the idea that smoking leads to lung cancer, to broader paradigms that emphasize

Figure 2.2: Social Determinants of Health

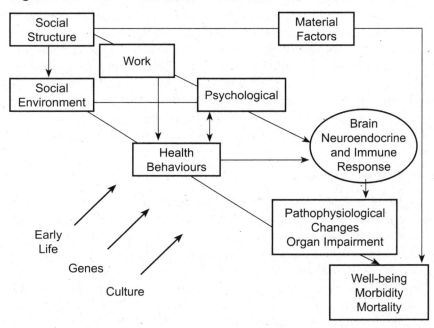

The model links social structure to health and disease via material, psychosocial, and behavioural pathways. Genetics, early life, and cultural factors are further important influences upon population health

Source: Brunner, E. & Marmot, M.G. (2006). Social organization, stress, and health. In M.G. Marmot & R.G. Wilkinson (Eds.), *Social determinants of health* (p. 9). Oxford: Oxford University Press.

how social environments and public policies shape health (Black & Smith, 1992; Labonte, 1993). More specifically, ways of thinking about health range from traditional concerns about clinical health care to an emphasis upon the economic, political, and social forces that shape the organization and delivery of health care services and related public policies that determine the health of a population (Raphael, 2008).

Understanding these different conceptions of health is important because these ideas can strongly influence how health care services are organized and delivered. They also can influence how health-related public policy is defined and implemented.

Four major paradigms for understanding health are available and these have influenced Canadian health policy to varying degrees. These are the medical, behavioural/lifestyle, socio-environmental, and structural/critical paradigms. The first three come from Labonte, while the fourth was added by Raphael (Labonte, 1993; Raphael, 2007). Each paradigm leads to different definitions of health problems, strategies for improving health, different target groups, and the delegation of responsibility to different people within society. In some models, health professionals are responsible for maintaining health while in others, responsibility falls to individual citizens. And in others the primary responsibility falls to citizens who become organized into political and social movements.

The Medical Paradigm

The medical paradigm is the traditional biomedical paradigm that defines health as the absence of disease and/or disability (Labonte, 1993). The primary health issues are defined in terms of disease categories and physiological risk factors such as a statistical deviation from the population average. Disease categories are professionally defined and include cardiovascular disease, diabetes, HIV/AIDS, obesity, arthritis, mental disease, and hypertension, among others. Moreover, the medical paradigm considers disease as having an independent existence from the individual's social environment and ideas (Wilson, 2000). It also embodies a cause-and-effect reasoning such that condition A does something to B, which results in effect C. The paradigm also focuses on the presence of risk factors for these same disease categories. For example, obesity becomes a concern of those working in this approach as it is hypothesized as increasing the risk of developing cardiovascular disease, high blood pressure, and diabetes, among other chronic diseases.

Defining health problems in terms of disease categories and risk factors highlights the need for professionally defined medical interventions to reduce individual risk and manage symptoms and disease. The paradigm is focused upon physical symptoms and clinical outcomes. The interventions can be surgery, drugs, and other therapies that usually require a referral from a physician. They also include medically managed behavioural change through patient compliance with diet and exercise regimens and ongoing patient education related to these factors.

The targets of such interventions are individuals identified as afflicted with a disease or those at higher risk for the disease. The general intervention approach is highly individualized. Physicians, nurses, and other allied health professionals are responsible for delivering these interventions to individuals one at a time. Monitoring of individuals' and their biomedical indicators is an important part of this process.

The organization and delivery of health care services are clearly organized within the parameters of the medical paradigm. Emphasis is upon the detection of disease and treatment by health care professionals. It is not surprising, given the vast expenditure on health care services, that governmental and public attention is focused upon these activities. Additionally, the medical paradigm is clearly the dominant manner by which the media, policy-makers, and the public think about the meaning of determinants of health and means by which health can be promoted (Gasher et al., 2007; Hayes et al., 2007).

Behavioural/Lifestyle Approach

The behavioural or lifestyle paradigm also provides an individualized concept of health (Labonte, 1993). Health is defined primarily in terms of individual energy, functional ability, and disease-preventing lifestyles. The primary health problems are seen as behavioural risk factors such as smoking, poor dietary habits, and lack of exercise. Drug and/or alcohol abuse, poor coping skills, and lack of life skills are also important health problems.

The principal strategies or interventions for changing these risk behaviours are health education, social marketing, advocacy for public policies that support and promote lifestyle changes such as smoking bans, prohibition on the use of trans fats in food products, and construction of bicycle paths to promote active lifestyles (Labonte, 1993). The targets for such interventions are groups of individuals deemed to be at high risk for health problems, usually children and youth.

The ones responsible for delivering these interventions are employees of municipal and regional public health departments; chronic disease advocacy groups such as the Canadian Cancer Society and the Lung Association; and city, provincial, and federal governments. Ultimately, however, individuals are seen as responsible for maintaining their health by taking these risk-reduction measures.

All three levels of government in Canada engage in social marketing that promotes individual responsibility for maintaining health. For example, public health departments develop anti-smoking campaigns that target young people, particularly adolescent girls. These campaigns admonish adolescents not to smoke, and focus on resisting peer pressure. Many health authorities engage in such lifestyle campaigns; an excellent example of such a paradigm is provided in the first part of Box 2.1.

Surveys indicate that the Canadian public clearly subscribe to many tenets of the behavioural/lifestyle paradigm. When asked what may be the best ways to promote health, the overwhelming tendency is to provide behavioural/lifestyle responses concerned with diet, exercise, and tobacco use (Canadian Population Health Initiative, 2004).

Although the behavioural paradigm shares some similarities with the traditional medical paradigm, it emphasizes prevention rather than treatment of

Box 2.1: Different Approaches to 10 Tips for Better Health

#1: The Traditional 10 Tips for Better Health

1. Don't smoke. Don't breathe others' smoke.
2. Follow a balanced diet with plenty of fruit and vegetables.
3. Keep physically active.
4. Manage stress by, for example, talking things through and making time to relax.
5. If you drink alcohol, do so in moderation.
6. Cover up in the sun, and protect children from sunburn.
7. Practise safer sex.
8. Take up cancer-screening opportunities.
9. Be safe on the roads: follow the Highway Code.
10. Learn the first aid ABCs: airways, breathing, circulation.

#2: The Social Determinants 10 Tips for Better Health

1. Don't be poor. If you can, stop. If you can't, try not to be poor for long.
2. Don't have poor parents.
3. Own a car.
4. Don't work in a stressful, low-paid manual job.
5. Don't live in damp, low-quality housing.
6. Be able to afford to go on a foreign holiday and sunbathe.
7. Practice not losing your job and don't become unemployed.
8. Take up all benefits you are entitled to, if you are unemployed, retired or sick or disabled.
9. Don't live next to a busy major road or near a polluting factory.
10. Learn how to fill in the complex housing benefit/asylum application forms before you become homeless and destitute.

Sources: L. Donaldson, *Ten Tips for Better Health* (London: Stationary Office, 1999); D. Gordon, *Ten Tips for Better Health*, 1999 (message posted on the Spirit of 1848 listserv).

existing health conditions. It does so primarily within an individualist approach (Labonte, 1996, 1997). Individuals are considered responsible for adopting healthy behaviours to promote good health, thereby reducing their risk of disease. While there is some effort to provide environmental supports to "make the healthy choice, the easy choice" (e.g., the imposition of sin taxes, changing food offerings in school cafeterias, and providing other incentives to "healthy living"), government interventions aim to improve individual behaviours by emphasizing personal responsibility for health.

Socio-Environmental Paradigm

The socio-environmental paradigm is concerned with risk conditions rather than risk factors (Labonte, 1993). Health is defined as a positive concept in terms of connectedness to family, friends, and one's community. It is concerned with people having control over their lives and having the ability to engage in activities that are important or have meaning for them. It directs attention to community and societal factors that support health. Health problems are defined in terms of psychosocial and socio-environmental risk factors such as poverty, residing in a district with high industrial pollution, isolation, stressful environments, and hazardous living and working conditions, among others. The approach can be seen as consistent with the second part of Box 2.1.

While attention is directed to the larger environments in which individuals live, some aspects of an individualized paradigm are present. The paradigm emphasizes building social supports for individuals to cope with problems in their lives. Joining organizations such as community centres or being with family and friends provide means for coping. The primary interventions promoted by this paradigm include small group development, community development, coalition building, political action and advocacy, and societal change (Labonte, 1993).

The target of these interventions is ultimately high-risk environments. The paradigm recognizes that the organization of communities and societies shape health and the importance of developing political and economic policies in support of health. Key agents of change are considered to be citizens, social development and welfare organizations, political movements such as the environmental and social justice movements, and political parties. This paradigm, however, does not explicitly direct attention to the influence of larger economic, political, and social forces that shape the local environments that influence health.

Structural/Critical

The structural-critical perspective is distinguished by its explicit concern with the organization of society and how it organizes and distributes social and economic resources within a population (Raphael, 2007). Structural-critical defines health in terms of an unequal distribution and control of economic and social power and resources within a society. The sources of this unequal distribution are attributed to the political ideology held by governing parties and an unequal distribution of political power (Armstrong et al., 2001; Coburn, 2006).

There are two aspects of the paradigm that have relevance for understanding health policy. The first focus is upon how these forces shape the organization and delivery of health care services in a society. How does political ideology and unequal distribution of resources and power determine the form of health care? Who gets to control how these institutions operate?

The second focus of the critical structural paradigm is that of examining how a society organizes the production and distribution of social and economic resources (i.e., income, employment, housing, and education) that shape health (Armstrong et al., 2001). The paradigm most closely related to this paradigm is the political economy approach.

In this paradigm, there is a focus on the collective, not the individual, as the instrument for change. There is particular attention given to the policy change process. Interventions or strategies for change involve mobilizing the population for political action to bring about desired public policy changes. Labour and other social movements (i.e., anti-poverty, feminist, labour, and cultural/racial) and social democratic political parties are seen as the catalysts for such mobilization and promoting public policies in support of health.

Implications for Health Policy

When one considers the decisions governments make about health, one has to consider which dominant paradigm of health is at play. One way to ascertain the dominant paradigm of a jurisdiction is to consider what attention governments are giving to various ways of promoting health. It should come as no surprise that in Canada, primary attention is given to the medical and behavioural/lifestyle paradigms. Why this is the case and the implications for understanding the scope of health policy constitutes much of the content of this book.

Ways of understanding the world are essential for understanding how knowledge exists in different forms, how these forms shape ways of thinking about health, and how they can be used by those attempting to influence health research and the health policy process. How these actors perceive or understand knowledge also influences how they use it in their activities. Moreover, the dominant knowledge approach also influences how policy-makers and elected representatives decide which are appropriate areas for health policy activity.

Perspectives on what constitutes knowledge about the world are also known as world views or paradigms. A knowledge paradigm can be defined as a set of basic beliefs or assumptions about knowledge and how it is created (Guba & Lincoln, 1994). More importantly, a paradigm sets parameters on what can be known. A paradigm consists of three components: ontology, epistemology, and methodology.

Box 2.2: A Larger Focus: Ways of Understanding the World

This leads to some important questions: How do certain assumptions influence governments' health policy? What processes lead to privileging certain types of understanding over others in the health policy change process? How does the research and policy development process in the health area reflect these differing approaches?

This consideration leads to the question: How do epistemological and political assumptions influence creating and disseminating knowledge to influence governments' health policy? What processes lead to privileging certain types of knowledge over others in the health policy change process? How does the research and policy development process in the health area reflect these differing epistemological approaches?

Ontology: Ontology refers to the form in which reality and its objects are said to exist. There are widely different views of what constitutes the nature of the world and this is particularly the case when issues such as health and health policy are considered. Ontology defines what can be known (Guba, 1990). For example, the ontology of the medical model described above is that reality consists of biomedical and physiological indicators of cell, organ, and body systems functioning. Patterns of bodily functioning are driven by natural laws and mechanisms. In the health sciences, this view is clearly dominant and reflects the understandings held by most health care professionals. The notion of reality—what health is and how to promote it—held by the other health paradigms (behavioural/lifestyle, socio-environmental, and structural-critical) are very different.

Epistemology: Epistemology refers to how the inquirer—that is, the one (doctor, nurse, or social scientist) who wishes to understand the world—creates knowledge through research and experience. What are the appropriate research approaches that can be used to learn about the world? Should one use the methodology of objective observation and experimentation developed in the natural sciences? Or, should knowledge be gained through understanding the personal experiences of individuals who are most affected by health issues? Perhaps knowledge can be gained by understanding the societal structures that shape the distribution of economic, political, and social resources among the population. What role do values play in shaping our inquiries and determining what is worthy of attention? Epistemology, therefore, represents a key aspect of the knowledge creation process since it shapes how knowledge is believed to be acquired and understood.

Methodology: Methodology is about the tool kit employed to acquire knowledge. The tool kit can contain experimental methodologies that focus on observation of the world, interactive approaches that examine the lived experiences of people, or critical analyses that consider the ways in which social institutions shape the distribution of resources.

All of these ways of understanding the world—through ontology, epistemology, and methodology—will shape our health care and profoundly affect health-related public policy action.

It is important to identify the epistemological assumptions of these various theories and what they say about health and health care. Since these theories reflect a view of how the world should be, including health care and health-related public policy, it is essential to explicitly consider their underpinnings and implications (Burrell & Morgan, 1979).

■ SOCIAL THEORY UNDERLYING THE APPROACHES TO HEALTH

Social theory can support the various approaches to health. We will examine three social theories that are particularly insightful. Each offers a different perspective, some with individualist orientations to health or micro analysis, and some socially based, or macro analysis. The three main theories are:

- Positivism (as well as structural functionalism)
- Interpretivism (with a short discussion of symbolic interactionism)
- Critical (including political economy)

■ POSITIVISM/RATIONALIST PARADIGM

Positivism is a philosophy that states that the only authentic knowledge is scientific knowledge, and that such knowledge can come only from positive affirmation of theories through strict scientific method. Traditional positivism holds that both natural phenomenon and human behaviour can best be explained through universal laws. In physics, for example, Newton's laws of motion explain the action of inanimate objects such as planets or falling apples (Brunner, 1991). The positivist approach emphasizes rational and linear concepts to explain the world with a focus on the observable and concrete.

The aim of positivist science is to predict and control conditions (Guba, 1990; Park, 1993). The physical and biological sciences and much of the health sciences are organized within this approach. There is an emphasis on the criteria of reliability, validity, and objectivity. The goal of inquiry is to search for truth, logic, generalizability, originality, and relevance (Albaek, 1995).

Positivism has been the dominant paradigm in social sciences and public policy studies, and this has especially been the case in health policy-related

---

Box 2.3: The Beliefs of Positivism

The essential beliefs of positivism as applied to knowledge and inquiry are: (1) there is an external world that exists independent of human interpretation, and (2) objective knowledge about the world can be acquired through direct sensory experience. Usually these experiences are identified and interpreted within the framework of the experimental scientific method (Fishman, 1991). Phenomena that cannot be observed either directly through experience or observation are excluded from this definition of credible knowledge.

---

studies. Positivism, applied to public policy analysis, depends on empirical testing of quantitative predictions that are logically deduced from hypotheses. Thus, knowledge creation involves developing a set of general principles that can explain and predict events. Why shouldn't these scientific methods, argue positivists, be applied to understanding health and health care, and the public policy processes that shape their form?

One reason it should not is that positivism holds that science is neutral and denies the influence of values on inquiry (Wilson, 1983b). It also neglects the study of power and fails to consider how inequalities in power shape the definition of what constitutes credible knowledge and the means by which such knowledge can be obtained and applied. Positivism, to state it bluntly, implicitly accepts the status quo (Woodill, 1992). In this way, it is thought to reinforce economic, political, and social inequalities.

Interpretations of the link between knowledge, health, and health policy have traditionally been informed by the positivist knowledge paradigm (Wilson, 1983b). The positivist paradigm grew out of the physical and natural sciences. This makes dealing with economic, political, and social forces and how they influence knowledge development and application somewhat difficult (Albaek, 1995; Gagnon, 1990).

Limitations of Positivism

Positivism tends to examine phenomena separately from the context in which they naturally exist or occur, a process that can be described as "context-stripping" (Lincoln & Guba, 1985). Indeed, the primary weaknesses of positivism stem from its linear assumptions about social reality and its need to remove all context (Bryant, 2001). Research is primarily about determining the form these fixed and constant processes take. There is frequently little consideration of the impact of broader economic, political, and social context on the phenomenon chosen to be

Box 2.4: Positivism and Policy Analysis

The introduction of positivism into the policymaking process was an attempt to make it more like traditional science. In the positivist-rationalist policy paradigm, politics is perceived as incongruent and competing with rational action (Albaek, 1995; Gagnon, 1990). Whereas science can be seen as driven by devotion to objective and open inquiry, reason, and truth, politics is concerned with power and interests, and therefore does not adhere to the claims of scientific rationality and objective inquiry. Thus, the methods and process of science are considered by some as essential to make public policy analysis and development a purely rational process.

Sources: Albaek, E. (1995). Between knowledge and power: Utilization of social science in public policy-making. *Policy Sciences, 28*(1), 79–100; Gagnon, A.-G. (1990). The influence of social scientists in public policy. In S. Brooks & A.-G. Gagnon (Eds.), *Social scientists, policy, and the state,* 1–18. New York: Praeger.

of interest. This is evident in the clinical health sciences and the lifestyle-related behavioural approach to disease prevention.

Linear assumptions about reality may blind the analyst to the many complex factors that shape social phenomena (Mills, 1959). In addition, the paradigm usually does not consider the importance of power relations in shaping social reality and policy development. In the health policy field it limits focus and understanding to biomedical and physiological indicators and behavioural risk factors. The focus is usually at the individual level. These understandings fit in with individualist interpretations.

Linking back to the earlier discussion, the biomedical and lifestyle approaches that emphasize individual risk factors and regimens and shape individual behaviours are informed primarily by the positivist approach. These approaches prefer to understand disease, its treatment, and disease prevention in terms of individual risk factors. They seek to discover predictable, usually narrow, cause-and-effect relationships. The concern with measuring and quantifying individual risk factors and specifying the impact of medical interventions on medical conditions reflect many assumptions of the positivist paradigm.

Attractiveness of Positivism for the Health Sciences and Health Policy Sectors

Despite the limitations of the positivist approach, researchers, health science professionals, and many health policy analysts value the research carried out in the positivist tradition because it emphasizes relationships between observable biomedical and behavioural risk factors and health outcomes.

This is a distinctively depoliticized approach as it emphasizes objectivity. It is also expert-driven as exemplified by top-down authoritative research and knowledge generating paradigms. In the health sciences, it is assumed that health can be maintained through medical interventions and by individuals following the recommendations of physicians, public health educators, and others who are deemed to be "experts" on appropriate medical and lifestyle regimens. Similarly, health policy activities focus on the capacity to quantify or measure impacts of various medical interventions.

Box 2.5: Poverty and Heart Disease

Poverty Is Main Predictor of Heart Disease, Says Canadian Report
By W. Kondro
The Lancet

Poverty is a greater predictor of heart disease than risk factors such as smoking, obesity, stress, or blood cholesterol concentrations, a Canadian sociologist says. In a review of more than 100 studies on the causes of heart disease, associate professor of health policy Dennis Raphael (York University, Toronto, Canada) suggests: "The economic and social conditions under which people live their lives, rather than medical treatments and lifestyle choices, are the major factors determining whether they develop cardiovascular disease." The report was published on May 3 by the Centre for Social Justice, a Toronto-based advocacy group. Lifestyle approaches to improvement of cardiovascular health, such as programmes to curb smoking or obesity, are counterproductive, Raphael said in an interview. They have the negative effect of pushing issues like income distribution, community services, and public transportation off the health-policy table. Poor people end up blaming themselves for their heart disease and "that's harmful because it diverts people from these main contributors to their heart disease, which is material deprivation, psychosocial stress, and the adoption of unhealthy behaviours (like using drugs) as a result of that stress."

Raphael's report, "Social Justice Is Good for Our Hearts," which is yet to be published in a peer-reviewed journal, suggests some 22% of life years lost before age 75 years (according to a Statistics Canada extrapolation) are because of income differences. "Were all Canadians' rates of death from cardiovascular disease equal to those living in the wealthiest quintile of neighbourhoods, there would be 6366 fewer deaths each year from cardiovascular disease," says Raphael.

The poor are at greater risk of developing heart disease because of "social exclusion," Raphael argues. "Individuals who suffer from material deprivation have greater exposures to negative events such as hunger and lack of quality food, poor quality of housing, inadequate clothing, and poor environmental conditions at home and work. In addition, individuals suffering from material deprivation also have less exposures to positive resources such as education, books, newspapers, and other stimulating resources, attendance at cultural events, opportunities for recreation and other leisure activities," he says.

Some of the political remedies Raphael advocates are: higher welfare and unemployment insurance outlays; improved pay equity; establishment of a national guaranteed minimum income; stronger antidiscrimination legislation; higher taxes on the wealthy, including an inheritance tax; a national housing strategy; and creation of national day care and pharmacare programmes. He also suggests "directing attention to the health needs of immigrants and paying attention to the unfavourable socioeconomic position of many groups and the particular difficulties many new Canadians face in accessing health and other care services."

The report "Social Justice is Good for Our Hearts" is available online at www.socialjustice.org/pdfs/JusticeGoodHearts.pdf.

Source: The Lancet (May 11, 2002), p. 1679.

Policy-makers are also oriented to a positivist approach to knowledge. They tend not to examine people's lived experiences or the root causes of social inequality. They tend to be dismissive of knowledge derived from critical analyses of structural social relations. The traditional approach, therefore, privileges some forms of knowledge above others, a process known as legitimization of knowledge. At the same time, it delegitimizes others, thereby shutting out some alternative perspectives from health policy debates.

■ STRUCTURAL FUNCTIONALISM

In practice, many inquiries that are grounded in structural-functionalist approaches tend to apply positivist notions of knowledge and methodology. Structural functionalism is a social theory developed by early sociologists after positivism. It can also support the medical approach to health. This theory views society as an organism, a system of parts, all of which serve a function together for the overall effectiveness and efficiency of society. It views society as a system of checks and balances. Structural functionalism is, at its core, a consensus theory. It is therefore a theory that sees society as built upon order, interrelation, and balance among parts as a means to maintain the smooth functioning of the whole.

Structural functionalism views shared norms and values as the basis of society, focuses on social order based on tacit agreements between groups and organizations, and views social change as occurring in a slow and orderly fashion. Functionalists acknowledge that change is sometimes necessary to correct social dysfunctions (the opposite of functions), but that it must occur slowly so that people and institutions can adapt without rapid disorder.

To sum up, structural functionalism makes specific assumptions about society:

- Societies are held together by co-operation and orderliness.
- Societies work best when they function smoothly as an organism, with all parts working toward the "natural" or smooth working of the system.
- Allocation and integration are two fundamental processes necessary for a state of equilibrium within a system.
- Each part interrelates to create efficiency and harmony; the most capable individuals must be motivated to fill the most important roles/positions.
- Systems tend toward self-maintenance involving control of boundaries and relationships of parts to the whole, control of the environment, and control of tendencies to change the system from within.

Limitations of Structural Functionalism

When applied to health and health policy, structural functionalism would have limited use. It would view health issues as "fixable" through medical intervention as each part of society would be successfully fulfilling a function. Effective change, in other words, is difficult in this model.

■ INTERPRETIVE PARADIGM

Interpretivism, or hermeneutics, is an approach that highlights how individuals understand themselves and others through shared systems of meaning (Wilson, 1983a). Meaning manifests itself through shared categories that help make sense of interpersonal relationships and social institutions (Park, 1993).

The intellectual partners in this paradigm include symbolic interactionism, ethnography, participant observation, and grounded theory, among others (Lincoln, 1994; Lincoln & Guba, 1985). This perspective clearly moves beyond many limitations of positivist epistemology, but may not explicitly address issues of unequal power relations created by societal institutions and economic, political, and social forces. One of the interesting aspects of the approach is that all views are considered equally valid. Individuals' understandings of how and why something occurs are accepted without critique. This may be a problem where there are clear issues of injustice and inequality that may not be perceived or understood by the individual being studied or the policy issue being considered.

The interpretive approach is typical of health studies that examine the experience of an individual with various health conditions. The focus is on describing and understanding the condition from the standpoint of the individual. Such studies provide important insights into the lived experiences of individuals and their interactions with the health care system. Results may help other individuals who have similar experiences and their families in providing support. Such studies also have their place in the body of knowledge on various medical conditions and their implications for coping and support. It is a fair conclusion, however, that these kinds of studies are clearly subordinate to positivist-oriented health sciences studies and rarely inform health policy decisions (Raphael et al., 2004).

Linking again to the earlier discussion, the socio-environmental approach to health presented earlier is related to the interpretive paradigm because it emphasizes the lived experiences of individuals. The socio-environmental approach also encourages the individual to engage in activities that allow individuals to find meaning in their lives. Social context becomes important as community structures such as community centres or organizations help to promote a sense of connectedness and community. Clearly understanding individuals' lived experiences would be a valuable addition when carrying out health sciences and health policy studies that aim to maintain and promote health.

Symbolic Interactionist Theory

As noted, symbolic interactionism dovetails with the interpretive approach. Symbolic interactionism is based on qualitative research, not quantitative figures and tables, and it is primarily concerned with individual experience and subjective analysis. Perception is everything. Meaning derives from social interaction. In other words, you can best understand a person's actions in relation to other (surrounding) people. Body language is a perfect example.

Limitations of Interpretive Approaches

The primary weakness of this way of knowing is its treatment of all perspectives as equally valid. It fails to take into account the impact of social relations. In particular, the approach does not consider social and other inequalities and how these shape the experiences and understandings of individuals concerning health issues and their experience of the health care system. Few of these kinds of analyses explicitly link the immediate experience of a health issue to the influence of larger systems on individual health outcomes and the experience of the health care system.

In addition, the interpretive approach fails to consider how differences in power and influence often define what may even be considered a health issue. Why do some health and health care issues arise at certain times while others do not? Who shapes the form that health care institutions take and the kinds of day-to-day aspects of life that individuals experience?

■ CRITICAL THEORY

An alternative approach is critical theory. Critical theory is social theory oriented toward critiquing and transforming society as a whole, in contrast to traditional theory, which is concerned only with understanding or explaining society as it is. Critical theory refers to a cluster of perspectives that challenge the bases of both the positivism/rationalism and interpretive/hermeneutics paradigms. These approaches inform the health sciences and health policy areas by locating actors (those involved in developing research and policy) within discourses (ways of talking about and understanding issues of concern) (Torgerson, 1996).

These approaches include critical realism, critique and deconstruction, and political economy (Torgerson, 1996). These perspectives vary in the degree to which they examine the interplay between power and public policy development.

Unlike the other approaches, critical theory considers the "haves" and "have-nots" of society. It also considers power relationships and social inequality. It frequently focuses on the socio-economic context in which institutions are shaped and individuals' lives are lived (Torgerson, 1996). Critical theorists focus on the nature and distribution of power among social institutions such as the state, the economic system, and citizens.

Critical theory explicitly links forms of knowledge to the existence and application of various degrees of power as a central organizing concept (Fay, 1987). By dealing explicitly with issues of power and domination within the social context of society, critical theory provides some of these categories of understanding. The approach considers the constructions of reality made by differentially positioned actors as resulting from the form that their social relations take. In its concern with issues of power and domination, it frequently focuses on the social, economic, and political context in which institutions are shaped and individuals' lives are lived (Torgerson, 1996).

Critical theorists, therefore, focus on the nature and distribution of power among societal institutions such as the state, the economic system, and citizens. The means by which these social relations can be understood is through analyses of the distribution of resources and the lived experience of individuals. Interpretivist or hermeneutic analyses can describe some of these relations, but conventional hermeneutic categories of meaning may not expose important categories related to the distribution of power and resources that are themselves shaped by societal institutions and systems.

Critical theory, by dealing explicitly with issues of power and domination within the social context of society, provides some of these categories of understanding. Critical theory also incorporates the idea that profound transformation of society may be necessary. The social order is characterized as having inherent political and social contradictions that reproduce themselves, thereby perpetuating social inequalities (Fay, 1987).

Political Economy Approach

The political economy approach falls under the umbrella of the critical theory. It focuses on the broader social, political, and economic context to analyze how objective living conditions help inform a variety of health-related issues. For example, a political economy considers how political and economic structures shape the form the health care system takes. It also examines how the distribution of economic, political, and social resources shape mortality and morbidity rates among the population. It carries out these analyses independent of the perceived meanings that citizens may have of these issues. It is beyond dispute that critical theory, in particular critical analytic frameworks such as political economy, has identified important questions about societies and how the organization of societies shapes the form of the health care system and the health of the population.

Limitations of Critical Theory

With their emphasis on power and domination, critical perspectives may neglect other important factors in their attempts to highlight inequalities in influence and power. It is important to highlight, however, that critical theory has a social action agenda that can democratize policy analysis. Its proponents argue that it provides the best opportunity for collaborative policy analysis between professional policy analysts such as those employed by professional think tanks and citizen activists (Fischer, 2000, 2003; Hawkesworth, 1988; Torgerson, 1996). It challenges the basic terms of conventional discussion and demands that authority and decision making be rooted in democratic principles.

Despite its limitations, the critical approach provides insights about power and domination in analyses of public policy and health issues, which provide a critical lens for framing and evaluating theories of public policy, and policy change.

This lens may be particularly relevant for analyzing knowledge issues and how they are deployed by particular groups to influence health policy in the provincial and federal policy arenas in Canada, and in the international political arena.

Box 2.6: Matching Approaches to Health with Research Paradigms

Approaches to Health		*Social Theory That Endorses the Approach*
Medical Approach	→→→	**Positivism**
- individual-based or micro		- objective, rational
Behavioural/Lifestyle Approach	→→→	**Positivism** (structural functionalism)
- individual-based or micro		- objective, rational
Socio-environmental Model	→→→	**Interpretive**
- both individual and environmentally based		- subjective
Structural/Critical Approach	→→→	**Critical (and Political Economy)**
- socially based, structural, macro		- both objective and subjective

---

■ APPLICATION OF THESE CONCEPTS TO THE SOCIAL DETERMINANTS OF HEALTH

As an example of how these concepts help explicate important health issues, consider the issue of the social determinants of health. An important development in understanding the sources of health has been recognition that living conditions are the primary determinants of health in nations such as Canada (Marmot & Wilkinson, 2006; Raphael, 2008).

The social determinants of health field is primarily about describing and understanding how living conditions—as indicated by such factors as social class, income level, employment security, quality of working conditions, adequacy of housing, levels of education, access to nutritious food, and availability of health and social services, among others—shape health. Informing these analyses is a concern with how the organization of production and distribution of social and economic resources influences health. As a result, various researchers and organizations have developed sets of social determinants that show marked similarities as well as some differences.

Table 2.1 shows four of the dominant conceptualizations of the social determinants of health. The Ottawa Charter in 1986, for example, identified various "prerequisites for health" (World Health Organization, 1986). For the first time, health was conceptualized as a resource for living rather than simply the absence of disease. People were identified as change agents who had the power to act on their social environments to improve the conditions of living.

Table 2.1: Various Conceptualizations of the Social Determinants of Health

Ottawa Charter[1]	Health Canada (CIAR)[2]	World Health Organization[3]	SDOH National Conference[4]
peace	income and social status	social gradient	Aboriginal status
shelter	social support networks	stress	early life
education	education	early life	education
food	employment and working conditions	social exclusion	employment and working conditions
income	physical environments	work	food security
stable ecosystem	social environments	unemployment	health care services
sustainable resources	healthy child development	social support	housing
social justice	health services	addictions	income and its distribution
equity	culture	food	social safety net
	gender	transport	social exclusion
			unemployment and employment security

1. World Health Organization (1986). *Ottawa Charter for Health Promotion*. Retrieved from http://www.who.dk/policy/ottawa.htm
2. Health Canada (1998).
3. Wilkinson & Marmot (2003).
4. Raphael, D. (2004).

The Canadian Institute for Advanced Research (CIAR) drew up its own list of health determinants, some of which are social determinants of health, which Health Canada has largely adopted. While on the surface, these determinants have similarities with the World Health Organization's "prerequisites of health," some argue that this list of health determinants represents a "re-medicalization of health promotion" (Labonte, 1996) as some of its terms, such as physical and social environments, derive from an epidemiological (that is, positivist) approach to health. In addition, there is frequently a refocusing upon biomedical risk factors and a neglect of issues concerned with the organization of society and the unequal distribution of economic, political, and social resources (Raphael & Bryant, 2002).

The CIAR population health approach considers population-based health status indicators such as infant mortality, morbidity, and mortality rates. It also recognizes the importance of available resources and various social determinants of health, but it betrays a tendency to apply a concern with the concrete and observable, typical of positivist notions at the cost of considering broader societal issues concerned with the unequal distribution of resources and the political and economic systems.

The CIAR approach frequently employs statistical tables of traditional biomedical and epidemiological indicators. One such example is provided by Labonte (1997), in which a CIAR publication argues for promoting "slight shifts in the overall distribution of serum cholesterol" to influence CVD (cardiovascular disease) rate (Labonte, 1997). They say little, however, about the forces that shape these distributions and the reason for inequalities among varying groups.

In contrast, social science research shows these indicators do not occur in a vacuum. They are influenced by the broader economic, political, and social contexts within which people live. These health indicators—and the living conditions that spawn them—are amenable to public policy action.

In this book, the opportunities provided by the political economy approach are taken to understand the forms that health policy takes in Canada. It is assumed that economic, political, and social forces shape the parameters within which health policy is defined and within which health policy action is taken. While each health and epistemological framework has an important role to play in this exercise, the organization and delivery of health care and health-related public policies can best be understood within a political economy framework.

■ CONCLUSIONS

This chapter has examined different approaches to understanding health and means of influencing it. Differing paradigms represent differing world views concerning the nature of health and define the "appropriate" realms for health care policy action. These approaches are themselves informed by different ways of knowing. Such epistemological analyses make explicit their assumptions about knowledge and how it is created.

By focusing on biomedical and behavioural/lifestyle factors, most of these health paradigms fail to consider how the distribution of economic, political, and social resources shape the form that health care services take and the health status of citizens. These paradigms also emphasize individual responsibility for health and fail to articulate how political power and public policy influence population health. Arguably, the medical and lifestyle/behavioural approaches to health, by not making explicit the nature of societal structures and their influence, lead to an acceptance of society as it is.

In contrast, the socio-environmental and structural/critical approaches provide a basis for societal change. The political economy approach especially recognizes how unequal distributions of resources and power influence policymaking and calls for the redistribution of such power in the service of health. These analyses suggest that improved health policy—both in the form of health care services and in the social determinants of health—requires policy approaches that address inequalities and provides means for their remediation.

■ REFERENCES

Albaek, E. (1995). Between knowledge and power: Utilization of social science in public policy-making. *Policy Sciences, 28*(1), 79–100.

Armstrong, P., Armstrong, H. & Coburn, D. (Eds.). (2001). *Unhealthy times: The political economy of health and care in Canada*. Toronto: Oxford University Press.

Black, D. & Smith, C. (1992). The Black Report. In P. Townsend, N. Davidson & M. Whitehead (Eds.), *Inequalities in health: The Black Report and the health divide*. New York: Penguin.

Brunner, R.D. (1991). The policy movement as a policy problem. *Policy Sciences, 24*(1), 65–98.

Bryant, T. (2001). *The social welfare policy change process: Civil society actors and the role of knowledge*. Unpublished PhD thesis, University of Toronto, Toronto.

Burrell, G. & Morgan, G. (1979). *Sociological paradigms and organisational analysis: Elements of the sociology of corporate life*. Portsmouth: Heineman Arena.

Canadian Population Health Initiative. (2004). *Select highlights on public views of the determinants of health*. Ottawa: CPHI.

Coburn, D. (2006). Health and health care: A political economy perspective. In D. Raphael, T. Bryant & M. Rioux (Eds.), *Staying alive: Critical perspectives on health, illness, and health care*, 59–84. Toronto: Canadian Scholars' Press Inc.

Epp, J. (1986). *Achieving health for all: A framework for health promotion*. Ottawa: Health and Welfare Canada.

Evans, R.G., Barer, M.L. & Marmor, T.R. (Eds.). (1994). *Why are some people healthy and others not? The determinants of health of populations.* Hawthorne: Aldine DeGruyter.

Fay, B. (1987). *Critical social science: Liberation and its limits.* Ithaca: Cornell University Press.

Fischer, F. (2000). *Citizens, experts, and the environment: The politics of local knowledge.* Durham: Duke University Press.

Fischer, F. (2003). *Reframing public policy: Discursive politics and deliberative practices.* New York: Oxford University Press.

Fishman, D.B. (1991). Epistemological paradigms in evaluation: Implications for practice. Evaluation and Program Planning 18:1, 351–363.

Gagnon, A.-G. (1990). The influence of social scientists in public policy. In S. Brooks & A.-G. Gagnon (Eds.), *Social scientists, policy, and the state,* 1–18. New York: Praeger.

Gasher, M., Hayes, M., Ross, I., Hackett, R., Gutstein, D. & Dunn, J. (2007). Spreading the news: Social determinants of health reportage in Canadian daily newspapers. *Canadian Journal of Communication, 32*(3), 557–574.

Grabb, E. (2002). *Theories of social inequality.* Toronto: Harcourt Canada.

Guba, E. (Ed.). (1990). *The paradigm dialog.* Newbury Park: Sage.

Guba, E.G. & Lincoln, Y.S. (1994). Competing paradigms in qualitative research. In N.K. Denzin & Y.S. Lincoln (Eds.), *Handbook of qualitative research,* 105–117. Thousand Oaks: Sage Publications.

Hawkesworth, M.E. (1988). *Theoretical issues in policy analysis.* Albany: State University of New York.

Hayes, M., Ross, I., Gasherc, M., Gutstein, D., Dunn, J. & Hackett, R. (2007). Telling stories: News media, health literacy, and public policy in Canada. *Social Science and Medicine, 54,* 445–457.

Labonte, R. (1993). *Health promotion and empowerment: Practice frameworks.* Toronto: Centre for Health Promotion and ParticipAction.

Labonte, R. (1996). *The population health/health promotion debate in Canada: The politics of explanation, economics, and action.* Toronto: University of Toronto Press.

Labonte, R. (1997). The population health/health promotion debate in Canada: The politics of explanation, economics, and action. *Critical Public Health, 7*(1 & 2), 7–27.

Lalonde, M. (1974). *A new perspective on the health of Canadians: A working document.* Retrieved from http://www.hc-sc.gc.ca/main/hppb/phdd/resource.htm

Lincoln, Y. (1994). Sympathetic connections between qualitative research methods and health research. *Qualitative Health Research, 2,* 375–391.

Lincoln, Y. & Guba, E. (1985). *Naturalist inquiry.* Newbury Park: Sage.

Marmot, M. & Wilkinson, R. (2006). *Social determinants of health* (2nd ed.). Oxford: Oxford University Press.

Mills, C.W. (1959). *The sociological imagination.* New York: Oxford University Press.

Park, P. (1993). What is participatory research? A theoretical and methodological perspective. In P. Park, M. Brydon-Miller, B. Hall & T. Jackson (Eds.), *Voices of change: Participatory research in the United States and Canada,* 1–19. Toronto: Ontario Institute for Studies in Education Press.

Raphael, D. (2007). Poverty and health. In D. Raphael (Ed.), *Poverty and policy in Canada: Implications for health and quality of life,* 205–238. Toronto: Canadian Scholars' Press Inc.

Raphael, D. (Ed.). (2008). *Social determinants of health: Canadian perspectives* (2nd ed.). Toronto: Canadian Scholars' Press Inc.

Raphael, D. & Bryant, T. (2002). The limitations of population health as a model for a new public health. *Health Promotion International, 17*, 189–199.

Raphael, D., Bryant, T. & Rioux, M. (Eds.). (2006). *Staying alive: Critical perspectives on health, illness, and health care*. Toronto: Canadian Scholars' Press Inc.

Raphael, D., Macdonald, J., Labonte, R., Colman, R., Hayward, K. & Torgerson, R. (2004). Researching income and income distribution as a determinant of health in Canada: Gaps between theoretical knowledge, research practice, and policy implementation. *Health Policy, 72*, 217–232.

Teeple, G. (2000). *Globalization and the decline of social reform: Into the twenty-first century.* Aurora: Garamond Press.

Teeple, G. (2006). Foreword. In D. Raphael, T. Bryant & M. Rioux (Eds.), *Staying alive: Critical perspectives on health, illness, and health care*, 1–4. Toronto: Canadian Scholars' Press Inc.

Torgerson, D. (1996). Power and insight in policy discourse: Post-positivism and problem definition. In L. Dobuzinskis, M. Howlett & D. Laycock (Eds.), *Policy studies in Canada: The state of the art*, 226–298. Toronto: University of Toronto Press.

Wilson, H. (2000). The myth of objectivity: Is medicine moving toward a social constructivist medical paradigm? *Family Practice, 17*(2), 203–209.

Wilson, J. (1983a). Idealism. In J. Wilson (Ed.), *Social theory* (pp. 106–121). Englewood Cliffs: Prentice Hall.

Wilson, J. (1983b). Positivism. In J. Wilson (Ed.), *Social theory* (pp. 11–18). Englewood Cliffs: Prentice Hall.

Woodill, G. (1992). *Independent living and participation in research: A critical analysis.* Toronto: Centre for Independent Living in Toronto.

World Health Organization (1986). *Ottawa charter for health promotion*. Retrieved from http://www.who.dk/policy/ottawa.htm

CRITICAL THINKING QUESTIONS

1. Which of the approaches to health is consistent with your own view of what health is and how it can be maintained? What approach do the media present in reports on health and health care issues?
2. What epistemological approach underlies Canadian health policy? What aspects of health do policy-makers emphasize?
3. How do the epistemology approaches of public policy-makers influence their receptivity to diverse approaches to health policy issues?
4. Which health approach provides an opportunity for marginalized populations to influence health policy?
5. How can shifts in health policy occur? Do we need a shift in health policy?

FURTHER READINGS

Brunner, E. & Marmot, M. (2006). Social organization, stress, and health. In M. Marmot & R.G. Wilkinson (Eds.), *Social determinants of health* (2nd ed.) 6–30. Oxford: Oxford University Press.

This chapter is one of a collection that examines different aspects of the social determinants of health. While there is an emphasis on quantitative studies, these all highlight the influence of social structures on health outcomes.

Evans, R.G. & Stoddart, G. (1990). Producing health, consuming health care. *Social Science and Medicine 31*(12), 1347–1363.

This article is an example of the population health approach of the Canadian Institute for Advanced Research (CIAR), an organization dedicated to research on population health. They present a framework to understand the evidence on population health and the various factors that influence health outcomes.

Labonte, R. (1993). *Health promotion and empowerment: Practice frameworks.* Toronto: Centre for Health Promotion and ParticipAction.

This landmark report helpfully outlines and explains the dominant approaches to health. It provides a critical assessment of each of the approaches.

Poland, B., Coburn, D., Robertson, A. & Eakin, J. (1998). Wealth, equity, and health care: A critique of a population health perspective on the determinants of health. *Social Science & Medicine, 46*(7), 785–798.

The authors critique Robert Evans and Stoddart's population health perspective. They provide a political economy analysis of key issues in Evans and Stoddart's "Producing Health, Consuming Health Care." This is a good example of a critical social science approach to health issues.

Raphael, D., Bryant, T. & Rioux, M. (Eds.). (2006). *Staying alive: Critical perspectives on health, illness, and health care.* Toronto: Canadian Scholars' Press Inc.

Staying Alive provides a fresh perspective on the issues regarding health, health care, and illness. In addition to the traditional approaches of health sciences and the sociology of health, this book shows the impact that human rights issues and political economy have on health.

Shaw, M., Dorling, D., Gordon, D. & Smith, G.D. (1999). *The widening gap: Health inequalities and policy in Britain.* Bristol: The Policy Press.

This volume is an excellent examination of the growing gap between low- and high-income groups in the United Kingdom and other advanced Western economies. The important message from this volume is that disadvantage clusters among a range of determinants such that some groups experience social and economic marginalization.

RELEVANT WEBSITES

Centre for Public Policy and Health, Durham University
www.dur.ac.uk/public.health
   Based in the United Kingdom, the centre conducts research on public health policy and management; evidence, decision making and policy implementation, inequalities in health, health effects of public policy, and work, and unemployment.

Politics of Health Group
www.pohg.org.uk
   This Politics of Health website is based at the University of Liverpool in the United Kingdom. The Politics of Health Group (PoHG) consists of people who believe that power exercised through politics and its impact on public policy is of critical importance for health. PoHG is a UK-based group, but has a clear international perspective and members throughout the world.

Politics of Health Knowledge Network
www.politicsofhealth.org
   The Politics of Health Knowledge Network is a forum for the exploration of the impact of political decisions on health. The network is concerned with how politics affect health on all levels, from individual organisms, to social groups, to the earth as a total ecological system.

Wellesley Institute
wellesleyinstitute.com/about-us/
   The Wellesley Institute is a Toronto-based, non-profit, and non-partisan research and policy institute. The institute is the former Wellesley Hospital. Their focus is on developing research and community-based policy solutions to the problems of urban health, including poverty and inequalities in health.

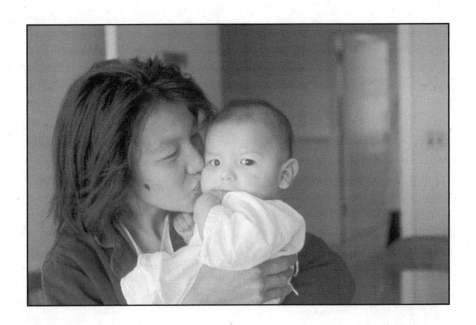

Chapter 3

THEORIES OF PUBLIC POLICY

■ INTRODUCTION: THE CONTRIBUTION OF PUBLIC POLICY THEORY TO UNDERSTANDING HEALTH POLICY

Health policy is a subset of public policy. As defined in Chapter 1, public policy is a course of action chosen by government to address what has come to be identified as a public issue (Pal, 2006). The political science literature provides a wide range of theories of public policy. Understanding the assumptions of these theories and how these are hypothesized to influence the development and implementation of public policy are important for understanding a range of health policy issues.

A theory is a framework for understanding how a set of facts or phenomena comes to be. It consists of a set of statements or principles developed to explain these facts or phenomena (Walt, 1994). Public policy theories are devised to help explain the nature of decision making in the public policy process (Brooks & Miljan, 2003). A variety of such theories exist and each emphasizes different features of the public policy process in an attempt to explain how governments make decisions and develop public policy.

These theories have different approaches to understanding the influence of power and how it is exercised in the public policy process (Brooks & Miljan, 2003). Not surprisingly, each theory has a particular set of values that inform their approaches. Each is also informed by a general model of society and how society is considered to function.

■ DEFINING THE CHARACTERISTICS OF DIFFERENT TYPES OF THEORIES

Theories of public policy may take a predominantly macro-view, meso-view, or micro-view of the public policy process. In addition, theories can also be distinguished as being either consensus or conflict models of public policy (Signal, 1998; Walt, 1994). Macro-view theories consider broad issues of the general shape of political systems and how power is exercised in these political systems. In relation to health policy, it has been argued that health policy consists of two types of public policy. The first is concerned with the organization and delivery of health care services. The second is concerned with the development and implementation of various health-related public policies.

Regarding the first type, health policy may be concerned with whether health care services are publicly or privately financed; that is, provided as entitlements through the rights of citizenship or made available as commodities to be bought or sold on the open market. When governments are involved in providing the financing and direction for the delivery of health care services to the population, the system is said to be publicly financed and managed. When government is not involved in financing and delivering health care services, it is said to be a private system. The value that underlies a public approach is that health risk should be shared across the population. The value that underlies a private approach is that of free enterprise and the commodification (or selling) of goods and services, including health care. Analysis of such profound differences in health policy is the focus of macro-level theories. In these analyses it is essential to understand how economic, political, and social forces both influence and reflect the predominant values present within a society.

The second type of health policy is that of health-related public policy. Societies that value—and have economic, political, and social structures concerned with promoting—equity and human rights usually create policies that assure economic and social security. Societies that have rather less concern with such values—and have less responsive societal institutions—may favour market-oriented approaches to provision of goods and services. In both cases, understanding the form these systems and related public policies take requires analyses of these macro-level forces.

Meso-view theories focus on the influence of advisory boards and departments within governments, government ministries, and other "middle-level" institutions upon public policy (Signal, 1998). Middle-level institutions can be organizations within governments charged with particular responsibilities or independent agencies that, while established by governments, operate at arm's-length. Ultimately, both types of agencies are still accountable to government for their decisions and public recommendations. These kinds of organizations may make recommendations of both types of health policy: health care-related and health-related public policy. The kinds of changes recommended may be profound or incremental.

Micro-view theories are concerned with the administrative routine and day-to-day government apparatus that shapes policymaking. Their concerns may include minor tinkering of public policy, but the focus is primarily on monitoring the operation of government operations, including spending allocations, monitoring operations, and revising guidelines for practice. Table 3.1 provides some examples of each type of policymaking activity in these two health policy spheres.

Table 3.1: Examples of Health Policy Issues at Differing Levels of Analysis

	Macro-Level	Meso-Level	Micro-Level
Health care policy	Creation of public-private partnerships	Creating a tele-health line	Increasing funding to community health centres
Health-related public policy	Creation of national daycare program	Changing eligibility requirements for social assistance	Increasing housing subsidy amounts for tenants

Three prominent theories of public policy with value for understanding the definition, development, and implementation of health policy are pluralism, new institutionalism, and political economy. These theories provide a lens through which the features of a health care system and health-related public policy come about and how they can be changed. Each theory has particular assumptions about the nature of society and how public policy is made. In addition, each theory tends to focus on some specific aspect as it attempts to explain the public policy process with its public policy outcomes.

■ PLURALISM

Pluralism or pluralist interest group theory considers society to consist of interest groups that vie for power and access to the state to realize their goals and objectives (Dahl, 1961; Latham, 1952; Signal, 1998; Walt, 1994). This viewpoint is consistent with the view that democratic societies are generally organized in the interests of the citizenry and that citizens are able to influence governmental directions. Policy emerges from competition in developing and advancing ideas among these different groups.

Since pluralism considers that all groups have equal opportunity to influence the policy change process, the resulting policy output reflects a rational balancing of costs and benefits. Pluralist policy analysis identifies the different interest groups and how they are organized. It also identifies their resources and strategies they apply to achieve their objectives. In the end, it documents the nature and success of their attempts to influence the public policy change process.

Box 3.1: The Pluralist View

1. Basic political rights to vote and free speech safeguard political equality and individualism. Citizens have access to government through regular competitive elections, trying to influence government through advocacy for particular policy changes and other activities.
2. Citizens gain power and influence by joining organizations and other groups to participate in the political process. Citizen engagement provides a means of challenging government decisions and influencing public policy.
3. The state in a pluralist society is defined as a complex of institutions that mediates diverse social and economic interests. The state is neutral and does not align itself with any one class or group, nor does it privilege particular interests over others.
4. The state is described as a "plurality" of elites. No single elite dominates at all times.

Source: Smith, B. (1977). *Policymaking in British government*. London: Martin Robertson. Cited in Walt, G. (1994). *Health policy: An introduction to process and power*, 36. London: Zed Books.

Pluralism and the Liberal Conception of Society

Pluralism is consistent with a liberal conception of society in which all citizens are considered to participate in numerous ways in the political process (Walt, 1994).

The state is considered to consist of a neutral set of institutions that mediate diverse social and economic interests. Pluralist theory developed alongside theories of Western democracy, specifically later theories of democracy that emphasize the importance of regular elections as part of the democratic process (Ham & Hill, 1984). Schumpeter defines democracy as "that institutional arrangement for arriving at political decisions in which individuals acquire the power to decide by means of a competitive struggle for the people's vote" (Schumpeter, 1947, 269). In democracies, interest groups are believed to compete to influence public policy decisions. Thus, pluralism was based on key features that characterize liberal democracy: political rights, citizens' access to political power, and the responsiveness of the political system to provide rational public policy outcomes (Smith, 1977).

For example, Easton's model of the political system shows the different inputs into the political system with government institutions at the centre. It presents the government as neutral and therefore receptive to all interests in society, including the business community, market forces, and civil society organizations such as social movements, unions, and other organizations.

Figure 3.1: Easton's Model of the Political System

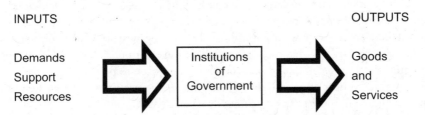

INPUTS   OUTPUTS

Demands   Institutions   Goods
Support   of   and
Resources   Government   Services

Source: Easton, D. (1965). *A framework for political analysis*. Englewood Cliffs, NJ: Prentice-Hall.

Limitations of Pluralism

Critics argue that pluralism fails to consider the role that political power or political ideology plays in the policymaking process (Signal, 1998; Walt, 1994). Pluralism seems to explain away these concepts, viewing the political process as essentially consensual and without conflict. It presents governments as neutral arbiters of diverse interests considered to be equal in their capacity to influence the political system. Pluralism does not focus on power relations and the existence of economic, political, and social inequalities. It says little about structural and societal factors that influence political power and how it is exercised.

Studies of policy change have demonstrated how governing parties privilege particular interests that are consistent with their own perspectives at the expense of other groups and interests (Rochon & Mazmanian, 1993). Governments operate under the control of these political parties that run in competitive elections on public policy platforms. Political parties always have a political ideology, but may not make their ideological commitments explicit in these electoral platforms. These platforms promise to address issues in particular ways, but ideology guides their selection of priorities and the types of public policies they enact to address issues they define as important.

Yet, in spite of these limitations, pluralism has remained the dominant understanding and approach of groups trying to influence politics and public policy in Western nations, particularly in North America. As a consensus approach to politics and governance, its avoidance of political conflict and neglect of social cleavages makes it an attractive approach for advocacy groups trying to change public policies.

For example, groups will work for years—with rather little effect—to convince government to enact particular policy solutions to address poor health outcomes. Since these groups have no other way of understanding the policy development and change process, they are limited to activities of advocating, educating, and attempting to influence governments to change policy. This may mean advocating for changes to the health care system, rather than considering other potential sources of poor health outcomes such as poverty. One way of thinking about this is that they strive to draw in government by making it "part of the solution," rather than recognizing that these governments and their policies may actually be the problem. In the end, pluralism's consensual approach to public policy change disguises the sources of groups' differences with the government and may stymie the development of the policy outcomes they seek.

As suggested in Chapter 1, the pluralist dominance may reflect a preference, particularly in North American politics, to depoliticize issues and to emphasize individualized approaches to health care and health-related policy formulations. In the UK and western Europe, policymaking and politics tend to be less pluralist and more conflict oriented. This can at times contribute to social cleavages along racial or income lines. It recognizes, however, that health care and health-related public policy are heavily politicized and require public solutions. While governments' responses do not always result in the implementation of progressive policies, governments may be more likely to recognize citizens' needs and respond to these needs proactively within such an explanatory framework.

◼ NEW INSTITUTIONALISM

Many political science models of public policy change adopt a consensus-driven political process. One influential model has been what is termed the new institutionalism. The new institutionalism has some pluralist features, but adds an interest in how institutions structure the nature of politics and political debate, and the policy change process. New institutionalism approaches to understanding public policy change have been prominently applied to explain the evolution of the health care system in Canada.

The focus of the new institutionalism is analysis of how societal institutions influence public policymaking (Hall & Taylor, 1996; Signal, 1998; Thelen & Steinmo, 1992). These institutions structure and manage the politics associated with policy change by determining the conditions and nature of political discourse (Coleman & Skogstad, 1990; March & Olsen, 1984). That is, what are the appropriate public policy domains that can serve as the targets of political action? The new institutionalism is seen as a reaction to the behavioural approaches that were dominant during the 1960s and 1970s (Hall & Taylor, 1996). In particular, there was seen to be a lack of theory to explain the manner by which institutions foster or impede policy change.

The new institutionalism consists of three frequently integrated theoretical approaches: (1) historical institutionalism, which traces how the past shapes the future; (2) rational choice institutionalism, which highlights the economic position of political actors; and (3) sociological institutionalism, which emphasizes culture and norms as determining influences (Fischer, 2003; Hall & Taylor, 1996). What they all share is a belief that institutions are primary in shaping or structuring the value and policy preferences of those working in the public policy realm (Coleman & Skogstad, 1990; March & Olsen, 1984).

Defining Political Institutions

Political institutions are state and governmental structures that develop over time and persist in their effects. These institutions can be formal rules of operation, organizational structures, and standard operating procedures as exemplified by the rules and regulations established by government institutions for obtaining services. The new institutionalism conceives these institutions as independent forces that promote particular ideologies and restrict the choices available to policy-makers. These political institutions therefore "structure" political reality and define the terms and nature of political debate. Institutionalist analysis can also examine advisory boards to government, government departments, and political institutions such as Parliament in order to understand their influence on the public policy process.

New institutionalists have contributed significantly to the understanding of the complexity of social and political change in modern societies. Their contribution is in analyzing the interaction between political elites, interest groups' demands, institutional processes, and ideas in political and policy analysis (Hall & Taylor,

1996). The focus for historical institutionalists is on both macro-level (higher level) and meso-level (middle level) processes. By doing so they provide analyses of some of the most important influences on the public policy process (Signal, 1998).

Historical Institutionalism: The Development of Public Health Care

Historical institutionalism provides one theoretical framework for examining health and health care policy issues by highlighting how the institutions of a political system structure policy discourse (Tuohy, 1992, 1999). One objective of the framework is to understand the uniqueness of national political outcomes. Another is to understand how the inequalities that characterize these outcomes come about (Eckstein & Apter, 1963).

Historical institutionalism identifies conflict among competing groups for scarce resources as key to understanding politics. An important focus is on how political and economic structures may interact with each other and with current situations to produce outcomes where some interests are privileged while others are demobilized or ignored.

For example, Carolyn Tuohy draws on historical institutionalism and rational choice approaches to explain health care decision making and varying policy outcomes in the United Kingdom, Canada, and the United States (Tuohy, 1999). Tuohy examines the logics of particular decision-making systems within which actors act rationally, or respond, to incentives and resources available to them. In other words, political goals and objectives, as well as the strategies to achieve these objectives, result from the incentives and resources available to policy-makers. She argues that the dynamics of change in decision-making systems must consider the temporal context. That is, policy change occurs when choices become available as a result of particular historical contexts. Structure allows change, but also sets limits to change:

> The structural dimension relates to the balance of influence across key categories of actors: in the case of health care, the balance across the state, the medical profession, and private finance. The institutional dimension refers to the mix of various instruments of social control—hierarchy, market, and collegiality. Change in the policy parameters establishing the structural balance and the institutional mix of the health care system requires an extraordinary mobilization of political authority and will. (Tuohy, 1999, 7)

Further, she argues that a key feature of the three health care systems and the logics that shaped them is how they have structured the relationship between the medical profession and the state. These systems are:

shaped by the climate of ideas and the constellation of interests that exist at the time that such a confluence occurs. Once established, the institutional mix and structural balance of these systems intersect to generate a distinctive logic that governs the behavior of participants and the ongoing dynamic of change. (Tuohy, 1999,7)

By way of illustration, Tuohy argues that the single-payer system, which has become synonymous with the Canadian approach to health care, operates according to the logic of an accommodation between the medical profession and the state (Tuohy, 1999). The provincial governments are the "single payers" for a comprehensive range of medical and hospital services that are provided on the basis of need to those living in the province. In the United Kingdom, the National Health Service involves an agency relationship between the government and the British medical profession (Tuohy, 1999). An agency relationship is one in which a prospective recipient of health care services assigns decision-making authority to particular health care providers. Providers in such relationships have wide discretion to decide the nature of and how much medical care an individual will receive. Mechanisms are put in place to protect against potential abuse that may stem from allowing wide discretion for providers.

In the United States, although proposals for national health insurance were unsuccessful, the immediate postwar era gave way to initiatives such as hospital construction grants from the federal government (Tuohy, 1999). Tuohy thus considers the institutional mix and the structural balance established in each country to understand how each arrived at their particular policy response to the provision of health care services (Tuohy, 1999).

As is evident, Tuohy is primarily interested in the roles of government and the medical profession in the development of the health care systems. Tuohy's focus on institutions seems to exclude other important factors and groups that helped to bring about a public health care system in Canada and the United Kingdom.

As noted, in this analysis, institutions are central to understanding policy outcomes. Some argue that while institutions are employed to explain all aspects of public policy development, in reality such an analysis says little about how public policies develop or change over time (Thelen & Steinmo, 1992). It may be that institutionalism as a policy framework minimizes the degree of policy change that is possible (Clemens & Cook, 1999). It does so by emphasizing that institutions can constrain and limit opportunities for change because they are enduring and embody the social, political, and economic values of a society. These, in turn, are influenced by structures and interests in a society over time.

Since they seem to constrain change, institutions may not be a useful analytic tool for explaining change. There is a need to consider institutions in relation to other factors that influence public policy outcomes. These may include various social, political, and economic forces than can be mobilized in the service of public policy change.

The new institutionalism is a middle-level theory about the evolution of health care systems. Ideas and knowledge are seen as driving policy responses. The new institutionalism can therefore be understood as a rational approach to public policy analysis. In contrast to the new institutionalism, political economy is a materialist perspective that considers living conditions as giving rise to ideas for social and policy change (Coburn, 2006).

The Political Economy Critique

Contrast Tuohy's view of the development of the Canadian health care system with the political economy perspective. The latter sees the creation of the public health care system as a victory for the working class, which made demands on the state to provide social security to citizens in the immediate postwar era (Armstrong & Armstrong, 2003; Teeple, 2000).

In this analysis, the public health care system, as well as many aspects of the welfare state in Canada, came about during the 1960s and 1970s when the economy was thriving and political and economic forces were able to pressure governments to provide a modicum of economic and social security to its citizens (Armstrong & Armstrong, 2003).

The seeds of these movements were planted at the end of the Second World War when citizens developed expectations that their efforts during the war required some responses. It took many years following the war to build this momentum, however, and this was especially the case concerning the public health care system. Ruling politicians, the media, and the medical profession were wary of public health care and what they perceived to be a socialist idea.

Nevertheless, the government of Tommy Douglas in Saskatchewan established the first publicly funded health care system in 1947, which was very well received. It wasn't until the 1960s that the federal government decided to model a national health care system on the successful health care program established in Saskatchewan. How can we explain the role played by economic, political, and social forces such as these in the policy development process?

■ OVERVIEW OF THE POLITICAL ECONOMY APPROACH

It is the premise of this book that the political economy approach offers the most useful means of understanding how public policy, including health policy, is created and implemented. To provide a means of applying these concepts to the study of health policy, the remainder of this chapter introduces a variety of political economy concepts and illustrations.

The political economy approach to understanding policy development and change is explicitly concerned with the economic, political, and social structures that influence the distribution of power and resources in a society (Armstrong & Armstrong, 2003; Armstrong, Armstrong & Coburn, 2001; Coburn, 2006). How a society organizes the production and distribution of economic and social resources is key to understanding policy outcomes. Political economists carry out these inquiries by looking at states, markets, power, ideas, discourses, and civil society and their impact on policy development.

There are a number of political economy perspectives (Coburn, 2006). One important political economy perspective is materialist. In contrast to the new institutionalist emphasis on the primacy of ideas, materialist political economists consider that how a society organizes production and distribution of social and economic resources shapes ideas and institutions.

Political economists use concepts such as the mode of production and social class to explain political events and phenomena (Grabb, 2002). The mode of production refers to the manner in which societal goods and services are produced and distributed. In Canada and most elsewhere, the current social formation is the capitalist mode of production. Political economy considers that this capitalism mode of production shapes all aspects of economic, political, and social life, including relations among different groups in society. Groups that are especially important include those that differ by social class, gender, and race, among others (Grabb, 2002).

There is also a feminist political economy. It is also concerned with the complex of institutions and social relations that operate through the political and economic systems to shape ideological and cultural systems (Drache & Clement, 1985). Feminist political economy focuses on gender and how it structures women's access to health care services and their opportunities for good health as compared to men (Armstrong, 2006). There is also interest in the power dynamic that shapes these relations and conditions of life for men and women such that men appear to have more opportunities than women.

Box 3.2: Focus of a Feminist Political Economy

Feminist political economy considers how the political, economic, and social organization of health structures opportunities for health for women. This focus is concerned with the role of political ideology in shaping health policy, indeed all public policies, with an attendant analysis of implications for women and other vulnerable populations. Thus, it is assumed that gender, race, and other social attributes such as class can increase vulnerability. Especially important is the increased likelihood of experiencing social and economic marginalization.

Political Economy as Critical Social Science Applied to Public Policy

Materialist and other political economy perspectives represent a critical social science perspective (Armstrong et al., 2001; Coburn, 2000, 2001, 2004). Political economy is concerned with issues of power, and as critical social theory it embodies a transformative component. This means that people are considered to have the power and the ability to change their environment, such as improving living conditions and health in the community in which they live. In addition, an important outcome of a political economy analysis is how power impacts policy change, which then impacts the health of populations. It considers the context in which events such as the creation of public policies or conflict among groups in society occur as important. Relations and power are considered to shape this context and the social, political, and economic institutions that develop in a society.

The Role of the State: Accumulation and Legitimation

Factored into the political economy perspective is recognition of the role of the state. O'Connor (1973) argues that the welfare state has critical roles of accumulation and legitimation. Accumulation refers to the state providing the conditions to enable private profits. States help foster the conditions to enable private profit-making by providing infrastructure such as roads, highways, and communication services, and an educated workforce. States also ensure social cohesion and mediating conflict among social classes by providing a justice system and services. Legitimation is the state's socially sanctioned right to use force in order to ensure social order and cohesion. Accumulation and legitimation are contradictory roles that require the state to vary its support for business and workers in order to maintain social cohesion and reduce the possibility of class conflict.

It does so in order to aid variations in the needs of organizations that seek profit. Health care and health are integral components of the welfare state. O'Connor argues that by the 1970s, states were paying for more of the costs of accumulation, yet at the same time allowed for the collection and control of profits by private interests. O'Connor attributes the oil crisis that developed in the 1970s to the private appropriation of state power to protect private interests (Armstrong & Armstrong, 2003; O'Connor, 1973). Within a political economy perspective, the processes of legitimation and accumulation have particularly adverse impacts on women and racial minorities in the formal economy. They foster large "surplus populations outside the market" (Armstrong & Armstrong, 2003; O'Connor, 1973).

Armstrong and Armstrong and others argue that O'Connor neglects the special impacts these processes have on households, particularly for women, who bear the larger burden of caregiving (Armstrong & Armstrong, 2003). For example, changes in the state's role that resulted in increasing market approaches to health care have impacted women as primary caregivers within families. Women frequently carry out health care responsibilities normally provided by trained health care professionals, such as nurses.

The Armstrongs argue that O'Connor's theory requires a third role for the state in addition to accumulation and legitimation and that is one of distribution. This is so since the state has a critical role "in structuring what is provided for publicly in the market and privately in households, in determining who does the work in these spheres and how it is done" (Armstrong & Armstrong, 2003, 8).

The Impact of Political Ideology on Health Policy

Of particular interest to political economists is the influence of the ascent of neo-liberalism as a governing political ideology. Neo-liberalism is a political ideology that favours the market as the vehicle for fostering economic growth and innovation (Coburn, 2000). Specifically, free enterprise policies are seen as key to economic growth and as the basis for the well-being of the population. Political economists trace the advent of neo-liberalism to events from the 1970s (Coburn, 2006; Teeple, 2000).

In later chapters the specific influence of neo-liberalism on the organization and delivery of health care will be examined. In these sections, the focus is on how neo-liberalism has been associated with growing inequalities in health between different groups in developed political economies such as Canada, the US, and the UK. Inequalities in health refer to unequal health outcomes that are based on some group characteristic of individuals.

▪ HEALTH INEQUALITIES, SOCIAL INEQUALITIES, AND HEALTH CARE

In Europe the focus has been on health inequalities as a function of social class or occupational status (Mackenbach & Bakker, 2002; Townsend, Davidson & Whitehead, 1992). In Canada, the primary focus has been on issues of income and poverty (Raphael, 2007b). A vast literature has established the link between low income and poverty with poor health status and status and outcomes (Auger, Raynault, Lessard & Choinière, 2004; Phipps, 2002; Raphael, 2007a).

Their belief in markets means that supporters of neo-liberalism tend to accept whatever the market produces, including social and health inequalities. These inequalities are seen as somewhat natural and stemming from personal failure to succeed in the market. These inequalities are not usually considered to be related

---

Box 3.3: The Main Tenets of Neo-liberalism

David Coburn considers that neo-liberalism refers to the dominance of markets and the market model. He identifies the main assumptions of neo-liberalism and the new right:

1. Markets are perceived as most efficient in the production and distribution of resources in a society.
2. Societies are comprised of autonomous individuals (producers and consumers) who are driven primarily by material or economic gain.
3. Competition is the primary source of innovation.

Coburn distinguishes between neo-liberalism and neo-conservatism because the latter is concerned with a particular social component supportive of traditional family values, certain religious traditions, among other issues, and is not only concerned with a laissez-faire economic doctrine. The essence of neo-liberalism is a commitment to the virtues of a market economy.

Moreover, neo-liberals tend not to be troubled by inequality, nor do they consider it as either positive or inevitable. If the market is "the best or most efficient allocator of goods and resources, neo-liberals are inclined to accept whatever markets bring."

Source: Coburn, D. (2000). Income inequality, social cohesion, and the health status of populations: The role of neo-liberalism. *Social Science and Medicine 51*, 135–146.

---

to public policies that allow increased skewing of the distribution of economic resources and to the social exclusion of some groups. Social exclusion is closely associated with social inequalities. Social exclusion is a process of marginalization of some groups, resulting in denying access to basic resources, such as sufficient income and affordable housing. This process is strongly influenced by a wide range of forces, as illustrated in Figure 3.2.

Coburn considers the relationship between income inequality and health within and among nations (Coburn, 2000, 136). He argues there is a need to consider the "basic social causes of inequality and health" by analyzing the social, political, and economic context within which income and health inequalities emerge. Coburn and others have linked inequalities to the welfare state and the class origins of different types of welfare state regime. Such a focus enables a consideration of the relationships among markets, states, and civil society. Coburn argues that it also presents a different causal configuration about national and

Figure 3.2: Social Exclusion in Context

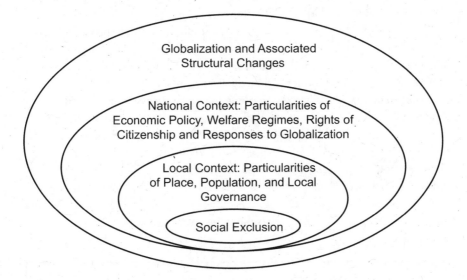

Source: Percy-Smith, J. (2000). Introduction: The contours of social exclusion. In J. Percy-Smith (Ed.), *Policy responses to social exclusion: Toward inclusion* (p. 5). Buckingham: Open University Press.

international differences in income inequality and in longevity than are usually acknowledged in the literature.

Neo-liberalism has undermined the welfare state, as reflected by Western governments such as Canada and the United Kingdom, by dismantling social programs that form the welfare states. As noted earlier in this chapter, the formation of the welfare state was intended as a way of sharing risk across the population and as means to redistribute income and access to programs from higher-income groups to lower-income groups.

There is much evidence to show that low-income groups especially benefit from these programs. Indeed, reduced poverty rates among different groups, particularly seniors, has been attributed to welfare state programs (Raphael, 2007b). Coburn and others have argued that the welfare state contributed to social cohesion or solidarity among social classes because it mitigated class differences. Coburn shows that the basic assumptions of neo-liberalism are consistent with higher levels of inequality and lowered social cohesion or increased class conflict attributable to accentuated differences among classes (Coburn, 2000).

Armstrong and Armstrong have shown how neo-liberal policies have led to reforms that have undermined health care through cutbacks in public financing and new approaches to managing health care services (Armstrong & Armstrong, 2003). They argue that hospital CEOs in particular have adopted new management strategies with a view to making hospitals more efficient. This approach results in reducing nursing and other hospital staff and providing care at the lowest unit cost (Bourgeault, 2006). This means that hospital staff who tend to be the least skilled in patient care usually end up providing greater amounts of patient care.

Some observers describe the deskilling of care whereby families are trained to insert catheters and other health equipment that is usually performed by registered nurses (Armstrong & Armstrong, 2003). Some hospitals trained cleaning staff to do the work of registered nurses as a way of reducing the cost of patient care. These processes have contributed to the decline in patient care, increased risk of infections in hospitals, and other problems that are preventable through proper cleaning of patients' rooms and other facilities in hospitals. These developments have been attributed to the under-resourcing of hospitals and the health care system as a whole.

Box 3.4: Political Economy Analysis: Social Exclusion, Gender, Race, and Health

A political economy approach can be applied to examine how social positions such as gender and race structure opportunities for health and the determinants of health such as income, employment, and access to a range of other resources. Political economy examines how race, gender, and others lead to social exclusion. Social exclusion is defined as both a process and outcome, whereby people experience social and economic marginalization on the basis of gender, race, or other characteristics (Galabuzi, 2006).

Political economists reject the view that the capitalist formation and the social relations that develop are inevitable (Coburn, 2006; Teeple, 2000). Rather, they consider capitalism and the social relations that emerge from the organization of society such as inequalities between women and men, White populations, and populations of colour, among others, to be social constructions. That is, society creates these processes and categories to make sense of differences within a population, and tend to reflect the dominant attitudes of a culture toward people of colour. Often, these differences are treated as pathologies or unattractive attributes and can become the basis of discrimination against various groups.

■ CONCLUSIONS

This chapter has examined the assumptions of three theories of public policy that represent the dominant political perspectives in the social science literature. These theories can be arranged along a continuum from consensus models to conflict models of the policy process. Consensus models tend to focus on group behaviours in the political process, whereas conflict theories are concerned with the influence of politics and economics on public policy outcomes. Institutionalist models take a middle course.

Pluralism has become one of the most influential theories of public policy and politics in Western societies such as Canada. It contends that politics consists of a "plurality" of interest groups that compete to influence public policy. No single interest group or political elite dominates the political process. Pluralism fails to recognize the inequality of access to the political system or the role of political power. The state is portrayed as a neutral arbitrator of interests that contributes to policy decisions arrived at by consensus.

The new institutionalism focuses on institutions as shaping policy behaviours and policy change outcomes. It is a structural approach that considers institutions to be primary in shaping the preferences and values of political actors. Institutions "structure" political reality and define the terms and nature of political debate. The focus on institutions tends to preclude a consideration of other forces that may be time-specific and important variables for understanding policy change outcomes.

Political economy is concerned with the interrelationship between politics and economics and how these structure policy change. Material conditions of societies are seen as primary in influencing ideas and institutions. Political economy considers political power and the influence of political ideology on policy change outcomes and health outcomes. It focuses on the broader political and economic context as being causal factors in influencing health outcomes. These theories also represent different levels of analysis. The application of theories reflects different perspectives on which factors can help explain political outcomes.

■ REFERENCES

Armstrong, P. (2006). Gender, health, and care. In D. Raphael, T. Bryant & M. Rioux (Eds.), *Staying alive: Critical perspectives on health, illness, and health care*, 287–303. Toronto: Canadian Scholars' Press Inc.

Armstrong, P. & Armstrong, H. (2003). *Wasting away: The undermining of Canadian health care*. Toronto: Oxford University Press.

Armstrong, P., Armstrong, H. & Coburn, D. (Eds.). (2001). *Unhealthy times: The political economy of health and care in Canada*. Toronto: Oxford University Press.

Auger, N., Raynault, M., Lessard, R. & Choinière, R. (2004). Income and health in Canada. In D. Raphael (Ed.), *Social determinants of health: Canadian perspectives*, 39–52. Toronto: Canadian Scholars' Press Inc.

Bourgeault, I. (2006). The provision of care: Professions, politics, and profit. In D. Raphael, T. Bryant & M. Rioux (Eds.), *Staying alive: Critical perspectives on health, illness, and health care*, 263–286. Toronto: Canadian Scholars' Press Inc.

Brooks, S. & Miljan, L. (2003). *Public policy in Canada: An introduction*, 22–49. Toronto: Oxford University Press.

Clemens, E.S., & Cook, J.M. (1999). Politics and institutionalism: Explaining durability and change. *Annual Review of Sociology, 25*, 441–466.

Coburn, D. (2000). Income inequality, social cohesion, and the health status of populations: The role of neo-liberalism. *Social Science & Medicine, 51*(1), 135–146.

Coburn, D. (2001). Health, health care, and neo-liberalism. In P. Armstrong, H. Armstrong & D. Coburn (Eds.), *Unhealthy times: The political economy of health and care in Canada,* 45–65. Toronto: Oxford University Press.

Coburn, D. (2004). Beyond the income inequality hypothesis: Globalization, neo-liberalism, and health inequalities. *Social Science & Medicine, 58*, 41–56.

Coburn, D. (2006). Health and health care: A political economy perspective. In D. Raphael, T. Bryant & M. Rioux (Eds.), *Staying alive: Critical perspectives on health, illness, and health care*, 59–84. Toronto: Canadian Scholars' Press Inc.

Coleman, W. & Skogstad, G. (Eds.). (1990). *Policy communities and public policy in Canada: A structural approach.* Toronto: Copp Clark Pittman.

Dahl, R.A. (1961). *Who governs?* New Haven: Yale University Press.

Drache, D. & Clement, W. (1985). *The new practical guide to Canadian political economy.* Toronto: James Lorimer.

Eckstein, H. & Apter, D. (1963). *Comparative politics.* Glencoe: Free Press.

Fischer, F. (2003). *Reframing public policy: Discursive politics and deliberative practices.* New York: Oxford University Press.

Galabuzi, G.E. (2006). *Canada's economic apartheid: The Social exclusion of racialized groups in the new century.* Toronto: Canadian Scholars' Press Inc.

Grabb, E. (2002). *Theories of social inequality.* Toronto: Harcourt Canada.

Hall, P.A. & Taylor, R.C.R. (1996). Political science and the three institutionalisms. *Political Studies, 44,* 936–957.

Ham, C. & Hill, M. (1984). *The policy process in the modern capitalist state.* Brighton: Wheatsheaf Books Ltd.

Latham, E. (1952). *The group basis of politics.* Ithaca: Cornell University Press.

Mackenbach, J. & Bakker, M. (Eds.). (2002). *Reducing inequalities in health: A European perspective.* London: Routledge.

March, J.G. & Olsen, J.P. (1984). The new institutionalism: Organizational factors in political life. *American Political Science Review, 78,* 734–749.

O'Connor, J. (1973). *The fiscal crisis of the state.* New York: St. Martin's Press.

Pal, L. (2006). *Beyond policy analysis: Public issue management in turbulent times.* Toronto: Nelson.

Phipps, S. (2002). *The impact of poverty on health.* Ottawa: Canadian Population Health Initiative.

Raphael, D. (2007a). Addressing health inequalities in Canada: Little attention, inadequate action, limited success. In A. Pederson, I. Rootman, M. O'Neill & D. S. (Eds.), *Health promotion in Canada: Critical perspectives,* 106–122. Toronto: Canadian Scholars' Press Inc.

Raphael, D. (2007b). *Poverty and policy in Canada: Implications for health and quality of life.* Toronto: Canadian Scholars' Press Inc.

Rochon, T. & Mazmanian, D. (1993). Social movements and the policy process. *The Annals of the American Academy of Political and Social Science, 528,* 75–85.

Schumpeter, J. (1947). *Capitalism, socialism, and democracy.* London: Allen & Unwin.

Signal, L. (1998). The politics of health promotion: Insights from political theory. *Health Promotion International, 13*(3), 257–263.

Smith, B. (1977). *Policymaking in British government.* London: Martin Robertson.

Teeple, G. (2000). *Globalization and the decline of social reform: Into the twenty-first century.* Aurora: Garamond Press.

Thelen, K. & Steinmo, S. (1992). Historical institutionalism in comparative politics. In S. Steinmo, K. Thelen & Longstreth, F. (Eds.), *Structuring politics: Historical institutionalism in comparative analysis,* 1–32. New York: Cambridge University Press.

Townsend, P., Davidson, N. & Whitehead, M. (Eds.). (1992). *Inequalities in health: the Black Report and the health divide.* New York: Penguin.

Tuohy, C. (1992). *Policy and politics in Canada: Institutionalized ambivalence.* Philadelphia: Temple University Press.

Tuohy, C. (1999). *Accidental logics: The dynamics of change in the health care arena in the United States, Britain, and Canada.* New York: Oxford University Press.

Walt, G. (1994). *Health policy: An introduction to process and power.* London: Zed Books.

CRITICAL THINKING QUESTIONS

1. Which of the public policy theories best explains recent developments occurring in health policy in Canada?

2. What are the specific issues of interest of each of the three main public policy theories?

3. What kinds of evidence do you think guide current health policymaking in Canada?

4. How do theories of public policy contribute to our understanding of health policies and their impact on the health of populations?

5. What considerations should be brought to bear on health policy discussions in order to improve health policy decisions?

FURTHER READINGS

Coburn, D. (2000). Income inequality, social cohesion, and the health status of populations: The role of neo-liberalism. *Social Science & Medicine, 51*(1), 135–146.

Coburn is one of the foremost political economy analysts in Canada. In this article, Coburn examines the impact of neo-liberalism on health policy, specifically the increase in inequalities in health in Canada and elsewhere.

Coleman, W. & Skogstad, G. (Eds.). (1990). *Policy communities and public policy in Canada: A structural approach.* Toronto: Copp Clark Pittman.

This text is a collection of essays on Canadian public policy examined from a new institutionalist perspective. The essays help to explicate the key areas of interest in the new institutionalism.

Hall, P.A. & Taylor, R.C.R. (1996). Political science and the three institutionalisms. *Political Studies, 44,* 936–957.
This article was among the first to explain the three variants of the new institutionalism. It defines the rational choice, historical institutionalism, and sociological institutionalism and key areas of interest of each with reference to American public policy.

Signal, L. (1998). The politics of health promotion: Insights from political theory. *Health Promotion International, 13*(3), 257–263.
This article examines three theories of pluralism, the new institutionalism, and political economy and their contributions to understanding and explaining health promotion.

Walt, G. (1994). *Health policy: An introduction to process and power.* London: Zed Books.
The book provides an overview of the health policy process and examines different theories of public policy. Walt examines international health policy issues. The author's interests are in power and politics in health policy.

RELEVANT WEBSITES

Canadian Centre for Policy Alternatives
www.policyalternatives.org
The Canadian Centre for Policy Alternatives is a think tank that publishes research papers and articles on current public policy issues in Canada. Its theoretical orientation on Canadian health policy and other public policies is political economy. Reports can be downloaded from this website.

Centre for Health Services and Policy Research, University of British Columbia
www.chspr.ubc.ca
This site provides research on current Canadian health care issues. It focuses on scientific enquiry into health care and population health policy research.

The Institute for Research on Public Policy
www.irpp.org
The Institute for Research on Public Policy was founded by Hugh Segal, former political aide to Ontario premiers and Canadian prime ministers. The institute publishes books on current Canadian public policy issues and also the journal, *Policy Options*. Current and back issues of *Policy Options* can be downloaded from its website.

School for Policy Studies, University of Bristol
www.bristol.ac.uk/sps/index.html
The school is renowned for its studies on public policies in the United Kingdom. Although not specifically focused on "health" policy, it addresses many issues related to health policy such as social exclusion and poverty.

World Health Organization
www.who.int/en
The World Health Organization addresses a wide range of health policy and health care policy issues. It is the directing and coordinating authority for health in the United Nations and provides leadership on global health issues. This site provides information on current global health issues and public policy.

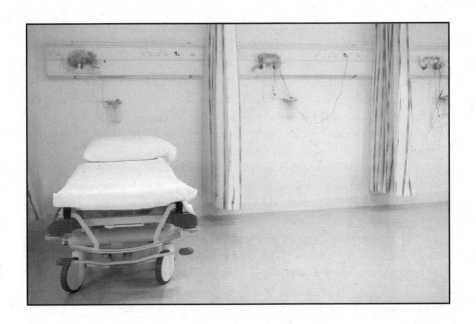

Chapter 4
UNDERSTANDING POLICY CHANGE

■ INTRODUCTION

Policy change is an adjustment to an existing public policy or set of related public policies. These adjustments can be incremental, leading to small changes in policy, such as increasing the fee schedule for physicians or adjusting the amounts of financial transfers to community health centres and hospitals. Adjustments can also be radical changes that lead to a fundamental shift in the underlying philosophy of a public policy area, such as a shift from institutional care to community-based care, or a shift from a biomedical understanding of health to a social determinants perspective that emphasizes living conditions as the primary influences on health.

While most theories of the public policy process address policy change, such as those examined in Chapter 3, they vary in their specificity about policy change, the roles different actors play, and the role of the state in the process (Mintrom & Vergari, 1996). A set of models termed learning models of policy change have been very influential in the policy studies area. These models show many conceptual similarities with the pluralist and new institutionalism approaches to understanding public policy presented in Chapter 3.

These models tend to de-emphasize the influence of conflict between interest groups and differences in the amount of, and exercise of, power in policy change. They focus instead on how the acquisition and application of knowledge influences policy-makers. The adherents of this view argue that such an emphasis produces better explanations of how public policies are developed and implemented than do conflict-based theories (Bennett & Howlett, 1992; Heclo, 1974).

Learning models, therefore, focus on learning as a potential source of policy change (Bennett & Howlett, 1992). Adherents of these views also argue that conflict-oriented theories neglect the role that information or knowledge plays in this process. Illustrating the focus on process over analyses of economic, political, and social forces, Heclo argues that policy change can arise from uncertainty: "men collectively wondering what to do …" (Heclo, 1974, p. 305). The learning approaches, therefore, focus on learning and assert that the state—and policy-makers—learn from experience and change public policies on the basis of their interpretations of how well previous policies have performed.

■ THE SCOPE OF LEARNING MODELS

The political science literature identifies several learning models of policy change (Bryant, 2001, 2002a, 2003, 2004b). This chapter is not intended to provide a definitive examination of all of these. Instead, this chapter focuses on two representative models: the Policy Paradigms (Hall, 1993) and the Knowledge Paradigms Policy Change models (Bryant, 2004b).

Building on the insights of historical institutionalism, Hall's model emphasizes the role that institutions and social learning play in policy change. He defines change as intentional efforts to adjust the goals or instruments of policy, given the experience of past policies and new information (Hall, 1993). Bryant's Knowledge Paradigms Policy Change Conceptual Framework builds on Hall's insights on knowledge and adds a concern with a political economy perspective on how power, conflict, and political ideology influence policy change. Apart from Tuohy's excellent analysis using historical institutionalism to explain the development of public health care, this approach is rarely applied to health policy issues. Bryant's model has been used in analyses of both health care policy and health-related public policy. This chapter explores the usefulness of both Hall's model and Bryant's conceptual framework for understanding how health policy develops and changes.

■ POLICY PARADIGMS

The new institutionalism discussed in Chapter 3 is an important contribution to understanding the role that institutions play in the policy change process. As enduring bodies in society with clear policy influence, they have the potential to shape policy changes. But of equal or more importance, they have the potential to constrain the policy change process and impede social and political change.

Hall integrated aspects of historical institutionalism and the literature on scientific paradigms to explicate the roles played by ideas and knowledge in public decision making (Kuhn, 1970). He acknowledges Anderson's observation that public policy discussion occurs within specific realms of discourse (Anderson, 1978). Policy-makers work within specific frameworks of ideas and standards that specify policy goals and the instruments or means by which these goals can be attained. These frameworks are grounded in the kinds of language through which policy-makers convey as well as carry out their work.

There exists, therefore, influential systems of ideas that guide both policy development and the policy-makers themselves. This may be problematic "because so much of it is taken for granted and is not amenable to scrutiny as a whole" (Hall, 1993, p. 279). These systems of ideas specify what types of problems will be defined as legitimate public problems requiring government action. These systems also specify the tools that government may apply to address these problems (Hall, 1993). Hall refers to these interpretive frameworks as "policy paradigms," which help to explain different patterns of policy change by linking these paradigms to specific instances of social learning.

Box 4.1: The Process of Social Learning

Hall draws on the work of Heclo to formulate the concept of social learning. He argues that a key factor affecting policy at time-1 is policy at time-0. Previous policy is an important influence on policy. In fact, Hall suggests that policy responds "less directly to social and economic conditions than it does to the consequences of past policy" (Hall, 1993: 277). Moreover, Hall agrees with Weir and Skocpol that the interests and ideals that policy-makers choose to follow are influenced largely by what are termed "policy legacies." In addition, experts in a policy field in which policy change is being considered tend to be very influential in the learning process. They may advise the state from a privileged and critical position at high-level meetings between the bureaucracy and intellectual leaders.

Hall's portrayal of the policy change process suggests a highly elitist activity from which many groups may be shut out. This suggests that policy changes reflect the interests of those attending such high-level meetings than those who are likely to be adversely affected by policy changes.

Source: Hall, P.A. (1993). Policy paradigms, social learning, and the state: The case of economic policy making in Britain. *Comparative Politics, 25*(3), 275–296.

Social learning refers to policy change that results from both new information about an issue as well as learning from past policy experience (Hall, 1993). Social learning, therefore, is primarily concerned with the role ideas play in policymaking. The social learning process is dominated by government officials and highly placed experts whose power is likely to be particularly influential. For Hall, this influence is especially the case in technical policy fields such as environmental or energy policy. The health policy area can also be added to these technical policy fields where the views of experts are especially valued. Hall's interest is also to examine how knowledge created by scientists and social scientists influence the policymaking process (Hall, 1993).

Different Types of Policy Change

A further aim of Hall's model is to analyze how policy-makers apply knowledge to effect different *types* of policy changes. Two such kinds of changes are routine (first- and second-order) or radical (third-order) policy changes (Hall, 1993). Hall terms these two kinds of policy change as normal and paradigmatic patterns of policy change (Hall, 1993).

First-order change has many elements of incrementalism, such as "satisficing" and "routinized" decision making (Hall, 1993). Such changes are usually minor adjustments to policy, such as increasing physicians' fees for various medical procedures, or increasing or lowering monthly social assistance payments. This constitutes much of the ongoing activities of governments and agencies.

Second-order change usually involves developing new policy instruments and moving toward strategic action (Hall, 1993). An example of second-order change would be a provincial government's decision to develop a telehealth line for the public to call for health advice from registered nurses to reduce inappropriate use of hospital emergency departments. Another instance might be modifying the means by which individuals could apply for social assistance and the means by which such applications would be processed. In both these first- and second-order policy changes processes, the overall goals of a policy area basically remain the same.

Third-order change is characterized by radical (paradigmatic) change in the overall terms of policy discourse. This change would result in diverging from the "received" or dominant paradigm (Hall, 1993). As defined in Chapter 2, a paradigm is a set of beliefs concerning the nature of an issue and the problems associated with the issues. For example one paradigm of health care is that it be seen as a commodity subject to being bought or sold on the market. A competing paradigm would be that health care is a basic human right and therefore should be an entitlement for citizens. Not all paradigmatic issues are as profound in their implications as this particular one, but paradigm disagreements usually involve a fairly significant discrepancy between sets of ideas as well as values.

Hall suggests that paradigmatic shifts involve simultaneous changes in all three components of policy: (1) the instrument settings; (2) the instruments themselves; and (3) the policy goals and objectives. For example, the creation of a national public health care system in Canada in 1961 represented a shift from a system based on ability to pay for health services to a system based on providing services in response to need (Romanow, 2002). Rather than health care being funded by individuals on an out-of-pocket basis, the government now pays for health care from general revenues. The policy goal of ensuring that all Canadian citizens receive care on the basis of need rather than ability to pay represents a paradigmatic policy change.

In the health-related policy area, government decisions to withdraw from providing affordable housing for those in need, which occurred federally during the 1990s, would represent a paradigmatic shift (Bryant, 2004a; Shapcott, 2004). Frequently, these kinds of profound shifts are made with little warning and with little, if any, public consultation.

Importance of Politics in Paradigmatic Policy Change

Noting the relative lack of attention in the policy change literature to the role played by politics in understanding third-order policy change, Hall argues that policy paradigms are never completely understandable solely in scientific or technical terms (Hall, 1993). Instead, the change from one paradigm to another may result more from political influences rather than the accumulation of scientific knowledge.

Indeed, the policy change outcome may also depend on the arguments of competing groups in a policy arena and from the advantages or disadvantages these various interest groups possess within this broader policy arena. In addition, resources available to competing political actors for advocacy activities may determine the shape of policy change. Sometimes external factors such as changes in the economy (the onset of a recession or surging economic growth) can affect the capacity of a group of actors to impose its ideas or policy paradigm on others.

Since each paradigm has its own explanation of how the world of policy-makers works, it is often difficult, if not impossible, for advocates of different paradigms to agree on a common body of knowledge on which to favour one paradigm over another. Yet sometimes paradigmatic change is a gradual process shaped by experiences accrued from policy experimentation and policy failure.

Paradigmatic shift can also occur as a result of an accumulation of inconsistencies in the old paradigm through testing of new forms of policy. The accumulation of problems associated with existing policy can weaken its dominance if its adherents are unable to explain new developments (Hall, 1993). For example, the outbreak

Box 4.2: Advocacy Coalition Framework

Like Hall's Policy Paradigms, Sabatier's Advocacy Coalition Framework is a learning model of policy change. The advocacy coalition framework of policy change is a conceptual framework for examining long-term policy change of a decade or more (Sabatier, 1993). This model attempts to explain the strategic interaction of political elites and policy experts in a policy community or subsystem. The policy subsystem consists of ideologically based advocacy coalitions that are involved in a particular policy area. Coalitions can include actors from both the public and private sectors, such as social scientists, senior civil servants, the media, politicians, and interest groups. The coalition can include actors from local and regional governments involved in policy formulation and implementation. These actors can all play a role in the generation, dissemination, and evaluation of policy ideas (Dunleavy, 1981; Heclo, 1978; Milward & Wamsley, 1984).

Sabatier agrees with Heclo that policy change occurs within a social, economic, and political context (Heclo, 1974). Policy change can also involve competition for power and conflicting activities within the community that arise to address a policy problem. Sabatier is particularly interested in the role of technical information and ideology throughout the policy process. Some key concepts require examination.

Belief system: Subsystem members can come from different advocacy coalitions and this shapes their activities (Sabatier, 1993). All share a set of normative and causal beliefs (ideology). Beliefs shape policy positions, instrumental decisions, and information sources chosen in support of specific policy positions. The belief system consists of three structural categories. These categories are termed "deep (normative) core," which comprises fundamental normative and ontological beliefs; "near (policy) core" or the coalition's policy positions; and "secondary aspects," which are instrumental decisions and information inquiries enlisted to support the policy core. The coalition's strategies (policy core) and secondary aspects respond to perceptions about the adequacy of governmental decisions in relation to the perceived problem. Changes in strategy can include lobbying for major institutional revisions at the broad policy level, or minor revisions at the operational level.

Change in the larger environment: Sabatier identifies a range of factors that can influence an advocacy coalition and its activities as well as its success in effecting policy change (Sabatier, 1993). Stable parameters and dynamic external events are identified as sources of new information that can affect perceptions of policy issues and lead to alterations in the belief systems of advocacy coalitions. Stable influences such as established policy parameters and the social, legal, and resource features of the society persist over a period of several decades. These influences frame and constrain the activities of advocacy coalitions. Dynamic influences such as changes in global socio-economic conditions (e.g., the 1973 Arab oil embargo or the election of Ronald Reagan in 1980) can alter the composition and resources of various coalitions. These influences also affect how public policy is carried out within the subsystem. Personnel changes at senior levels within government ministries can also affect the political resources of various coalitions and the decisions that are made at the collective choice and operational levels.

Policy-oriented learning: A key component of the framework is policy-oriented learning. This refers to relatively enduring changes in thought or behavioural intentions that are based on previous policy experience (Sabatier, 1993). Learning occurs through internal feedback mechanisms and includes perceptions of external dynamics and increased knowledge of problem parameters. Such learning is instrumental, since it is assumed that members of the various coalitions seek to improve their understanding of the world in order to further the achieving of their policy objectives. This notion is the enlightenment function of public policymaking, which implies that political actors are more committed to improving the quality of public policy decisions than to furthering their own political interests.

of severe acute respiratory syndrome (SARS) in Toronto was recognized as resulting from lack of a central institution to monitor disease outbreaks in various jurisdictions (National Advisory Committee on SARS and Public Health, 2003). In response, the Public Health Agency was established with one centre given responsibility for monitoring infection outbreaks in Canada and elsewhere.

Another example is that the spread of SARS in Toronto from hospital to hospital was identified as resulting from many nurses having only part-time employment and having to move from hospital to hospital on any given day (National Advisory Committee on SARS and Public Health, 2003). A response was to review the employment situation of nurses and the development of public policy to address the part-time employment situation of nurses.

Therefore, policy failures such as the SARS outbreak or others such as an explosion of homelessness or food bank use can bring about a shift in paradigmatic authority. These changes in policy can heighten conflict between competing paradigms (Hall, 1993). Efforts to explain these new and potentially problematic phenomena by persisting in using an old paradigm can further undermine its intellectual coherence. Politicians may be especially instrumental in deciding whose knowledge claims—and whose paradigm—becomes authoritative and will prevail in a policy arena.

Hall's most widely quoted application of his model was his explanation of the shift from Keynesianism welfare state economic policy in Britain to a monetarist approach during the 1970–1989 period (Hall, 1993). Keynesianism had led to the development of the welfare state and hence significant government intervention to provide publicly funded health care. However, economic stresses led to a questioning of the value of such a paradigm.

British politicians intervened when social scientists were unable to resolve the dispute between these Keynesian and monetarist paradigms (Hall, 1993). The politicians, who happened to be Conservatives, favoured monetarism because it was consistent with their neo-liberal ideology of wanting to advance the role the market played in allocating resources at the expense of the state.

The British government thus launched a new era in economic policymaking that, while drawing on social science, did so in a selective manner to support the very right-wing inclinations of Margaret Thatcher, the leader of the Conservative Party. Monetarists successfully attributed rising unemployment and other economic problems to perceived failures of Keynesianism. Hall concludes that social science ideas in this case and others enter policy debates through the broader political system rather than through the traditional knowledge contributions of a narrow network of experts and officials.

Hall therefore shows how understanding of changes such as shifting economic policy from Keynesianism to monetarism requires analysis of the influence institutions to impede or help bring new ideas into the policy discourse and into public policy decisions (Fischer, 2003). Changes in the British economy, specifically an unemployment crisis and high levels of inflation, by challenging the principles of Keynesianism, contributed to the paradigm shift to monetarism. These changes therefore provided an opportunity for application of new paradigmatic ideas from the Conservative Party (Fischer, 2003).

Limitations of Policy Paradigms

Hall provides a compelling explanation of the shift to monetarism and shows how institutions can structure outcomes. The focus on institutions, however, precludes other considerations. For example, his model fails to consider how structures and interests influence political, economic, and social change. He seems unconcerned about the close association between certain interests such as social scientists and the political system.

Moreover, Hall does not consider how the Thatcher government deliberately excluded particular groups from the political process. For example, after her election as prime minister, Thatcher undermined trade unions in the United Kingdom, thereby increasing class conflict (Krieger, 1987; Towers, 1989). This increase in class conflict distorted the policy change process by weakening the ability of information and knowledge supportive of the working class to influence policy change. More overtly, she also abolished the Greater London City Council since it appeared to oppose her policies. These actions represented clear exercise of political power that limited the ability of opposition groups to challenge these policy changes.

Hall does identify the influence of political elites on the policy change process, but does so in a manner that implies that this relationship and its impact on the policy change process is unproblematic. This close relationship between elites and policy-makers may serve to see policy development in the service of particular segments or interests of the population to the detriment of others.

In addition, Hall articulates a single path to paradigmatic change. Paradigmatic change occurs in response to a series of policy failures, a shift in political power, or in response to external shocks. But there is another trajectory for paradigmatic policy change. It has also been argued that paradigmatic policy change can also result from a series of incremental policy changes over several years (Coleman, Skogstad & Atkinson, 1997).

Hall recognizes political considerations as having a significant role in bringing about change (Hall, 1993). He demonstrated how Thatcher's contingent within the Conservative Party contributed to shifting state machinery toward monetarism. The model provides some useful analytic tools for classifying different types of policy change. The model, however, depicts the public policy arena as being almost exclusively the purview of senior civil servants, policy analysts, and academics.

While much policy debate occurs at this level, other interests mobilize to try to influence policy change outcomes. Hall describes state and societal actors as the chief agents of learning, but does not consider the relationship between the civil service and the public, or the relationship between the state and civil society.

Identifying these concerns is important to draw attention to inequalities in the distribution of power and opportunities to influence policy change outcomes. In Hall's model, the shift from one policy paradigm to another emerges as a largely academic debate in which politicians seem to arbitrate over whose paradigm will dominate in a given policy arena. There is a need for a model that considers the impact of an unequal distribution of political power, a broader range of political actors, and defines the role of the state involved in public policy debates.

■ KNOWLEDGE PARADIGMS POLICY CHANGE FRAMEWORK

The Knowledge Paradigms Policy Change Framework builds on Hall's insights into policy change and the role of political ideology by incorporating a concern with inequality, conflict, and power in the political process (Bryant, 2002a, 2002b). It also explicitly considers how various forms of knowledge can influence the different types of changes contained in Hall's models. Figure 4.1 shows the framework and its key components.

Figure 4.1: Model Informing the Policy Change Process

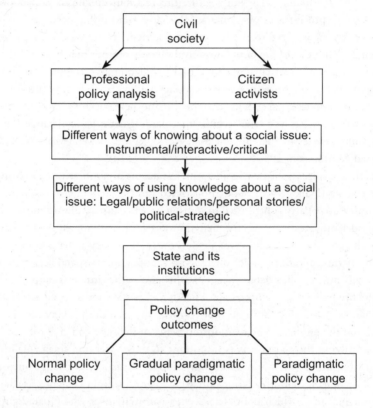

Source: Bryant, T. (2004). Housing and Health. In D. Raphael (Ed.), *Social determinants of health* (p. 229). Toronto: Canadian Scholars' Press Inc.

Policy Actors

The first component of the model considers the various actors in the policy change process. While Hall focused on technical experts, policy-makers, and elected officials, other segments of the population can be involved in the policy change process.

Civil society: Beginning at the top of the figure, civil society encapsulates the values and beliefs of the citizenry, as well as its institutions and traditions, thereby providing a context for the policy change process.

Professional policy analysts and citizen activists: Civil society consists of many groups, including the market, trade unions, professional associations such as the medical and nurses associations, and faith communities, among others. The groups of interest identified in the figure are professional policy analysts, the experts in Hall's policy paradigms, and citizen activists because these are the groups that try to act on the political system to influence public policy.

Some political actors constitute a hybrid. That is, they possess post-secondary degrees and specialized knowledge in a particular policy field. They may work as policy analysts for trade unions in social and health policy think tanks. These aggregates are politically engaged groups in civil society and are not necessarily mutually exclusive. Nor are they intended to be representative of all groups in civil society. These groups represent different political entities in the public policy process.

Box 4.3: Editorial: Flawed Premise on Health Care

Toronto Star

In his inaugural address to the Canadian Medical Association's annual convention on Wednesday, new CMA president Dr. Brian Day started out offering some welcome advice for making Canada's publicly funded health-care system better at meeting patients' needs.

He said governments must address the "critical shortage of doctors" in the country and the reasons why too many leave Canada. He talked about the high student debt that young doctors must assume to complete their studies and the pressures it puts on some of them to seek the higher incomes available in privatized health-care systems elsewhere. He also said other doctors leave Canada because they are not getting what they need, like sufficient time in operating rooms.

And he warned that Canada is not investing nearly enough in new technologies, such as electronic medical records, that could make the health-care system both more efficient and effective.

But after raising these important issues that would help make Canada's publicly funded health-care system work even better, Day then did a complete about-face, arguing that the public system would never be able to provide top-notch health care to all Canadians unless it was combined with a parallel system of privatized medicine available to those who could afford private insurance.

That point of view was not unexpected from Day, who owns Canada's largest private hospital, based in Vancouver, which lets those who can afford to pay privately jump to the front of the queue.

In his speech, Day says, "Those who have studied or worked in other countries know there are systems with universal coverage and no wait lists. They do deliver better care at less cost than here in Canada."

He is talking, of course, about countries such as Britain that have parallel public and private health-care systems.

So just how good is the British system? And how low are its costs?

A recent letter to Day from a group of senior British doctors offers some insights. In advising Day and his Canadian colleagues not to follow Britain down the road to privatization, they note that the significant reduction in wait times that accompanied the "English Experiment" with a dual public-private system "is hardly surprising given that health spending has more than doubled since 1997."

What this doubling of spending reflects, they say, "is that money has been lavished on politically sensitive wait lists for elective surgery through expansive and unsustainable deals with the private sector ... to the detriment of many patients with more long-term needs."

Pointing out that the British counterpart of the CMA, the British Medical Association, "has repeatedly voiced its opposition to the competitive model," the letter provides a scathing indictment of privatized health care. Because the private sector's objective is profits, "it selects fit patients for high-volume, simple procedures, leaving the medically complex and expensive care to the (public) National Health Service. The result is overdiagnosis and overtreatment of some patients and neglect and undertreatment of others."

Similarly, experience in Australia and New Zealand has shown that parallel private insurance and dual practice reduces cost efficiency and increases wait times in the public system.

And just last year, a CMA position paper found the introduction of parallel private insurance would not lower costs or improve quality of care and could increase wait times for those not privately insured.

At the heart of Day's argument is his flawed assumption that medicare is broken and cannot be fixed. But as former Saskatchewan premier Roy Romanow concluded in 2002 after his exhaustive 18-month review of Canada's health-care system, medicare is far from broken and the problems that do exist can be fixed at reasonable cost.

Indeed, since Romanow's report, both the federal and provincial governments have invested heavily in addressing the bottlenecks in the system. Those investments have already resulted in shorter wait times in many key areas, a rise in sophisticated diagnostic equipment, and the introduction of programs of enhanced primary care.

Although there is still more to be done, the vast majority of Canadians continue to support our publicly funded medicare system. What Day has failed to recognize is that their opinions count for far more than his. Not only are they the people who pay for medicare, polls consistently show that those who have received treatment through our universal system are generally quite satisfied with the care they got.

Source: Editorial, Flawed premise on health care, *Toronto Star* (August 24, 2007), AA6.

An important element here is the inequality in the capacity of each group to influence the political process. Both kinds of groups engage in knowledge creation and advocacy activities (see Box 4.3).

Professional policy analysts are perceived as having specialized knowledge that gives them an aura of objectivity and authoritativeness, which can enhance their credibility in the public domain. In contrast, citizen activists may be seen as lay experts. The wider public may perceive citizen activists as addressing issues that affect them personally and therefore as self-interested. For example, a university professor or policy analyst speaking out against barriers to accessing health care for marginalized communities may be considered to have more credibility in the public domain than someone who is actually experiencing barriers to accessing health care services. Many activists sometimes advocate on issues that do not directly affect them. Citizen activists may also advocate on behalf of communities that experience barriers in their access to health care services, yet not actually experience such barriers themselves.

Different ways of knowing about a social issue: Instrumental/interactive/critical: One typology of knowledge—the Habermas-Park typology—represents different ways of knowing about or understanding an issue. There are three types of knowledge: instrumental, interactive, and critical knowledge (Habermas, 1968; Park, 1993). The different types of knowledge represent different approaches to understanding the nature of knowledge and how it is created.

Box 4.4: Habermas's Typology of Knowledge

Habermas devised three categories of knowledge that Park has refined as instrumental knowledge, interactive knowledge, and critical knowledge. Park's interest in these categories is to understand the role of lay knowledge to engage in participatory research that helps to give marginalized populations a voice.

Instrumental knowledge is knowledge produced by the traditional sciences through systematic research and hypothesis testing. Instrumental knowledge involves detachment and objectivity on the part of the research. This knowledge aims to control external events and create explanatory theories of causal relationships. An example is carrying out an experiment on a new pharmaceutical product or medication to test its efficacy in treating a health condition. The experiment would consist of an experimental group with the health condition who would receive the drug and a control group that would have the same characteristics as the experimental group such as age, income level, education, etc., in addition to having the same health condition. The control group does not receive the drug. The researcher carries out statistical analysis to compare the results for the two groups. Did the experimental group improve their symptoms as a result of taking the medication? Or, did the control group experience similar improvements in their symptoms?

Interactive knowledge is created through exchanges or conversations with other people. People exchange information and actions supported by common experience, tradition, history, and culture. This knowledge builds connections among members of a community and enables the formation of community. An example of interactive knowledge would be lived experience such as asking people what they would do for their children if they are unable to find a space in child care, or understanding the culture of nurses working in a particular ward of a hospital. What is the nurses' informal understanding of their work, and their relationships with each other, physicians, and patients?

Critical knowledge is derived from reflection and action. Citizens acquire critical knowledge by questioning or challenging their life conditions and identifying what they wish to achieve as self-determining social beings. Through critical knowledge, they can mobilize others to challenge existing public policies and programs that govern their lives. Thus, critical knowledge has a transformative element. An example of critical knowledge would be the relative power of nurses and doctors and how this developed. Nurses would acquire a critical understanding of why they are subordinate to doctors and hence undervalued for their contribution to patient care.

Source: Park, P. (1993). What is participatory research? A theoretical and methodological perspective. In P. Park, M. Brydon-Miller, B. Hall & T. Jackson(Eds.), *Voices of change: Participatory research in the United States and Canada*, 1–19. Toronto: Ontario Institute for Studies in Education.

Instrumental knowledge represents a positivist-rationalist approach to problem solving as exemplified by the biomedical approach defined in Chapter 2. It is usually associated with experts such as social scientists, physicians, or others in the health field, for example, with specialized knowledge perceived as objective and value-free.

Interactive knowledge develops from people's daily interactions with one another or perceptions and understandings of a health condition, for example. This type of knowledge can be stories or concepts that people can create in order to make sense of something. For example, nurses in a hospital may discuss with one another how doctors treat them poorly and do not respect their professionalism. They may, however, lack insight into why doctors treat them disrespectfully. Another example might be someone trying to make sense of why they have a particular disease or health condition. They may attribute their affliction to exposures to toxins, but may not consider that it may have something to do with their housing or the wider public policy arena. They would not see this as a problem of low income, which means they can afford only housing with poor conditions that impair their health.

Both instrumental and interactive knowledge may tend to depoliticize issues. Interactive knowledge is similar to the interpretive research paradigm discussed in Chapter 2 in which all perceptions and understandings are treated as having equal validity. There is rather little recognition of the societal tendency to privilege certain types of knowledge and understanding of issues.

Critical knowledge reflects an awareness of power and its influences on society and an explicit interest in initiating political action to change life conditions. Thus, unlike instrumental and interactive knowledge, critical knowledge has a transformative component. Critical knowledge is consistent with the structural-critical and political economy perspective defined in chapters 2 and 3.

For example, members of the Chalk River community in Ontario opposed the reopening of the nuclear plant for fear of increasing the incidence of cancer diagnoses among residents in the local community. They see a potential relationship between the incidence of cancer and the presence of a nuclear plant, and will lobby the state, which they see authorizing the reopening of the plant with little concern about the potential impact on the health of the local community.

Another example is the recovery process in the aftermath of Hurricane Katrina in New Orleans. This process revealed that poverty in the United States is highly racialized and gendered. In a CNN report, the reporter remarked that residents were "very Black and very poor."

Both aggregates of policy actors may draw upon all three ways of knowing in their political activities. They all engage in processes to decide what kind of evidence they need to convince the government of their position.

Box 4.5: Feminist Policy Analysis: A Form of Critical Knowledge

Rational policy analysis, heir to positivism, attempts to imbue political action and policy activity with the attributes of science (Albaek, 1995). Science is concerned with a methodical, detached approach to data collection and analysis of policy options. Rational policy analysis has been the dominant approach to policy analysis.

From a feminist perspective, Hawkesworth (1988) criticizes positivism as having a "misplaced concern with objectivity" about the influence of personal experiences. Biases and perceptions of the observer are seen as hampering the understanding of the phenomenon under study. Hawkesworth argues that this concern with objectivity conceals "the real ... which is the role of social values" as exercised by feminism to reveal how social values such as racism and sexism "filter perception, mediate arguments, and structure research investigations" (Hawkesworth, 1994, 21). Positivism separates social phenomena from their social and political context, a process known as context-stripping. Feminism is a form of critical knowledge that attempts to explain the power dynamic between women and men and inequality between men and women. The economic and political structures are considered to reinforce inequality between women and men.

Different ways of using knowledge to lobby—legal, public relations, political-strategic, personal stories approaches: Professional policy analysts and citizens use different activities and strategies to convince policy-makers to make policy changes. Lobbying is political pressure that aims to achieve a particular policy change. These approaches—legal, public relations, political/strategic, and personal stories—are strategies. They all have elements of the three ways of knowing and involve processes of knowledge dissemination to promote a policy position. The legal approach is the use of legal knowledge, cases, and legal analysis.

Public relations refers to how advocates market or present their ideas to government. The political-strategic approach is knowledge about the political process and how to work one's way through it to lobby government and present policy ideas. Finally, personal stories refer to the use of narratives about experiences as a result of public policies. For example, former patients may present information to a legislative committee about how laying off registered nurses affects the quality of care they received when they were in hospital. Fewer nurses mean that patients may not have their needs addressed as quickly as may be necessary.

All of these approaches are about how to present information to government in order to influence public policy decisions. They are therefore informed by political considerations and questions of how advocates can effectively make their case on proposed policy changes and draw media attention to their efforts. Knowledge dissemination and issue promotion are also inherently political activities. Civil society actors present their policy ideas to government officials and opposition parties. They also attempt to influence other civil society actors. They may form new alliances to enhance their political power. Media presence can help groups enhance their political power by increasing their visibility and may arouse public sympathy for their cause.

The state: The state consists of the government of the day and state institutions responsible for a policy domain. In Canada, state institutions consist of legislative bodies, including Parliament, the Senate, legislative committees, law-making institutions such as the courts, as well as ministries or government departments run by civil servants (Ham & Hill, 1984). These different components of the state exist at different levels. In Canada, for example, there are municipal, provincial, and federal levels of government with varying degrees of responsibility for enacting and enforcing laws in public policy areas. The state represents the legitimate use of force to achieve certain objectives and outcomes (Ham & Hill, 1984). The state is led by a political party that is elected by citizens every four years in most jurisdictions.

The state is not always well conceptualized in many models and is often presented as one-dimensional. It is often presented as an essentially neutral or apolitical organization that mediates among competing interests. In this manner it is consistent with the pluralist view of policymaking presented in Chapter 3.

The state has numerous roles within the many areas that constitute health policy in modern capitalist societies such as Canada, the United States, and the United Kingdom. The economic system is integrally related to the political system, and state roles are often contradictory. It must promote economic development while at the same time ensure social order and solidarity among different social classes and other groups in society (Teeple, 2000). Thus, in addition to identifying the institutions that the state comprises, the linkages between the state and the social system—including hierarchies of class, gender, and race—must be clearly articulated.

With the creation of medicare, the federal and provincial governments assumed significant roles in health policy. The federal government developed legislation to use its spending power to help finance health care programs in each province and territory. As discussed in Chapter 1, the British North America Act and the Canadian Constitution assign responsibility for the administration of health care to the provincial and territorial governments.

Since the 1980s, the federal and many provincial governments have attempted to reduce the role of government in health care and related health policy areas. Few governments appear willing to address inequalities in health outcomes in the Canadian population. This retreat of government has occurred in other areas of health policy. For example, Lexchin shows how government has ceded its responsibility for regulating the pharmaceutical industry by allowing the industry to regulate itself, to test its own products for consumer safety, and by not conducting its own independent tests of new drug products (Lexchin, 2006). Many consider this approach as providing inadequate protection for consumers and as a conflict of interest for the industry to regulate itself.

Civil servants, such as deputy ministers and senior policy analysts, interact with both groups of civil society actors in policy discussions. An assumption of this framework is that the state or government of the day is not neutral, but has its own political agenda. The government as a political actor can try to exclude civil society actors from the process by selecting or filtering out knowledge provided by specific civil society actors.

Policy outcomes: The knowledge paradigms framework incorporates Hall's typology of policy change. Hall identifies first- and second-order change as normal policy change, and third-order change as paradigmatic change that involves a fundamental change in overall policy goals (Hall, 1993). The framework identifies two potential paths to paradigmatic change. The first is a series of incremental changes that result in a paradigm shift. The second is an accumulation of policy failure and anomalies in the received paradigm that result in a sharp paradigmatic shift (Coleman et al., 1997). Deciding not to change policy is also a policy decision. The government always makes these decisions on the basis of what they perceive as valid reasons.

This framework can serve as a template for analyzing the policy change process on a case-by-case basis. It can also be used to understand a government's general approach to policy change over time. The framework was applied to a case study of Women's College Hospital during the hospital restructuring process in Ontario, Canada, in 1996. It was also applied to a study of government changes to a health-related public policy—rent control in Ontario—around that same period.

■ THE CASE OF WOMEN'S COLLEGE HOSPITAL AND THE HEALTH SERVICES RESTRUCTURING COMMISSION

The case study focused on the 1995 to 1998 experience of Women's College Hospital during the hospital restructuring process in Toronto (Bryant, 2003). The purpose of the study was to learn about the knowledge activities used by individuals attempting to influence the health policy change process to see whether and how knowledge influenced the outcome. The specific policy goal of the hospital was to forestall its proposed closure by the Health Services Restructuring Commission during a period of economic retrenchment and health care service rationalization.

Box 4.6: Case Study of Women's College Hospital: Methodology and Data Analysis

Document review and in-depth interviews with key informants explored the relationship between knowledge and the influence of civil society actors on the policy change process through the exemplar of the Health Services Restructuring Commission. The document review identified key issues in health policy and the motivations of state and civil society actors and their epistemological assumptions. Friends of Women's College Hospital provided copies of all of the hospital's and Friends' submissions to the Health Services Restructuring Commission and access to materials on the campaign against the proposed merger with Toronto Hospital in 1989–1990. This information supplemented the data provided by in-depth interviews. The in-depth interviews provided insights about participants' perceptions of knowledge, and how they selected the information and evidence to use in their briefs. Interviews were recorded and transcribed. Themes and issues contained within the data were identified.

The data were organized using concepts and categories identified in the policy change model. For example, civil society actors were organized into the categories of professional policy analysts and citizens. Additional categories were created for activists who are paid employees of interest groups. The categories of interactive, rational/scientific, and critical were used to classify the knowledge used by actors. Policy change patterns were identified and coded using the typology in the policy change framework: normal, paradigmatic, and gradual paradigmatic change. These initial concepts and categories were tested on emergent understandings. New categories were developed to fit the data.

Analysis involved identification of key ideas associated with the use of knowledge in political advocacy and policy change. Inductive analysis was used to analyze notes taken during the document review. Comments from the interviews were used to develop additional categories to reflect accurately emerging themes and patterns in the data. This approach allows consideration of alternative explanations and understandings. Participants identified a range of issues on knowledge and its uses in political advocacy. The focus here is on issues relating to the types of knowledge brought to bear on the hospital restructuring process by Women's College Hospital.

Of all the Toronto hospitals facing closure, Women's College Hospital presents one of the most interesting cases. Women's College Hospital grew out of the Ontario Women's Medical College established in 1911 (Kendrick & Slade, 1993). The founding of the college was a response to the refusal of the University of Toronto to accept women as medical students in the late 19th century. The college provided an opportunity for women to study and practise medicine. The hospital retained the word "College" in its name as a reminder of this history. In 1960, Women's College Hospital sought affiliation with the University of Toronto and became a teaching hospital.

Since the late 1980s, Ontario governments grew increasingly concerned about controlling hospital expenditures. One of several hospitals running a deficit during this period, Women's College received one-time-only bridge grants of CDN $2 million for the 1988–1989 and 1989–1990 fiscal years on the condition that it eliminate its deficit (Lownsbrough, 1990). In October 1989, the hospital board voted in favour of pursuing a merger with the larger Toronto Hospital, which had already merged with its western division, Toronto Western Hospital.

Women's College Hospital's medical staff association and other staff opposed the proposed merger. Friends of Women's College Hospital was formed to oppose the merger and worked with the medical staff association in this aim. By reframing the issue as a stakeholder debate, these combined forces defeated the merger at a public meeting where 648 of 700 hospital shareholders voted against the merger.

In November 1995, the newly elected Conservative government introduced legislation—Bill 26, the Savings and Restructuring Act (also referred to as the Omnibus Bill)—that created the Health Services Restructuring Commission (HSRC) (The Caledon Institute, 2001). The bill empowered the commission to close and merge hospitals across Ontario in order to eliminate $1.3 billion from the hospital budget within two years. In Metropolitan Toronto, the goal was to close 12 of 44 hospitals. The commission recommended closing Women's College Hospital and merging its in-patient services with Sunnybrook Health Sciences Centre.

In the end, Women's College Hospital applied sufficient pressure to force the HSRC to reverse its decision to close the hospital. Specifically, it threatened to sue the commission, which helped to secure the outcome the hospital sought. Not only did the hospital avert closure, it legally secured its existence in legislation—a first in any jurisdiction—and was reconfigured as an ambulatory care centre for women's health programs. It has since reclaimed its independent status, as the Ontario Liberal government severed the merger in 2006.

Through document review and interviews with key strategists for the hospital, policy analysts among others, Bryant examined how Women's College Hospital influenced the health policy change outcome (Bryant, 2001, 2003). Of key interest was whether knowledge brought to bear on the political process by Women's College Hospital was the decisive factor in the commission's final decision.

> ## Box 4.7: Case of Women's College Hospital during the Hospital Restructuring Process in Ontario, 1995
>
> "[W]ithout the word being used, it was defined as woman-driven and woman-centred and woman-positive at its founding ... in direct response to discrimination from the University of Toronto ... you wouldn't necessarily use the term "feminist" ... if you look at what was said and you look at the values and whatever the defining term was, it was about equal opportunity."
>
> —Participant Interview
>
> *Source:* Bryant, T. (2003). A critical examination of the hospital restructuring process in Ontario, Canada. *Health Policy, 64*, 193–205.

■ FINDINGS FROM THE WOMEN'S COLLEGE HOSPITAL STUDY

The detailed findings from this case study are available (Bryant, 2003). Generally, it was found that advocates for Women's College Hospital used various forms of evidence to avert closure in its dealings with the Hospital Restructuring Commission. By doing so, it mobilized women across the province to help fight the closure.

Yet, while there was careful selection and deployment of various forms of knowledge in its submissions to the commission, and to inform its supporters, it was the combination of political skills and access to the government that may have clinched the outcome for the hospital. The hospital's strategists arranged meetings with Cabinet ministers in the Ontario government through contacts of board members. Some of the themes that emerged from this analysis have direct implications for understanding the policy change process.

HSRC's Emphasis on Quantitative Evidence

The commission was identified as being focused on objective, quantitative indicators such as the condition of the physical plant of a hospital, the number of patients receiving care, and the number of procedures carried out at a given hospital rather than information about the experiences that women had when they were patients at the hospital. This focus led to the exclusion of quality-of-care issues and neglect of women's health issues.

Feminist Issues and Feminist Policy Analysis

The strategists used gender and gender issues to market the hospital. They viewed the hospital as committed to feminist principles, a pioneer in women's health research, and as having a history of providing quality health services to women. The uniqueness of the hospital was also expressed in terms of its organization of power and its collaborative approach to care.

Use of Legal Arguments and Analysis

Legal arguments and analysis were applied in both the 1989 and 1995 anti-merger campaigns. During the 1989 campaign the issue was defined as a shareholder fight. Advocates sought legal advice on litigation options, although litigation was not pursued. Participants perceived legal arguments and analysis as strengthening the case of the hospital in the restructuring process.

Knowledge Is Political

It was concluded that knowledge and its use were profoundly political. Each piece of information provided was seen through the lens of political ideology by both the government and the advocates. When considering the hospital's outcome, some advocates considered the hospital unsuccessful since it lost its independence, while others saw it as being a success since it maintained its existence. As one interview participant argued, it may have been not lack of knowledge but lack of power that determined the outcome in the restructuring process.

In summary, the use of various forms of knowledge was consistent with the conceptual framework presented. The findings add to an understanding of how different forms of knowledge can influence the health policy development process. Particularly important was not only the gender and abilities of the hospital strategists but also their close association with the governing Conservative Party at Queen's Park. Many were lawyers and highly skilled, and therefore knew how to strategize to meet their political objectives. In other words, specific interests drove the process. The elite did not achieve the outcome it sought, which was retaining the independence of Women's College Hospital. Thus, in the end, the outcome can be attributed not so much to knowledge and its uses during the restructuring process, but rather to the dominance of specific interests and structures that ensured particular policy outcomes.

Women represented an important constituency that the Ontario Conservative government did not wish to offend. Women's College Hospital represented the health interests of predominantly white, middle-class, professional women. There was little concern with the health issues of marginalized women, such as women of colour, women who are homeless, and other communities of women who also use the health care system, but lack a political voice to assert their interests in the political arena.

Different Ways of Knowing about a Social Issue

Different ways of knowing was used to influence policy change. The approach of Women's College Hospital to the selection of knowledge and evidence was affected by the emphasis of the Health Services Restructuring Commission and the commitments of the hospital's board.

Since the commission emphasized instrumental knowledge in its use of objective indicators such as volume of care issues, program levels, clinical activity, and the state of the physical plants of hospitals, the strategists provided these kinds of information as well as interactive and critical. They are developed through legal cases. Legal arguments are made using verifiable evidence and judicial rulings. Rulings arising from legal cases are considered authoritative and demand discipline in the construction of cases.

■ HEALTH SERVICES RESTRUCTURING PROCESS: A CLASH OF WORLD VIEWS

The differences in approaches to knowledge used by the commission and Women's College Hospital can be understood as a clash of world views. The hospital emphasized quality of care and women's perspective, while the commission emphasized objective indicators such as the number of procedures carried out at a hospital to justify hospital closures. The effect of this framing was to limit debate and depoliticize the process, and potentially silence opposition to the restructuring process and how it was carried out.

The case of Women's College Hospital demonstrates the use of instrumental, interactive, and critical ways of knowing in political advocacy. While knowledge was important and helped to establish the credibility of the hospital, it did not emerge as the decisive factor in the case. Political considerations were more important in determining the outcome.

The relative success of the hospital can be attributed to a number of factors. Among these is its use of gender, its status as an institution, its capacity to initiate legal action to force a policy change to achieve its objectives, and the political connections of some board members to the Ontario Conservative government. Some board members were card-holding members of the Ontario Conservative Party. The hospital and women represented a constituency that the government did not wish to offend and identified as important to its future electoral success.

■ THE CASE OF THE TENANT PROTECTION ACT

The second case provides an example of analysis of a health-related public policy change. The case study on housing policy change focused on the Tenant Protection

Act (Government of Ontario, 1997). This study systematically examined the context within which the new provincial regime changed rental housing policy from 1995–1998. The case study focused on how tenant advocates in Toronto, the largest urban centre in Ontario, attempted to influence the policy change process. A particular focus was how oral presentations that challenged the provisions of the legislation were constructed through the selection of specific forms of knowledge and evidence. These oral briefs were means by which tenant advocates constructed their arguments and selected evidence, and the epistemological commitments within which these decisions were made, in attempts to influence the government.

There were many other activities taking place at this time: media campaigns, speeches, and material distribution by advocates and Opposition party activities. Use of briefs provided a selected sample of information-rich exemplars of the processes used to influence government policy by civil society actors.

Canadian provincial governments have constitutional responsibility for providing social housing and rent control. Most provide some form of housing subsidy, but fiscal conservatism in recent years has reduced these subsidies. In Ontario through the 1970s until 1995, successive provincial governments were committed to rent regulation to protect an affordable rental housing stock in the private rental housing market, and to increase the number of social housing units.

In 1975 the Conservative government introduced rent-control legislation as an anti-inflation strategy. In 1995 the Conservative Party won a majority government on a Common Sense Revolution platform (Progressive Conservative Party of Ontario, 1995).This platform reversed many long-held commitments to social housing and rent control. The new platform emphasized cutting taxes and increasing efficiencies to reduce the provincial deficit. The document proposed shelter allowances for low-income populations, but did not identify the government's intention to eliminate rent control.

The 1996 Tenant Protection Act replaced all existing legislation related to rental housing and introduced vacancy decontrol to remove rent control one unit at a time (Government of Ontario, 1997). Vacancy decontrol allows landlords to increase rent without restriction when a tenant vacates a rental unit. The tenant is protected from large rent increases provided she or he does not move.

The Act also amended the Ontario Human Rights Code to allow landlords to use income criteria to screen potential tenants. This amendment sharply reduced the access of low-income groups to housing. An Ontario court judge later struck down the amendment as unconstitutional. In addition, the government imposed a moratorium on social housing construction, ending the prospect of 18,000 planned social housing units. Shortly after its election, the government also reduced social assistance by 22 percent. These changes severely affected low-income populations dependent on these programs for shelter and income.

■ FINDINGS FROM THE CASE OF THE TENANT PROTECTION ACT

Detailed findings from this case are available (Bryant, 2004b). Findings were very similar to that seen for the Women's College Hospital case study. The advocates were all professional policy analysts, yet described a participatory process in which they drew upon their professional work as lawyers and community workers. They emphasized the use of a variety of forms of knowledge. Some collected primary data through systematic research processes consistent with positivist assumptions about knowledge and evidence. They also provided evidence that considered the lived experiences of people and provided a critical analysis of how the proposed legislation would affect an especially vulnerable group of people.

Uses of Evidence

Empirical evidence applied in the briefs was grounded in the lived experience of tenants. Advocates emphasized the need for empirical data to support their claims and to persuade politicians and the public of the validity of their positions. Advocates also used legal analysis and arguments that contain elements of instrumental, interactive, and critical ways of knowing.

Getting on the Public Record

Participants did not believe that their presentations would change the legislation to address their issues. However, participating in public hearings provided means of mobilizing tenants, and planning for future changes in government that would be more likely to address the concerns of low-income tenants.

Different Ways of Using Knowledge about a Social Issue

Participants used various strategies. They used legal knowledge and interpretation of the provisions of the Act. They used personal stories drawn from their professional and clients' experiences with landlord and tenant issues. They also used political-strategic approaches to work the political system by meeting with senior civil servants in the ministry of housing to influence the government. Finally, they met with Opposition parties to help the Opposition to develop amendments. While the knowledge and evidence they presented did not influence the government, it assisted Opposition parties in developing their positions. In the end, participants described the government as interested only in evidence that reinforced its ideological commitments.

The Role of Political Ideology

Participants identified how government ideology was a barrier to their effectiveness in the policy change process. Political ideology drove the legislation and therefore affected their ability to protect the interests of their constituencies. Advocates considered the current regime in Ontario to be unreceptive to perspectives that did not agree with its own. They considered the government to be motivated solely by ideological considerations.

■ CONCLUSIONS FROM BOTH CASE STUDIES

It was clear that political ideology and influence play a particular role in both health care and health-related public policy change. The political ideology of the state shapes perspectives on health care and health-related issues and determines, in large part, the policy responses developed to address these issues. Political influence shapes government receptivity to information. Although knowledge came to the government from diverse sources inside and outside government, political influence and ideology emerged in the housing case study as one of the most important dynamics influencing housing policy change in Ontario.

The case studies also identified the complex of actors who can work to influence policy. It confirmed the existence and application of various forms of knowledge in the policy change process. It also allows for specifying the kinds of change that eventually occur. In both case studies, the political and economic structures and interests shaped the outcomes.

■ CONCLUSION

This chapter examined two approaches to understanding and explaining the policy change process. Hall's Policy Paradigms is primarily a rational model concerned with the role of ideas in shaping public policy change outcomes. Policy paradigms refer to the system of ideas in which policy-makers work. They determine the policy instruments and goals of policy, as well as define the issues that will be recognized as public issues requiring government action.

Policy paradigms focuses on the role of social learning whereby policy-makers make decisions based on experience with previous public policies and on new information on a given issue in a policy field. As such, it is concerned with the role of experts such as social scientists in the public policy process. Hall applied the model to understand the ascendance of neo-liberalism led by Margaret Thatcher in the United Kingdom in the late 1970s. The model builds on the insights of historical institutionalism. It emphasizes how institutions can structure politics and thereby influence political outcomes. Above all, it demonstrates how institutions are basically conservative and can obstruct policy change.

The model considers a limited range of participants in the public policy process and seems to consider the close association between experts and policy-makers as unproblematic. The model does not seem to recognize inequality in access to the political system and in the distribution of political power as being important factors in shaping the policy change process.

The Knowledge Paradigms Policy Change Framework builds on Hall's insights into knowledge. The framework is also concerned with the role of political and economic structures such as political ideology, inequality, political power, and the privileging of information and groups in the political process. Applied to the case of Women's College Hospital during the hospital restructuring process and changes to the Tenant Protection Act in Ontario, Canada, the framework highlights the influence of political issues upon knowledge development, the receptivity of the state, and its eventual application.

Policy change, especially health care and health-related public policy, can be politically charged. Many areas of health policy are contentious. Dominant health interests attempt to hide behind a veil of objectivity and intellectual detachment from issues. The aura of scientific inquiry can sometimes draw attention away from the highly conflictual nature of the health policy field. In the next chapter the various actors who attempt to influence health policy are examined.

■ REFERENCES

Albaek, E. (1995). Between knowledge and power: Utilization of social science in public policymaking. *Policy Sciences 28(1)*, 79–100.

Anderson, C. (1978). The logic of public problems: Evaluation in comparative policy research. In D. Ashford (Ed.), *Comparing public policies*. Beverley Hills: Sage.

Bennett, C. & Howlett, M. (1992). The lessons of learning: Reconciling theories of policy learning and policy change. *Policy Sciences, 25*(3), 275–294.

Bryant, T. (2001). *The social welfare policy change process: Civil society actors and the role of knowledge*. Unpublished PhD thesis, University of Toronto, Toronto.

Bryant, T. (2002a). The role of knowledge in progressive social policy development and implementation. *Canadian Review of Social Policy, 49*(50), 5–24.

Bryant, T. (2002b). Role of knowledge in public health and health promotion policy change. *Health Promotion International, 17*(1), 89–98.

Bryant, T. (2003). A critical examination of the hospital restructuring process in Ontario, Canada. *Health Policy, 64*, 193–205.

Bryant, T. (2004a). Housing and health. In D. Raphael (Ed.), *Social determinants of health: Canadian perspectives*. Toronto: Canadian Scholars' Press Inc.

Bryant, T. (2004b). The role of political ideology in rental housing policy in Ontario. *Housing Studies, 19*, 635–651.

The Caledon Institute. (2001). The Harris record. In R. Cohen (Ed.), *Alien invasion: Ontario politics and government 1995–2003*. Toronto: Insomniac Press.

Coleman, W.D., Skogstad, G.D. & Atkinson, M.M. (1997). Paradigm shifts and policy networks: Cumulative change in agriculture. *Journal of Public Policy, 16*(3), 273–301.

Dunleavy, M. (1981) The politics of mass housing in Britain, 1945–75. Oxford: Clarendon Press.

Fischer, F. (2003). *Reframing public policy: Discursive politics and deliberative practices*. New York: Oxford University Press.

Government of Ontario. (1997). Tenant Protection Act (Bill 96). Toronto: Queen's Printer.

Habermas, J. (1968). *Knowledge and human interests*. (J.J. Shapiro, Trans.). Boston: Beacon Press.

Hall, P.A. (1993). Policy paradigms, social learning, and the state: The case of economic policy making in Britain. *Comparative Politics, 25*(3), 275–296.

Ham, C. & Hill, M. (1984). *The policy process in the modern capitalist state*. Brighton: Wheatsheaf Books Ltd.

Hawkesworth, M.E. (1994). Policy studies within a feminist frame. *Policy Sciences 27*: 97–118.

Hawkesworth, M.E. (1988) *Theoretical issues in policy analysis*. Albany: SUNY Press.

Heclo, H. (1978). Issue networks and the executive establishment. In A. King (Ed.), *The new American political system*. Washington: American Enterprise Institute.

Heclo, H. (1974). *Social policy in Britain and Sweden*. New Haven: Yale University Press.

Kendrick, M. & Slade, K. (1993). *Spirit of life: The story of Women's College Hospital*. Toronto: Women's College Hospital.

Krieger, J. (1987). Social policy in the age of Reagan and Thatcher. *Socialist Register, 23*, 177–198.

Kuhn, T.S. (1970). *The structure of scientific revolutions*. Chicago: University of Chicago Press.

Lexchin, J. (2006). Pharmaceutical policy: The dance between industry, government, and the medical profession. In D. Raphael, T. Bryant & M. Rioux (Eds.), *Staying alive: Critical perspectives on health, illness, and health care*, 325–345. Toronto: Canadian Scholars' Press Inc.

Lownsbrough, J. (1990). The insurrection: How the anti-merger troops seized control of Women's College Hospital. A blow-by-blow account. *Toronto Life, 1990*, 24:10, 43–93.

Milward, H.B. & Wamsley, G. (1984). Policy subsystems, networks, and the tools of public management. In R. Eyestone (Ed.), Public policy formation and implementation (pp. 105–130). New York: JAI Press.

Mintrom, M. & Vergari, S. (1996). Advocacy coalitions, policy entrepreneurs, and policy change. *Policy Studies Journal, 24*(3), 420–434.

National Advisory Committee on SARS and Public Health. (2003). *Learning from SARS: Renewal of Public Health* in Canada. A report of the National Advisory Committee on SARS and Public Health. Ottawa: Health Canada.

Park, P. (1993). What is participatory research? A theoretical and methodological perspective. In P. Park, M. Brydon-Miller, B. Hall & T. Jackson (Eds.), *Voices of change: Participatory research in the United States and Canada*, 1–19. Toronto: Ontario Institute for Studies in Education Press.

Progressive Conservative Party of Ontario (1995). The Common Sense Revolution. Toronto: Progressive Conservative Party of Ontario.

Romanow, R.J. (2002). *Building on values: The future of health care in Canada*. Saskatoon: Commission on the Future of Health Care in Canada.

Sabatier, P.A. (1993). Policy change over a decade or more. In P.A. Sabatier and H.C. Jenkins-Smith (Eds.), Policy change and learning: An advocacy coalition approach, 13–40. Boulder: Westview Press.

Shapcott, M. (2004). Housing. In D. Raphael (Ed.), *Social determinants of health: Canadian perspectives*, 201–215. Toronto: Canadian Scholars' Press Inc.

Teeple, G. (2000). *Globalization and the decline of social reform: Into the twenty-first century.* Aurora: Garamond Press.

Towers, B. (1989). Running the gauntlet: British trade unions under Thatcher, 1979–1988. *Industrial and Labour Relations Review, 42*(2), 163–188.

CRITICAL THINKING QUESTIONS

1. What do you think are critical determinants of recent health policy changes?
2. Which of the two policy change models presented in this chapter explain recent health policy changes that have occurred in Canada or elsewhere?
3. How can we understand the role of institutions, gender, or social class in health policy change outcomes?
4. How does political ideology influence public policy change?
5. How can civil society actors have greater influence on the health policy change process?

FURTHER READINGS

Bennett, C. & Howlett, M. (1992). The lessons of learning: Reconciling theories of policy learning and policy change. *Policy Sciences, 25*(3), 275–294.

The authors provide an excellent assessment of the learning models of policy change and compare conflict-based theories with new institutionalist approaches. In particular, they highlight some of the limitations of these approaches to understanding policy change.

Bryant, T. (2003). A critical examination of the hospital restructuring process in Ontario, Canada. *Health Policy, 64*, 193–205.

Building on some of the insights of Hall's policy paradigms, Bryant presents the *Knowledge Paradigms Policy Change Framework* to examine the case of Women's College Hospital during the hospital restructuring process in Ontario, Canada, in 1996. One of the key findings was that although knowledge was important, political considerations were more decisive in the final outcome for the hospital.

Bryant, T. (2004). The role of political ideology in rental housing policy in Ontario. *Housing Studies, 19*, 635–651.

A case study of the Tenant Protection Act in Ontario, Canada, is presented. The findings revealed that while different forms of knowledge—scientific, anecdotal, and critical—had some influence on the process, the political ideology of the government played a significant role in determining the influence of opponents on legislation. It was concluded that while the neo-liberal political ideology of the government did not consistently influence policymaking in all areas, housing policy was found to be particularly sensitive to political ideology.

Fischer, F. (2003). *Reframing public policy: Discursive politics and deliberative practices*. New York: Oxford University Press.

Frank Fischer appraises Hall's *Policy Paradigms* model. While he extols Hall's efforts to demonstrate the influence of institutions the public policy change process, he provides a post-positivist alternative that focuses on policy discourse and argumentation.

Hall, P.A. (1993). Policy paradigms, social learning, and the state: The case of economic policy making in Britain. *Comparative Politics, 25*(3), 275–296.

Hall introduces the policy paradigms model and applies it to explain the rise of neo-liberalism in the United Kingdom in the mid-1970s. Although he did not apply the model to a health policy change, he clearly shows how institutions structure political outcomes.

Hawkesworth, M.E. (1988). *Theoretical issues in policy analysis*. Albany: State University of New York.

This book provides an excellent discussion about gender in public policy analysis. Hawkesworth articulates a convincing case for feminist policy analysis and its key elements.

RELEVANT WEBSITES

Centre for Health Policy Improvement
www.healthpolicyguide.org/advocacy.asp?id=23

This website provides tools for policy change, as well as definitions of policy and how communities can engage to change health policies. Although based in the United States, the site focuses on civil society as a key actor in the health policy change process.

Centres of Excellence in Women's Health
www.cewh-cesf.ca/en/index.shtml

The CEWH conducts research on health issues with the aim of improving the health of women and girls through health policy change. The site provides links to its regional centres in Atlantic Canada, Manitoba, British Columbia, and Quebec, and other links on women's health issues in Canada.

The Change Foundation
www.changefoundation.ca

The Change Foundation was founded and endowed by the Ontario Hospital Association. It is a health policy think tank that focuses on research and information on health care policy issues to promote health care policy change.

The Health Communications Unit
www.thcu.ca/workshops/hpskills.htm

The Health Communications Unit is located in the Centre for Health Promotion at the University of Toronto. Its mandate was recently expanded to include health policy change. The site provides tools and workshops to help communities and public health authorities work for health policy change.

The Policy Project
www.policyproject.com/about.cfm

The Policy Project is based in the United States and provides another approach to health policy. Its focus is helping governments and civil society organizations in developing countries to develop policies on family planning, HIV/AIDS, and promote human rights and gender equality through multisectoral activity.

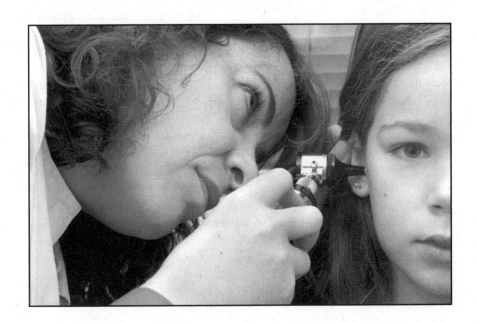

Chapter 5
INFLUENCES ON PUBLIC POLICY

■ INTRODUCTION

Numerous influences impinge upon the public policy change process. At a broad level, political, economic, and social forces related to the workings of the economic system, the state or government, and the attitudes and beliefs of the citizenry shape policy development. Closer to the ground, various groups and interests compete to influence the public policy change process. Advocacy organizations play an important role in the public policy change process by drawing attention to and informing the public about issues and offering policy solutions. These advocacy organizations differ widely in the resources they possess to further their aims. They also do not possess equal political clout to realize their health policy goals.

Specific groups' ability to influence policy development depends on the area in which they are engaged. There may be some policy areas where the interests that support opposing policy options are more entrenched than is the case in others. Ability to influence policy will also be shaped by the extent to which specific policy areas—and the potential for policy change—are informed and consistent with the political ideology of the government of the day.

Political ideology is important because it provides a context for understanding state receptivity, as well as resistance, to some perspectives rather than others. Receptivity to policy options is clearly going to be less when policy advocates challenge components of the ruling governments' ideological commitments and beliefs. In short, most governments tend not to be receptive to criticism of their policies and programs. Any government of the day can privilege some interests over others, such that some groups can be deliberately shut out of the policy change process (Gamson & Wolfsfeld, 1993). This chapter considers some of the dynamics and influences on health policy in Canada. These influences include the state itself and various groups that are part of civil society. The chapter also examines different frameworks by which these influences on public policy development can be classified. The assumption guiding this examination is that the public policy process in general and the health policy arena in particular are heavily influenced by politics (Rachlis, 2004).

■ POLICY INFORMED BY POLITICS

Many theories of public policy present a rational process in which governments receive inputs such as information on an issue from a variety of sources, calculate the benefits and liabilities of various policy options, and then make a carefully reasoned decision about public policy. The issue of the politics of policymaking provides a challenge to this view by implying that public policy decisions are not based solely on what is usually termed as evidence. In reality, policymaking is part of the political process that can be characterized as a struggle in which different groups in civil society such as the corporate, labour, and health and social service sectors, among others, vie to influence the policymaking process. The objective of these activities is to ensure policy change that favours their interests.

In the health policy field, these forces include the health professions (physicians, nurses, psychologists, and others), citizen activists organized into social movements such as the Canadian Health Coalition and Citizens for Medicare, professional policy analysts, policy institutes such as the Caledon Institute of Social Policy, the Fraser and C.D. Howe Institutes, and the Canadian Centre for Policy Alternatives, among others.

Corporate influences such as the nursing and home care industry, pharmaceutical companies, medical testing business, and insurance industry are well organized and well resourced to carry out advocacy activities. They lobby governments to develop policy approaches that support their interests.

These varied interests themselves are associated with or even embedded within ideological ideas that both shape and result from the political, economic, and social institutions; the economy; the state or government; and citizen beliefs and values that structure society. Together these institutions and ideas shape the context and form of public policy discourse and debate. Understanding where these groups come from and their policy goals are critical for understanding the process of policy change as well as those instances where policy does not change.

What are the motivations for such advocacy actions? In many cases, advocacy groups work for policy goals that clearly benefit their economic interests. One example is that of a major pharmaceutical company lobbying governments to make available a vaccine, Gardasil, manufactured by Merck, against a virus, the human papilloma virus, which is said to cause cervical cancer. Clearly, economic interests in the form of substantial profits for pharmaceutical companies shape these activities.

In other cases, advocacy groups seek policy changes that are consistent with a set of values and beliefs. For example, advocacy groups may work to ensure that socially disadvantaged populations have greater access to health care services. Members of these advocacy groups may themselves not be socially disadvantaged, but pursue these efforts in support of their values and beliefs about what the nature of society should be. Similarly, members of housing-related advocacy groups may work to end homelessness, but may not be at risk of becoming homeless themselves.

These groups present different types of evidence to convince governments of the need for policy changes that reflect their understanding of the issue and means by which they could be addressed. While it would be hoped that these groups would advocate for policy change based on available evidence, frequently such information is not available. These groups must, however, carry on with their efforts even in the face of these limitations. Not surprisingly, it has been commented that even governments frequently make policy decisions in the face of limited available evidence (Lindblom, 1959).

These are all critical factors that ensure that the public policymaking process is an explicitly political process. And this process also involves economic and social forces such as values and beliefs that shape the state and governments' public policy decision making (Walt, 1994). They all play a role in the policy development process, but vary in their influence on the health policy process.

■ KEY INFLUENCES ON THE PUBLIC POLICY PROCESS

As discussed in Chapter 3, there are macro-, meso-, and micro-level theories that attempt to explain different inputs or factors that influence public policy outcomes. For example, the pluralist model offers a generally micro-level perspective of the political process that considers how rival interest groups vie to influence the public policy process. Pluralism focuses on how interest groups act as inputs into the policymaking system with the assumption that no one group or set of groups will always dominate policy discussion and action.

New institutionalism is primarily a meso-level perspective concerned with the role that institutions such as governments, organizations, and agencies play in shaping policy discourse and debate. It emphasizes how institutions and their associated ideas influence public policy outcomes. Political economy is primarily a macro-level perspective concerned with how the organization of production and distribution of economic and social resources influences public policy decisions related to the organization of the health care system and public policy that shapes citizens' living conditions.

A number of models have been developed to identify and explain the important influences on policy change. Some theories provide category systems or typologies to make sense of these various influences on public policy. For example, Leichter (1979) identified four groups of factors that influence the public policy change process:

- Situational factors
- Structural factors
- Cultural factors
- Environmental factors

Leichter's Framework and Its Implications

In Leichter's framework, *situational factors* can be sudden or violent events such as the 9/11 attack on the US, Hurricane Katrina, the oil price crisis of the 1970s, or the onset of wars that are associated with policy development and change. These events can sometimes enable governments to introduce policy changes leading to innovations or other policy responses that might otherwise be unacceptable to the public or usually dominant groups (Walt, 1994). For example, during the Second World War, the UK government annexed private, voluntary hospitals to ensure a coordinated and national health service (Walt, 1994). This experience during the war showed that it was feasible to provide publicly organized health care that ensured that all citizens had access to health care services on the basis of need. That this policy innovation was positively received helped to make this experience a template for the post-Second World War creation of the National Health Service in Britain and public health care systems in other developed countries. The taking advantage of such governmental upheavals or shocks to introduce policies that may not normally be easily implemented is receiving increased attention (see Box 5.1). That these policy innovations may also benefit some groups at the expense of others is also being examined.

Box 5.1: Shocks and Public Policymaking

Review of *The Shock Doctrine: The Rise of Disaster Capitalism*, by Naomi Klein
By Lenora Todaro
Village Voice

In *The Shock Doctrine*, journalist Klein trains her sharp investigator's eye upon the flaws of neo-liberal economics. This meticulously researched alternative history, ranging from economist Milton Friedman's "University of Chicago Boys" to George W. Bush, brings Klein's argument into the present. Using stirring reportage, she shows the ways that disasters—unnatural ones like the war in Iraq, and natural ones like the Asian tsunami and Hurricane Katrina—allow governments and multinationals to take advantage of citizen shock and implement corporate-friendly policies: Where once was a Sri Lankan fishing village now stands a luxury resort. *The Shock Doctrine* aims its 10-foot-long middle finger at the Bush administration and the generations of neo-cons who've chosen profits over people in war and disaster; the effect is to provide intellectual armor for the now-mainstream anticorporatist crowd.

Source: The Best of 2007, *Village Voice* (November 27, 2007),
http://www.villagevoice.com/books/0749,asdf,78504,10.html/3

Sometimes situational factors enable governments to introduce changes that are unpopular, such as cutbacks to funding of social programs. The budget and debt crisis of the early 1990s in Canada was used to justify profound cuts in federal transfers to the provinces in both health care and other health-related areas. Sometimes what seems like a progressive policy change can come around to justify not-so-progressive changes. For example, in 1974, Minister of Health and Welfare Marc Lalonde published *A Report on the Health of Canadians* (Lalonde, 1974). This was the first federal report to discuss factors such as the environment and health-related behaviours as important influences upon health.

In practice, health professionals seized upon lifestyle factors as means to promote better health to the exclusion of environmental factors (Legowski & McKay, 2000). More importantly, another effect of the report was to justify changes brought about by the Established Programs Financing Act (1977). The shift away from the sole focus of the role of health care on health allowed the federal government to consider withdrawing from some of its health care financing commitments (Rachlis, 2004). This act shifted the federal government's contribution to health care from the 50:50 cost-sharing mechanism to a block-funding arrangement between the federal and provincial governments.

This change represented a profound shift in health policy. The previous cost-sharing arrangement had helped the provincial governments accept medicare at its inception in 1961. This 1977 act effectively ended cost-sharing as the mode of financing health and social services and increased the provincial governments' financial burden for these services. Lalonde's report—usually seen as a progressive advance in health policy—may have inadvertently justified the federal government's decision to reduce its contribution to provincial health care insurance plans (Rachlis, 2004).

Structural factors can also lead to policy changes (Walt, 1994). A radical change in political leadership can trigger health policy change. Following his election in Venezuela, for example, socialist Hugo Chavez initiated health reforms to ensure the provision of health care to poor and marginalized citizens (Muntaner, Salazar, Benach & Armada, 2006). The reforms signified a move away from health as a commodity to be bought in the marketplace to the provision of health care as a social right by means of a public health care system. This shift was especially important for the marginalized poor living on the periphery of large urban centres who previously did not have access to health care (see Box 5.2).

Box 5.2: Structural Change and Health Policy in Venezuela

Upon election in 1998, Hugo Chavez embarked on health care reforms that would ensure the provision of health care as a social right particularly to marginalized populations. Muntaner et al. argue that the reforms signified a movement away from health as a commodity to be bought in the marketplace to the provision of health care as a social right. This social right would be provided by means of a public health care system that provides care to all, including the marginalized poor, who live on the periphery of large urban centres in the country.

During the 1980s, most Latin American countries had reduced health and social programs significantly. These deep funding cuts characteristic of structural adjustment policies during this period gradually led to conditions that fostered neo-liberal reforms and the destabilization of the welfare state and erosion of social services such as health care. In Venezuela, the erosion of welfare institutions throughout the 1990s fuelled calls for health care reform. During the election campaign, Chavez campaigned vigorously against further neo-liberal reform. Once in office, Chavez called for a referendum on a new "Bolivarian" constitution, prepared by a special constituent assembly. Three articles in the new constitution contained important implications for health care reform. First, health was viewed as a fundamental human right that the state was obliged to ensure (Article 83); second, the state has the duty to create and manage a universal, integrated public health system providing free services and prioritizing disease prevention and health promotion (Article 84); and third, this public health care system must be publicly financed through taxes, social security, and oil revenues, with the state regulating both the public and private elements of the system and developing a human resource policy to train professionals for the new system (Article 85).

Source: Muntaner, C., Salazar, R.M., Benach, J. & Armada, F. (2006). Venezuela's barrio Adentro: An alternative to neoliberalism in health care. *International Journal of Health Services 36*(4), 803–811.

As another example of how structural factors can affect the organization of the health care system, consider the United States, which has a private health care system rooted in its free market economic system. Instead of having a public health care system primarily organized by the state, which is the case in every other developed nation, the US has numerous private insurance plans that provide differing levels of health coverage. Most Americans have some form of insurance coverage, but many must pay additional health care costs that are not covered by their plans.

During his term in office (1993–2001), US President Clinton attempted health reform with the intent of introducing some form of universal public health care. His efforts failed, but had they succeeded, in all likelihood they would have resulted in a system that merely extended the existing system of health care plans provided by different private health insurance companies, albeit with a greater breadth of coverage for Americans (Navarro, 1994).

Vicente Navarro served on Clinton's National Health Care Reform Task Force and describes the theoretical framework for the reforms as "the purest form of managed competition" (Navarro, 1994, 206). The proposed reforms would have required health care providers to work in managed care plans controlled by large insurance companies. The reforms would have transformed health care providers into employees, or contractors to the insurance companies. Navarro suggests that the reforms would have required providers to offer services in a cost-efficient manner. Controllers were to enrol in a managed care plan.

Generally, the reforms would have perpetuated much of the existing system, including the attendant inequities related to the presence of many uninsured citizens. Clinton's plan would have done little to change the basic organization of the privately organized American health care system, which would have continued to be closely aligned within the American free enterprise approach to health policy.

Demographic and social factors are also structural determinants that can affect public policy (Leichter, 1979). The extent to which a country is urbanized affects the structures that are developed to provide health and other services. The age structure of the population affects the type of health services (Walt, 1994). For example, depending on the perceived health of seniors, governments might move to ensure provision of long-term care and palliative services. These kinds of issues clearly inform current debates about wait times, especially as hip replacement appears to be an emerging issue. Such surgeries are more prevalent among the elderly.

Culture affects policy. The political and cultural environment can influence levels of participation and trust in government and the possibility of political change (Leichter, 1979). In a situation where the populace does not trust government, their subsequent disengagement from the political system can hinder policy change. Believing that they have no influence on the political process, more and more people decline to vote at election time. Lack of interest and delays between elections may make it unlikely that a government will do anything to change public policies.

It has also been suggested that the dominant religions of a country can influence policy positions and policy change (Walt, 1994). For example, some analysts identified the tenor of the US presidential election in 2004 as being strongly influenced by conservative Christian issues and perspectives (Hillygus & Shields, 2005). There were several reasons for this development. Membership in these groups had been increasing, and the George W. Bush campaign seized on this demographic. By highlighting his Christian faith, this demographic was put to his advantage. Indeed, exit polls from the election found that among voters who considered morals to be a pressing issue for the country (about 22 percent of the total number of voters), 80 percent of these indicated they had voted for Bush.

In addition, the same study notes that campaigns organized around defeating same-sex marriage proposals in 11 US states seemed to provide further evidence of the importance of conservative moral issues for many voters (Hillygus & Shields, 2005). Issues such as the war in Iraq and the economy were downplayed by a perception that voters were concerned with a need to reinforce and protect traditional nuclear family values. These issues have been rarely studied in Canada.

Finally, *environmental factors* can affect policy (Leichter, 1979). Walt suggests that these factors may be better understood as external or international factors (Walt, 1994). Some of these factors are changes in the international political and economic arena that can affect the domestic policies of states. These forces sometimes result in radical changes to national policies.

For example, the economies of states are increasingly interdependent as a result of international trade treaties such as the General Agreement on Trade in Services (GATS) (Grieshaber-Otto & Sinclair, 2004). These agreements integrate their economies and enhance the mobility of international capital to move from location to location. The North American Free Trade Agreement (NAFTA) is signed by Canada, the US, and Mexico, and integrates the economies of these countries (Grieshaber-Otto & Sinclair, 2004; Walt, 1994). These agreements may help commodify different goods and services by identifying them as sites for investment. Such trade agreements have implications for national policy-making and this is especially the case for health care and health-related policy. These issues are taken up later in this book.

Some analysts suggest that increasing interdependence between nations may be jeopardizing democratic processes. This may be occurring because civil society actors are losing the ability to influence national policies, which are becoming increasingly required to meet the requirements of international trade and capital mobility agreements (Teeple, 2000).

Leichter's framework therefore provides a useful conceptual tool for identifying and classifying various types of influences on the political system and its related public policymaking. It enables both identification and examination of broader factors that can influence the public policy process and public policy change outcomes.

Leichter does not explicitly consider the important role that civil society actors play in policy change or the impact of political ideology on public policy. Nor does he consider how structures and interests influence public policy outcomes. For example, the development of medicare in Canada was not solely about the forging of an agreement between the medical profession and the government as Tuohy suggests (Tuohy, 1999). The establishment of medicare was also an achievement for the working class, which pressured for social change in the immediate postwar period (Armstrong & Armstrong, 2003; Teeple, 2000). Returning Second World War veterans wanted something in return for their sacrifices and governments felt obliged to respond to these demands. In addition, Canadians who had suffered deprivations as a result of the Depression of the 1930s wanted increased security during periods of unemployment. These civil society actors advocated for social change that would improve their living conditions.

And while many changes in the international and national political arenas have impeded the capacity of civil society actors to influence health policy, these individuals continue to try to influence public policy, and this is particularly so in the health policy field. As will be seen, the motivations and interests of civil society actors are increasingly in conflict with international market forces. The outcomes of these conflicts will shape national health policy as well as the health status of a population.

Easton's Framework and Its Implications

Easton presents an analytic framework that contains many institutions and processes concerned with what he terms the authoritative allocation of values for society (see Figure 3.1) (Easton, 1965). Values refer to those objects that have meaning for people. These can be material consumer goods, such as home appliances or cellphones, or services, such as educational opportunities or health care. They can also be symbolic or spiritual entities, such as the right to speech or a fair trial, or other citizen rights expected by citizens in a democratic society.

Inputs

Easton identifies inputs into the political system as demands, support, and resources. Governments select which of these inputs—values, demands, supports, resources—to afford greater attention to and which to deny. These choices then shape its process of making or changing policies.

More explicitly, demands represent the expressed wishes of groups who desire particular policies implemented that address their own objectives and interests. In the health care area, for example, this could be a health coalition demanding that governments not allow public financing to private health care providers or that governments ensure universal access to all health care services. It could also include efforts to have the government develop a policy to provide universal access to prescription medications and dental care services.

Resources refer to the means available to governments to address the demands made by these interest groups. Does the government have the financial resources or policy levers to gain such resources in order to provide these services? Support refers to the public acceptance of these demands. Is there any reason that the government needs to respond to these requests?

The State

The middle box of Easton's model represents the institutions of government. The insights he initially provided concerning the various forms of the welfare state seem especially relevant here. Social democratic, conservative, and liberal welfare states are guided by fundamentally different sets of structures and interests that shape the development of institutions, values, and ideological principles in each regime. These factors come to influence state receptivity to various policy directions.

Briefly, Figure 5.1 lays out the fundamental forms that the welfare state takes in wealthy industrialized nations. Of particular interest are their guiding principles and dominant institutions. Canada is a liberal welfare state (Saint-Arnaud &

Figure 5.1: Ideological Variations in Forms of the Welfare State

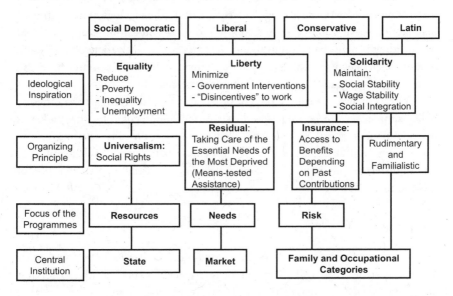

Source: Saint-Arnaud, S. & Bernard, P. (2003). Convergence or resilience? A hierarchical cluster analysis of the welfare regimes in advanced countries. *Current Sociology, 51*(5), 504.

Bernard, 2003).The dominant institution is the marketplace. Liberal welfare states generally provide the least support and security to its citizens.

Within liberal welfare states, the dominant ideological inspiration is that of liberty, which leads to minimal government intervention in the workings of the marketplace (Saint-Arnaud & Bernard, 2003). Within this framework, the increasing receptivity of governments in Canada to the marketplace as a source for health care policy ideas can be understood. In terms of meeting needs of citizens, the greatest focus is upon the most deprived. Canada, the US, the UK, and Ireland are the best exemplars of this form of the welfare state.

The opposite situation is seen among social democratic welfare states. The ideological inspiration for the central institution of these nations—the state—is the reduction of poverty, inequality, and unemployment. Rather than being concerned with governments meeting the basic needs of the most deprived, the organizing principle here is universalism and providing for the social rights of all citizens. Denmark, Finland, Norway, and Sweden are the best exemplars of this form of the welfare state. In these nations, private involvement in health care delivery has been strongly resisted.

The conservative and Latin welfare states provide somewhat superior economic and social security to its citizens than do liberal welfare states, but rather less so than social democratic nations (Esping-Andersen, 1999). The ideological inspiration of maintaining social stability, wage stability, and social integration is accomplished by providing benefits based on insurance schemes geared to a variety of family and occupational categories (Saint-Arnaud & Bernard, 2003). These states have also tended to resist private involvement in health care delivery.

Within the welfare state typology, differences in state receptivity to differing policy approaches can be understood. Nations already focused on the market as the dominant institution in society will have greater difficulty resisting private involvement in health care delivery. The issue of welfare states and their influence on health-related public policy is considered in greater detail in a later section of this volume.

Outputs

The outputs in Easton's model are those goods and services that the government agrees to provide. These will involve all the issues related to how health care services are organized and delivered. They will involve macro-, meso-, and micro-level decisions that concern all aspects of how health care is delivered within a nation. The details of the history and present configuration of the health care system are described in the next chapter.

Evaluation of the Leichter and Easton Models

Like Leichter, Easton provides useful tools for identifying and assessing inputs and policy outcomes. However, Easton's model focuses primarily on state institutions and too little on categories of actors and other influences on the political system. These models are primarily concerned with the political advocacy activities of experts with a focus on state responses. There is little consideration of the structures and interests that influence policy outcomes. In addition, the models seldom consider the political activities of other civil society actors as contributing to and influencing the policy process. Civil society organizations, such as social movements, are either absent from these theories, or they are described in generally apolitical terms, strangely unattached to the political process.

The health policy field comprises a wide range of government, corporate, health professions, and citizen activists and groups that bring their knowledge of issues and policy proposals for consideration and implementation. Citizen coalitions form to address pressing political issues and have been particularly influential in directing attention to issues of access to care and the sustainability of the public health care system. Such groups play an important role by informing and educating the public about key health issues usually related to access and advocating policy solutions to ensure universal access to health care services.

■ CIVIL SOCIETY AND HEALTH POLICY

Civil society refers to politically engaged citizens, professional policy analysts, and associational networks such as unions and other social movements that attempt to influence public policy decisions (Walzer, 1995). Social movements are organizations formed with the explicit purpose of carrying out collective action. They may come to exist for extended periods of time with some good examples being those of the environmental, labour, and women's movements.

Civil society also includes associations and relational networks such as churches and educational institutions (Bryant, 2001). These institutions may form outside the state and act in partnership with larger social movements to promote health policy change. Informal organizations that advocate and champion policy change can also form within the state apparatus among senior civil servants. An especially relevant type of social movement is that of health coalitions that have come together in support of a public approach to health care organization and provision. Few theorists consider the important role played by these civil society organizations in the political process (see Box 5.3).

Box 5.3: Civil Society and Social Capital

Smith examines Putnam's controversial work on social capital and his arguments concerning the decline of social capital in the United States, and Foley and Edwards's response to Putnam. Putnam's definition of social capital refers to social networks, connections between individuals, and norms of reciprocity and the sense of trust that develops between them (Putnam, 1995,1993). He notes that some equate social capital with "civic virtue" [*sic*]. Putnam argues that social capital highlights civic virtue becomes "more powerful when it is embedded in a dense network of reciprocal social relations" (Putnam, 1993: 173, 176). In contrast, a society with many virtuous but isolated individuals does not also necessarily have abundant social capital. Putnam laments the decline of social capital in American society as fewer people join community organizations in droves as they once had in previous generations.

In response to Putnam, Foley and Edwards identify two concepts of civil society (Foley & Edwards, 1996). Civil Society I is based on de Tocqueville's work on the contributions of American associational life to democratic governance. This approach argues that apolitical associations

---

that intersect with major lines of conflict within a society help to cultivate "moderation and the compromising spirit" that are essential for efficient democratic governance. Civil society, then, solely comprises organizations that mediate social and political divisions, and excludes organizations that foster social and political cleavages. Civil Society II is defined as consisting of politically mobilized social actors outside the usual political associations. Foley and Edwards argue: "Indeed, Tocqueville ... identified specifically political associations" as essential features of the rich associational life that he observed in the United States in 1832 (Foley & Edwards, 1996:42). Foley and Edwards argue that both versions of civil society fail to consider the political factors that influence and explain where or how civil society meets the political order. Both exclude "the nature and form of explicitly political institutions—including electoral systems and political parties—that structure relations between citizens and the state" (Smith, 1988: 93). Moreover, excluding political organizations from conceptualizations of civil society seriously downplays critical sources of civil engagement and social formation.

Smith suggests that this observation can also apply to studying transnational political associations that function in an increasingly global political arena. She argues that transnational social movement organizations similarly play an important role in fostering social capital even in the event that they do not engender face-to-face contact among members.

Taking issue with Smith's content about transnational movements fostering social capital at the global level, the concept of social capital has been poorly defined in the literature. Much has been attributed to social capital to the point that it has little meaning and is not a useful analytic tool. But, as Muntaner compellingly argues, the issue is not social capital, but class solidarity in identifying the public good and working together to change public policies to achieve social and political change (Muntaner, 2004).

Sources: Foley, M. & Edwards, B. (1996). The paradox of civil society. *Journal of Democracy 7*(3), 38–52; Smith, J. (1998). Global civil society? Transnational social movement organizations and capital. *American Behavioral Scientist 42*(1), 93–107.

Muntaner, C. (2004). Commentary: Social capital, social class, and slow progress of psychosocial epidemiology. International Journal of Epidemiology 33: 4, 674–680.

■ ADVOCACY GROUPS AND THE OPPORTUNITY STRUCTURE

A fundamental problem with much theory and research is their failure to consider the outcomes and consequences of social movements (Giugni, 1998). In other words, few studies consider the impact of social movements or politically engaged civil society organizations on public policy. This is an odd gap in the literature, given that many social movements become politically engaged in their efforts to promote policy change.

A focus of early work on social movements and their impacts is the political opportunity structure (Burstein, Einwohner & Hollander, 1995). The political opportunity structure refers to the larger context of social support and alliances that can form as a political resource to achieve political objectives, including policy change. Social movements devise many different strategies to increase their impact and this theoretical perspective analyzes their capacity to broker activities with allies and opponents as means to achieve their objectives.

Other perspectives consider how social movements achieve their ends through comparisons of their efforts in different countries. How is it that health systems evolve differently in response to the same pressures? What role do social movement activities play in shaping public policy in differing jurisdictions? What lessons can we learn by studying these differing scenarios?

Giugni argues that this approach enables explicating how the political context mediates, and perhaps mutes, the impact of movement on policy outcomes (Giugni, 1998). It is important to identify and understand the strategies social movements employ to achieve their impact.

Social movements may influence health policy discourses and shape what issues will even be addressed in the political system. For example, the emphasis on anti-smoking bans in Canada and in other jurisdictions reflects the ability and success of the anti-smoking lobby in having the evidence of the negative health impact of tobacco use on human health put into policy development. Where 20 years ago, smoking was permitted in most public places, current bans prevent smoking inside public buildings, public vehicles, or on commercial flights.

Contrast this success with that of the anti-poverty community and related social movements' failure to have the health impacts of poverty integrated and applied in the service of policy development. A poverty and health discourse in Canada is very rare and reflects numerous difficulties in having a structural approach to health determinants integrated into health policy development and application (Raphael, 2007b).

■ MEDIA

The media are a critical influence on public policy activity within a society. The media play an important role in identifying what issues are health policy issues. The media usually claim to be impartial and would have us believe that they take seriously their responsibility to present a variety of perspectives. In reality, the media rarely present all views on an issue, especially when dealing with health policy issues. It has been argued that their selective coverage of health care issues has been instrumental in creating numerous health care crises where in reality such crises do not exist. And as with most institutions in modern society, media activities—like those of the state—are more likely to reflect the views of ruling elites rather than an objective presentation of the evidence available.

A recent set of articles on media coverage and understanding of health determinants demonstrates not only the persistent biases of the media but also their ability to shape public perceptions. Of 4,732 stories from 13 Canadian daily newspapers that considered the determinants of health and disease, 65 percent of these stories were on health care topics, such as disease treatments, service provision, and health care research. Only 13 percent of stories were concerned with physical environments and their effects upon health, and only 6 percent considered the effects of socio-economic circumstances on health (Hayes et al., 2007).

Issues such as income, housing insecurity, and working conditions and their impacts upon health are unmentioned. Considering the explosion of research demonstrating that these issues are the primary determinants of health and disease, the results of the study are rather disturbing (Marmot & Wilkinson, 2006; Raphael, 2004). The understandings of health reporters of these issues were either lacking or undeveloped (Gasher et al., 2007).

The media's focus on health care contributes to public perceptions concerning the determinants of health. Canadians are strikingly unaware of the primary influences upon their health (Canadian Population Health Initiative, 2004). It is not surprising, then, that the health policy discourse is strikingly devoid of any mention of socio-economic circumstances as being important determinants of health (Legowski & McKay, 2000). With such ignorance and the associated lack of public activity to raise these issues, it is not surprising that health policy in Canada is undeveloped in addressing these issues as compared to activities in other developed nations (Mackenbach & Bakker, 2002; Raphael, 2007a).

Another effect of the media preoccupation with health care has been increasing concern about the sustainability of the public health care system. In reality, health care spending in Canada is clearly not out of control and satisfaction levels with the system in some accounts have been stable during the past decade (Organisation for Economic Co-operation and Development, 2005).

Yet, frequent front-page headlines that highlight wait times as a grave health care crisis have led to the preoccupation of Canadian politicians on reducing wait times as a health policy priority. Statistics Canada suggests that public perceptions regarding wait times for care may be influenced by the "intense focus and attention paid to this issue by both policymakers and the media" (Statistics Canada, 2006, 5). This perception may fuel support for the development of a parallel private system. The rationale for a parallel health care system is to relieve pressure on the public system. While there is evidence that indicates that such a system will do the opposite—that is, it will increase wait times—such a perception serves the interests of those who wish to introduce private, for-profit health care.

■ POLITICAL IDEOLOGY

In addition to activities of social movements and embedded interests, political ideology can play a role in shaping health policy. Existing at an abstract level, societal acceptance of one political ideology over another can serve as a potent stimulus to policy development. This may especially be the case in the health policy areas (see Box 5.4).

Box 5.4: Private Health Care in Quebec

Private Health Care Flourishes in Quebec's Under-funded System; The Three Major Parties Either Advocate More Private Care or Ignore It, While Professing Support for the Public System
By Josée Legault

MONTREAL—Here's my hypothesis on why Jean Charest ordered a report on health-care financing only to have his health minister shoot it down like an enemy plane.

The report was ordered in June 2007. Charest's minority government was facing Mario Dumont, who had just become leader of the official Opposition and was seen as the premier-in-waiting. The media were full of musings on voters shifting to the right.

This created what I called the "adéquisation" of Quebec politics, with Charest cozying up to Action démocratique policies. So it was no surprise when the premier called on Claude Castonguay, an advocate of user fees and private health-care services and insurance. He was a shoo-in to produce an ADQ-clone report. Predictably enough, Dumont just called the report the best thing since sliced bread.

But things have changed since 2007. The ADQ is in trouble and Charest is in better shape.

This pro-business report was too hot to handle. Health Minister Philippe Couillard was thus sent out to sound like he was shredding it. But did he really?

The fact is that private health care has been on the rise in Quebec for a decade and nobody's stopping it.

The Parti Québécois created the conditions for it when it weakened public health care with its zero-deficit policy. Since 2003, the Liberal government has turned a blind eye to the growing number of privately paid-for services and tests.

Result: Quebec is now the province with the highest rate of private health-care spending, at 30 per cent.

The *Gazette*'s Aaron Derfel also reported that while the public sector is short 800 family doctors and 650 specialists, the number of doctors who have gone private has tripled in the past 10 years.

Meanwhile, Ontario stopped allowing doctors to opt out of medicare in 2004.

Who hasn't been told by a doctor to get a test done in a privately run clinic where you pay out of pocket or through private insurance?

Some family doctors ask first-time patients for a battery of tests to be done privately for $500 to $1,000 before they'll even see them.

This week's *Globe and Mail* reported that Quebec, in violation of the Canada Health Act, refuses to give Ottawa its data on extra-billing or user fees.

Ottawa has turned its own blind eye by refusing to penalize the province for this. Like the three monkeys, nobody sees, hears, or says anything.

It is no wonder private care flourishes in Quebec.

In fact, the three major parties either advocate more private care or ignore it, while professing support for the public system.

PQ leader Pauline Marois's own silence on the Castonguay report said it all.

Even Couillard couldn't fake it that well. He said he wanted a "dialogue" on a user fee based on revenues and use of services, he was open to privately run hospitals and allowing doctors to move between the private and public sectors under certain conditions.

His Bill 33 could also extend private-insurance coverage to a number of surgeries through a simple change of regulation.

He also said a final no to the only equitable way to finance public health better: increase the sales tax.

This government cut income taxes by $900 million and now gives up $1.5–$2.5 billion a year if it took back one or two of the GST points that Ottawa vacated.

But isn't money what is needed to train, hire, and give better conditions to more doctors and nurses, and to get better technology, more home and long-term care?

By saying no to the tax revenue that would strengthen public health care, it means the private sector will be called upon more and more. Keeping the public system starved of cash also scares the public into wanting more private services. It's called agenda setting.

> The private sector is persevering. It knows that profit-based medicine will continue to grow here as governments and political parties fail to protect public health care and voters are told the public system can't do the job without even more private services.
> Future generations will pay a very dear price for that.
>
> *Source: Edmonton Journal* (February 24, 2008), p. A18.

Political ideology is a system of ideas and meanings that guides interpretation of events and political action (Hofrichter, 2003). Ideology becomes embedded in the social and political structures such as public policies and institutions of a society. It plays a key role in legitimating and obscuring structures of political power that are related to class, race, and gender (Deetz, 1992; Metzaros, 1989). If policy-makers and the public come to believe that the market is the best source of the means to carry out health care organization and provision, policy development will increasingly move toward the creation of private systems of delivery. If policy-makers and the public believe that the primary determinants of health are biomedical indicators and healthy lifestyle choices, little policy development in support of improved living conditions will be seen.

Interestingly, few political theories consider the influence of political ideology and power on public perceptions of health issues, on public policy change, and on the influence of different civil society organizations on public policy. As noted in Chapter 3, political economy emphasizes these dimensions of health policy as it considers how the organization of production and distribution of social and economic resources influence the organization of the health care system and the living conditions to which the population is exposed. The political economy approach also places these issues within the context of dominant political ideologies and how they shape policy understandings and policymaking.

For example, political economists have identified the rise of neo-liberalism as a significant force in bringing about economic globalization (Armstrong, Armstrong & Coburn, 2001; Coburn, 2000, 2006; Grieshaber-Otto & Sinclair, 2004; Poland, Coburn, Robertson & Eakin, 1998). These studies attribute increasing attention to private delivery of health care, as well as growing inequalities in health between rich and poor within advanced nations such as Canada, to neo-liberal policies that emphasize a reduced state role in policymaking and social provision.

As an example of a political economy analysis, a study of the Canadian Centre for Policy Alternatives examines the potential implications of the General Agreement on Trade in Services (GATS) and the North American Free Trade

Box 5.5: Neo-liberalism: A Political Ideology of the Market

As another example, neo-liberalism is defined as a political ideology that advocates the market as the best vehicle for the production and distribution of resources in what is termed the post-industrial capitalist economy, which is economic globalization. Economic globalization requires the liberalization of trade and the mobility of capital across national borders, and increased interdependence between nations. Interdependence means that national economies are more open to foreign investment and trade. Neo-liberal ideology provides the rationale for economic globalization (Coburn, 2000; Teeple, 2000).

Increased economic interdependence among countries has raised concerns about the capacity of civil society actors to influence public policy outcomes. This issue is particularly salient in the social and health policy fields, which have experienced radical changes (Laxer, 1997; McQuaig, 1993; Teeple, 2000). In response to changes in the global economy, Canadian governments at all levels have undertaken measures to balance budgets and reduce deficits often at the expense of social programs. Social programs such as the Family Allowance Program and the Canada Assistance Plan have been replaced by the Canada Health and Social Transfer. The Transfer provides block funding for health and social services. Some observers perceive such changes as enhancing international economic activity (Laxer, 1997; Teeple, 2000). Others perceive increased global interdependence as undermining the capacity of domestic governments to make domestic policy, thereby diminishing the influence of both state and civil society actors (Teeple, 2000). Both perspectives reflect different ideological commitments. Those who support enhancement of international economic activity support neo-liberalism. Opponents to neo-liberalism reflect another political ideology, such as social democracy, which is pro-redistribution, and are committed to reducing inequalities between groups and maintaining a public voice in public policy decisions. The spectre of neo-liberalism as an ideology has influenced the decline of social programs in Canada and elsewhere.

This perspective highlights the role that ideology can play in legitimating and reinforcing systems of inequality (Howe, 1994). Political ideology is conceived as tied to economic relations. Ideology can help to promote a sense of inevitability of existing economic relations. For example, the power of neo-liberalism lies in its ability to promote economic globalization as somehow inevitable. A dominant political ideology can suppress other ideologies or explanations of social situations, particularly those that conflict with the ideas promoted by the dominant ideology. Harden's (1999) examination of health care restructuring in Ontario during the 1990s shows how the agenda of the Common Sense Revolution radically altered health care and politics in the province. The government appropriated common sense to market their policies and make them more palatable and acceptable to Ontario voters. It promoted what Howe terms an ideology of individualism that he describes as so influential "that it is commonsensically true" (Hutson & Jenkins, 1989, 115). Equating a political ideology with common sense makes it especially powerful.

The broader political context takes into account what is presented as fact versus opinion. As demonstrated here, ideology can influence what is defined as fact. For example, while globalization and the perceived need for deficit reduction can be presented as inevitable, they may be seen as constructions of the social world asserted by certain groups in society. By examining specific cases of social policy change, the role of civil society in the policy change process can be identified and explained. Other structural factors, such as the economic base of a country or the way in which the labour force is organized and the role of the state, can affect the types of policy changes that occur. For example, if a country's economy is mixed as it is in countries with a welfare state, the role of the state is larger than in a country with a laissez-faire or market approach. With the advent of the welfare state in Western countries such as Canada, the UK, and western European countries following the Second World War, the state became involved in health, housing, social welfare, and other social policy areas that had been considered the responsibility of private charity or the market. Problems such as poverty or the inability to find appropriate, affordable housing had shifted from being private problems to public issues, and hence it became the responsibility of the state to respond.

Agreement (NAFTA) on medicare (Grieshaber-Otto & Sinclair, 2004). Coburn attributes the decline of the welfare state and changing class structures in advanced capitalist societies to neo-liberalism (Coburn, 2000). Political economy presents issues concerning the system of production and distribution as social processes that reflect the dominant political ideology. We live in a capitalist society and the dominant ideology reflects the interests of the capitalist class—that is, those who own the means of production and distribution and employ those who will produce goods and services to earn an income.

Although Chapter 11 will pick up these issues related to the impact of globalization on health care and health policy in general, it is important here to note the importance for civil society groups to understand the influence of political ideology, particularly neo-liberalism, and its implications for domestic health policy and their ability to influence national health policy.

■ THE INFLUENCE OF HEALTH COALITIONS AND HEALTH PROFESSIONS

The Canadian Health Coalition and related provincial health care coalitions have lobbied government about the importance of maintaining a public rather than private approach to the provision of health care. They have prepared studies and reports to document their concerns about medicare and the problems that people face trying to access health care services.

They have been joined in their concern by numerous nurses associations such as the Canadian Nurses Association. Such support, however, has not been forthcoming from mainstream physician organizations, including the Canadian Medical Association, which have increasingly stressed private approaches to health care organization and delivery.

Proponents of medicare now often compete with powerful lobbies such as the corporate sector and these physicians' associations. The influence of these powerful groups on the public policy process cannot be underestimated. Although all health professions have associations that protect the interests of the professions they represent, the health professions are not equal in their ability to influence public policy.

The corporate sector and physicians' associations are powerful lobbies that have already significantly influenced the direction of health discourses. Both of these sectors possess substantial resources that enable them to mount effective lobbies to protect their interests.

Corporate and physician groups sometimes work in tandem to achieve a particular health policy outcome. For example, the new program to innoculate all 13-year-old girls in Canada against the human papilloma virus with Gardasil reflects the capacity of the corporate sector to lobby the political system and create new markets for its products. In spite of the lack of definitive evidence of the cost effectiveness of the vaccine as compared to other approaches to disease prevention, the federal government is financing provincial programs to vaccinate all adolescent girls against the virus believed to cause cervical cancer (see Box 5.6).

Box 5.6: How Politics Pushed the HPV Vaccine
By Andre Picard

Globe and Mail

Not since the Salk vaccine was triumphantly unveiled in 1955 as the miracle drug that would end the scourge of polio has there been as much hoopla surrounding a vaccine as there is today about one that is being touted for having potential to eradicate cervical cancer.

Unlike polio, where children were dying and crippled in large numbers and immunization stopped an epidemic in its tracks, cervical cancer develops slowly, and the positive or negative effects of a vaccine for human papillovirus (HPV), which can cause cancer of the cervix, will not be seen for decades.

There remain many unanswered questions about the vaccine: Will it actually prevent cervical cancer or just prevent infection with some strains of the virus?

... Conservative politicians have embraced the drug as a means of bolstering their street cred, and winning women's votes.... [O]n March 19, during his budget speech, Finance Minister Jim Flaherty short circuited the scientific and economic discussions by announcing $300-million to kickstart an HPV vaccination program.

Ottawa's move stunned public health officials, as well as the provinces.... "Aside from the polio vaccine in the fifties, it was the first time that the federal government made a direct medical decision," said Noni MacDonald, an infectious disease specialist and professor of pediatrics at Dalhousie University in Halifax. "Why are politicians making medical decisions? This is not how health-care delivery should be decided."

Anne Rochon Ford, coordinator of Women and Health Protection, agrees. The lack of transparency in a program that could have a dramatic impact on women's health is troubling, she said, and doubly so because governments to have succumbed to backroom lobbying from the massive marketing campaign of Gardasil's maker, Merck Frosst Canada Ltd., and its international parent.... Ms. Rochon Ford said the rhetoric about the vaccine with no long-term track record has been unbelievable, and the media has mindlessly and uncritically parroted outrageous claims, while ignoring the importance of proved measures of reducing cervical cancer like Pap testing.

The result of all the attention to Gardasil has been to drive public demand. A poll released earlier this week showed that 81% of parents want their daughters to get the vaccine and 77% favour a universal, school-based program.... "What has happened here is a milking of public sentiment around the fear of cancer and politicians, along with some other well-meaning people, have bought into it," Ms. Rochon Ford said.

Source: Globe and Mail (August 11, 2007), A1, A11.

Also, in recent years, both sectors have publicly expressed their acceptance of private sector involvement in the financing and delivery of care. At its recent annual meeting in 2007, the Canadian Medical Association (CMA) voted to support allowing physicians to practise in both the public and the private systems (Canadian Broadcasting Corporation, 2007; Priest, 2007). Although the motion violates the provisions of the Canada Health Act, this decision fuels governments' efforts to accelerate activities to increase private sector involvement in health care delivery.

The Registered Nurses Association of Ontario (RNAO) opposed the CMA's motion, noting the vast research on the high costs associated with private health care. Conflicts arise between health professions, and such developments provide additional support for the view that health policy development and implementation is a highly contested area. Such conflict between physicians and other groups is not new and represents only one example of a situation where physicians clearly have greater influence in policymaking than the allied health professions.

■ THE CORPORATE SECTOR

The corporate sector is well organized in Canada. Through a strong network of institutes, media outlets, and policy analysts, it advocates for greater private involvement in all aspects of public policy, especially with regard to health care organization and delivery. The idea of public-private partnerships or P3s—in health care provision is one such focus and is taken up in later sections of this book. Box 5.7 summarizes the corporate policy advocacy network in Canada (Langille, 2004).

Box 5.7: The Network of Corporate Advocacy Groups in Canada

Business Associations

Canadian Bankers Association: The leading lobby group for the chartered and foreign banks. Nancy Hughes Anthony is president and CEO.

Canadian Manufacturers and Exporters: Canada's oldest business lobby group represents large manufacturers and exporters. Jayson Myers is president.

Canadian Chamber of Commerce: A coalition of local chambers of commerce representing the interests of many large and small businesses. Perrin Beatty is president and CEO.

Canadian Council of Chief Executives: The voice of big business, representing the 150 CEOs of the major transnational corporations, formerly known as the Business Council on National Issues. Tom D'Aquino is president and CEO.

Think Tanks

C.D. Howe Institute: The voice of the Bay Street business elite, led by president and CEO William B.P. Robson.

Fraser Institute: Founded in 1974 by Michael Walker to represent the "new right" devotion to free markets. Mark Mullins is the current executive director.

Institute for Research on Public Policy: A liberal response to the economic challenges of the 1970s, allowing more scope for government. Mel Cappe is president.

Citizens' Front Groups

Canadian Taxpayers Federation: A watchdog for the well-to-do against the "special interests" responsible for "runaway spending." John Williamson is the federal director.

National Citizens Coalition: Funded by business leaders to defend individual freedom against government intervention. Peter Coleman is president and CEO.

Lobbyists

Lobbyists are "government relations consultants" hired to help firms increase their influence and gain favours from government; lobbying has become a growth industry in recent years as dozens of firms enter the market. Examples include Earnscliffe, GCI, Hill and Knowlton, and Strategy Corp.

Source: Adapted from Langille, D. (2008). Follow the money: How business and politics define our health. In D. Raphael (Ed.), *Social determinants of health: Canadian perspectives* (2nd ed.) 305–317. Toronto: Canadian Scholars' Press Inc.

■ CONCLUSIONS

Numerous complex factors influence the public policy development process, particularly in the development of health policy. Important determinants of health policy are the structures of government itself; the extent of organization and the activities of civil society actors; dominant political ideologies and the understandings concerning health care and the determinants of health held by policy-makers and the public; media activities; and the influence of health professions. It is clear that health policy is a highly contentious policy area.

Of particular concern should be the impact on health policy of media coverage, neo-liberal political ideology, the corporate sector, and the dominant health professions. Media coverage is a concern because of its narrow emphasis on health care and biomedical approaches to health and its tendency to highlight health care crises. Neo-liberal ideology is a concern as it clearly represents a policy approach known to threaten universal health care and overall population health.

The corporate sector is primarily concerned with generating profits and such a concern may be a threat to the public health care system and public policies that support health. And, finally, physician receptiveness to private organization and delivery of health care is a cause for concern as physician influence upon public policymaking is clearly stronger than may be the case for the allied health professions, which tend to support public approaches to health care organization and delivery.

Few models of the public policy process capture all of the forces that shape health policy. Numerous forces play a role in shaping the health discourses and public perceptions about key health issues within which policymaking is made. These forces can prey on public fears about health care and health maintenance, and shape the responses of policy-makers to perceived health policy issues. As with other policy areas, health policy can be manipulated to serve particular interests in a society. The best means of avoiding this is to be aware of the wide range of forces that influence policy change and recognizing that these forces will usually advocate an agenda that support their interests. Whether these interests represent the views of a majority of Canadians requires careful analysis and reflection.

■ REFERENCES

Armstrong, H. & Armstrong, P. (2003). *Wasting away: The undermining of Canadian health care.* Toronto: Oxford University Press.

Armstrong, P., Armstrong, H. & Coburn, D. (Eds.). (2001). *Unhealthy times: The political economy of health and care in Canada.* Toronto: Oxford University Press.

Bryant, T. (2001). *The social welfare policy change process: Civil society actors and the role of knowledge.* Unpublished PhD thesis, University of Toronto, Toronto.

Burstein, P., Einwohner, R.L. & Hollander, J.A. (1995). The success of political movements: A bargaining perspective. In J.C. Jenkins & B. Klandermans (Eds.), *The politics of social protest,* 275–295. Minneapolis: University of Minneapolis Press.

Canadian Broadcasting Corporation. (2007). Ontario nurses condemn CMA's health-care plan. *CBC News,* July 31. Online at www.cbc.ca/health/story/2007/07/31/nurses-privatehealth.html.

Canadian Population Health Initiative. (2004). *Select highlights on public views of the determinants of health.* Ottawa: CPHI.

Coburn, D. (2000). Income inequality, social cohesion, and the health status of populations: The role of neo-liberalism. *Social Science & Medicine, 51*(1), 135–146.

Coburn, D. (2006). Health and health care: A political economy perspective. In D. Raphael, T. Bryant & M. Rioux (Eds.), *Staying alive: Critical perspectives on health, illness, and health care,* 59–84. Toronto: Canadian Scholars' Press Inc.

Deetz, S.A. (1992). *Democracy in an age of corporate colonization: Developments in communication and the politics of everyday life.* Albany: State University of New York.

Easton, D. (1965). *A framework for political analysis.* Englewood Cliffs, NJ: Prentice-Hall.

Esping-Andersen, G. (1999). *Social foundations of post-industrial economies.* New York: Oxford University Press.

Foley, M. & Edwards, B. (1996). The paradox of civil society. *Journal of Democracy 7*(3), 38–52.

Gamson, W. & Wolfsfeld, F. (1993). Movements and media as interacting systems. *Annals of Political and Social Sciences, 528,* 114–125.

Gasher, M., Hayes, M., Ross, I., Hackett, R., Gutstein, D. & Dunn, J. (2007). Spreading the news: Social determinants of health reportage in Canadian daily newspapers. *Canadian Journal of Communication, 32*(3), 557–574.

Giugni, M. (1998). Was it worth the effort? The outcomes and consequences of social movements. *Annual Review of Sociology, 24*(1), 371–393.

Grieshaber-Otto, J. & Sinclair, S. (2004). *Bad medicine: Trade treaties, privatization, and health care reform in Canada.* Ottawa: Canadian Centre for Policy Alternatives.

Harden, J.D. (1999). The rhetoric of community control in a neo-liberal era. In D. Drache and T. Sullivan (Ed.), *Market limits in health reform.* London: Routledge.

Hayes, M., Ross, I.E., Gasher, M., Gutstein, D., Dunn, J.R. & Hackett, R.A. (2007). Telling stories: News media, health literacy, and public policy in Canada. *Social Science & Medicine, 64,* 1842–1852.

Hillygus, D.S. & Shields, T.G. (2005). Moral issues and voter decision making in the 2004 presidential election. *PS: Political Science and Politics, 38*(2), 201–209.

Hofrichter, R. (2003). The politics of health inequities: Contested terrain. In *Health and social justice: A reader on ideology and inequity in the distribution of disease,* 1–56. San Francisco: Jossey Bass.

Howe, L. (1994). Ideology, domination and unemployment. *Sociological Review 42*(2), 315–340.

Hutson, S. & Jenkins, R. (1989). *Taking the strain: Family unemployment and the transition to adulthood.* Milton Keynes: Open University Press.

Lalonde, M. (1974). *A new perspective on the health of Canadians: A working document.* Retrieved from http://www.hc-sc.gc.ca/main/hppb/phdd/resource.htm

Langille, D. (2004). The political determinants of health. In D. Raphael (Ed.), *Social determinants of health: Canadian perspectives,* 283–296. Toronto: Canadian Scholars' Press Inc.

Laxer, J. (1997). *In search of a new left: Canadian politics after the neoconservative assault.* Toronto: Penguin.

Legowski, B. & McKay, L. (2000). *Health beyond health care: Twenty-five years of federal health policy development.* CPRN Discussion Paper No. H04. Ottawa: Canadian Policy Research Networks (CPRN).

Leichter, H.M. (1979). *A comparative approach to policy analysis: Health care policy in four nations.* Cambridge: Cambridge University Press.

Lindblom, C.E. (1959). The science of "muddling through." *Public Administration Review, 19*(2), 79–88.

Mackenbach, J. & Bakker, M. (Eds.). (2002). *Reducing inequalities in health: A European perspective.* London: Routledge.

Marmot, M. & Wilkinson, R. (2006). *Social determinants of health* (2nd ed.). Oxford: Oxford University Press.

McQuaig, L. (1993). *The wealthy banker's wife: The assault on equality in Canada.* Toronto: Penguin.

Metzaros, I. (1989). *The power of ideology.* New York: New York University Press.

Muntaner, C., Salazar, R.M.G., Benach, J. & Armada, F. (2006). Venezuela's barrio Adentro: An alternative to neoliberalism in health care. *International Journal of Health Services, 36*(4), 803–811.

Muntaner, C. (2004). Commentary: Social capital, social class, and the slow progress of psychosocial epidemiology. *International Journal of Epidemiology 33*(4), 674–680.

Navarro, V. (1994). *The politics of health policy: The US reforms 1980–1994*. Cambridge: Blackwell Publishers.

Organisation for Economic Co-operation and Development. (2005). *Health at a glance: OECD indicators 2005*. Paris: Organisation for Economic Co-operation and Development.

Poland, B., Coburn, D., Robertson, A. & Eakin, J. (1998). Wealth, equity, and health care: A critique of a population health perspective on the determinants of health. *Social Science & Medicine, 46*(7), 785–798.

Priest, L. (2007). Debate among doctors builds over CMA health-care proposal. *The Globe and Mail*, August 1.

Putnam, R.D. (1993). *Making democracy work: Civic traditions in modern Italy*. Princeton: Princeton University Press.

Putnam, R.D. (1995). Bowling alone: America's declining social capital. *Journal of Democracy* 6(1), 65–78.

Rachlis, M. (2004). *Prescription for excellence: How innovation is saving Canada's health care system*. Toronto: HarperCollins.

Raphael, D. (Ed.). (2004). *Social determinants of health: Canadian perspectives*. Toronto: Canadian Scholars' Press Inc.

Raphael, D. (2007a). Canadian public policy and poverty in international perspective. In D. Raphael (Ed.), *Poverty and policy in Canada: Implications for health and quality of life*, 335–364. Toronto: Canadian Scholars' Press Inc.

Raphael, D. (2007b). The politics of poverty. In D. Raphael (Ed.), *Poverty and policy in Canada: Implications for health and quality of life*, 303–333. Toronto: Canadian Scholars' Press Inc.

Saint-Arnaud, S. & Bernard, P. (2003). Convergence or resilience? A hierarchical cluster analysis of the welfare regimes in advanced countries. *Current Sociology, 51*(5), 499–527.

Statistics Canada. (2006). *Access to health services in Canada*. January to June 2005. Ottawa: Minister of Industry.

Teeple, G. (2000). *Globalization and the decline of social reform: Into the twenty-first century*. Aurora: Garamond Press.

Tuohy, C. (1999). *Accidental logics: The dynamics of change in the health care arena in the United States, Britain, and Canada*. New York: Oxford University Press.

Walt, G. (1994). *Health policy: An introduction to process and power*. London: Zed Books.

Walzer, M. (1995). The civil society argument. In R. Beiner (Ed.), *Theorizing citizenship*, 153–174. New York: State University of New York.

CRITICAL THINKING QUESTIONS

1. What is it about the current political system that citizens feel disengaged from the process and having any influence on the political process?

2. What are some ways that citizens can influence health policy? What resources do they need to make their voices heard?
3. What do you think are the dominant influences on the political process? How can citizens challenge these forces in the interests of saving the public health care system?
4. How can citizens contribute an alternative discourse on health policy and key health issues affecting citizens?
5. What kind of model would you devise to show how the health policy development process works?

FURTHER READINGS

Armstrong, P. & Armstrong, H. (2003). *Wasting away: The undermining of Canadian health care*. Toronto: Oxford University Press.

Armstrong and Armstrong examine the rationalization of health care from the perspective of health care workers and family caregivers. The book is based on research they have carried out based on interviews with these two groups.

Gamson, W. & Wolfsfeld, F. (1993). Movements and media as interacting systems. *Annals of Political and Social Sciences, 528*, 114–125.

This article considers how the media influence social movements and their impact on the political process in the US. A key finding is that the message of a movement plays a significant role in determining their overall impact on the political process.

Hayes, M., Ross, I.E., Gasher, M., Gutstein, D., Dunn, J.R. & Hackett, R.A. (2007). Telling stories: News media, health literacy, and public policy in Canada. *Social Science & Medicine, 64*, 1842–1852.

This article examines the literacy of the media on social determinants of health.

Hofrichter, R. (2003). The politics of health inequities: Contested terrain. In R. Hofrichter (Ed.) *Health and social justice: A reader on ideology and inequity in the distribution of disease*, 1–58. San Francisco: Jossey Bass.

Hofrichter writes cogently about the political economy of inequalities in health. The entire volume pulls together important essays on current political economy issues in health and the current influences on health policy and population health such as economic globalization.

Rochon, T.R. & Mazmanian, D.A. (1993). Social movements and the policy process. *Annals of the American Academy of Political and Social Science 528*, 75–87.

This article discusses the importance of social movements in the political process. The authors argue that participating in the public policy process is essential for social movements to influence public policy outcomes.

Tarrow, S. (1994). *Power in movement: Social movements, collective action, and politics.* Cambridge: Cambridge University Press.

This book is one of the most cited works on social movements. Although not specifically focused on social movements in the health sector or in Canada, the book discusses the historical development of social movements and theories of social movements and collective action.

RELEVANT WEBSITES

Canadian Centre for Policy Alternatives
www.policyalternatives.ca

The Canadian Centre for Policy Alternatives is an independent, non-partisan research institute concerned with issues of social and economic justice. Founded in 1980, the CCPA is one of Canada's leading progressive voices in public policy debates.

Canadian Council for Public-Private Partnerships
www.pppcouncil.ca

The newly established Crown corporation, PPP Canada Inc., pledges to work with the public and the private sectors toward increasing the presence of P3s in Canada. The development of such an agency within the federal government reflects the growing interest of Canadian governments in increasing the presence of the private sector in health care.

Canadian Health Coalition
www.healthcoalition.ca

The Canadian Health Coalition is a not-for-profit, non-partisan organization dedicated to protecting and expanding Canada's public health system for the benefit of all Canadians. The CHC was founded in 1979 at the Canadian Labour Congress-sponsored S.O.S. medicare conference attended by Tommy Douglas, Justice Emmett Hall, and Monique Bégin. The coalition includes organizations representing seniors, women, churches, nurses, health care workers, and anti-poverty activists from across Canada.

Douglas-Coldwell Foundation
www.dcf.ca/en/about_us.htm
Founded in 1971, the Douglas-Coldwell Foundation was formed to support the movements on the political left in Canada and to stimulate discussion on key public issues such as health care. The foundation provides scholarships and publications on poverty, health, and other public policy issues.

Fraser Institute
www.fraserinstitute.org
The Fraser Institute examines the impact of competitive markets and government interventions on Canadians and Canada as a whole. Its peer-reviewed research on the impact of economic policy is internationally renowned.

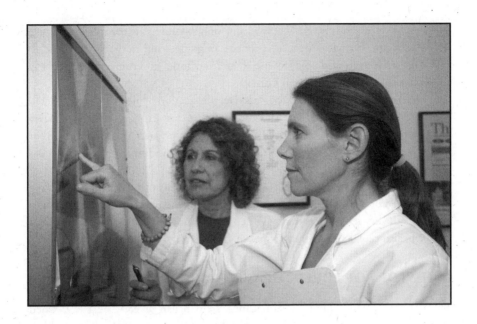

Chapter 6
OVERVIEW OF THE CANADIAN HEALTH CARE SYSTEM

■ INTRODUCTION

Canadians are proud of medicare. For many, it symbolizes what it means to be Canadian. Medicare distinguishes Canada from the United States where, in 2005, about 47 million (approximately 15 percent of the US population) Americans lacked any form of health care insurance coverage (National Coalition on Health Care, 2007). Under medicare, Canadians share the cost of risk (Armstrong & Armstrong, 2003). Health care is provided on the basis of need, not income.

Health care is an important public policy area in the 21st century. A convergence of social, economic, and political factors brought about medicare in Canada. A particularly important determinant of medicare is Canadian federalism. From a new institutionalist perspective, medicare signifies the impact of institutions in shaping social policy. Health care is a politically contentious policy area involving intergovernmental co-operation, and has become a political football as the federal and provincial governments wrangle over the financing of provincial health care programs (McIntosh, 2004). This is so not only because it is the most expensive social program, but also because it reflects ongoing conflict that is intrinsic to relations between the federal, provincial, and territorial governments, particularly in the health care policy arena in Canada.

From a critical social science perspective, the creation of medicare is considered a compromise between the state and the capitalist class (Teeple, 2000). Medicare is a welfare state program in the health field, and represented a significant gain for the working classes, and therefore is seen as reflecting an implicit or explicit class struggle (Teeple, 2006).

This chapter examines the important role of federalism and other factors in the development of medicare, and the nature of the Canadian health care system. It also examines the key federal acts that have determined financing and administration of public health care, and emerging issues in Canadian health care policy.

■ HISTORY OF PUBLIC HEALTH CARE IN CANADA

Political interest in a public health care system began as early as 1919, when then federal Liberal leader William Lyon Mackenzie King pledged to establish public health care in his party's election platform (Rachlis, 2004). In fact, the federal government did not act immediately to implement a national health care program. In 1947, Premier Tommy Douglas and his newly elected Co-operative Commonwealth Federation (CCF) government in Saskatchewan established the first universal hospital health care plan in Canada, indeed in North America (Health Canada, 2005). The health program had the support of the province's doctors and hospitals because they received regular remuneration in contrast to the past, when more than 10 percent of hospitals' and physicians' bills were unpaid (Rachlis, 2004).

During the 1950s, a change in the leadership at the federal level and in Ontario in the immediate postwar era contributed to more conciliatory relations between the federal and provincial governments (Tuohy, 1999). Prior to this time, there were few policies and programs in which the two levels of government agreed to co-operate. The positive intergovernmental relations thus contributed to a political climate that was more favourable to developing innovative social programs such as medicare, which required co-operation between the two levels of government. Out of these negotiations, the single-payer system, which has become synonymous with Canadian health care, emerged.

In 1957, Paul Martin Sr. introduced a national hospital insurance program. The medical profession, insurance companies, and business opposed the program. In 1960, the Canadian Medical Association, a powerful lobby that represents all physicians in Canada, opposed all publicly funded health care. In 1962, the

NDP government of Premier Tommy Douglas in Saskatchewan met opposition from doctors and citizens who associated public health insurance with socialism (Rachlis, 2004). More than 90 percent of the doctors in the province went on strike in opposition to the introduction of public medical care insurance in the province (Tuohy, 1999). The dispute between the doctors and the Saskatchewan government went to arbitration. In 1960, the settlement that emerged from the strike, known as the Saskatoon Agreement, permitted doctors to charge patients above fees negotiated with the provincial government. In other words, the agreement allowed doctors to extra-bill their patients for services they provided. Both parties agreed to private fee-for-service medical practice. This agreement became a template for the national program when it was established in 1966 with the federal government's passage of the Medical Care Act (Rachlis, 2004; Tuohy, 1999). Under the federal plan, the provincial governments became single payers of a comprehensive range of physicians' and hospital services, with Ottawa cost-sharing 50 percent of provincial health care costs and the provinces paying 50 percent of their health care costs.

The Canadian Medical Association lobbied then Prime Minister John Diefenbaker to appoint a Royal Commission to study health care, hoping the commission would highlight the problems associated with a publicly financed health care system (Rachlis, 2004). In 1965, Justice Emmett Hall's commission not only supported a national medical insurance program, it also recommended expanding the program to include home care, mental health, pharmaceuticals, and dental and optical programs for children. These programs are still not covered by medicare.

The provinces were required to comply with the five principles of medicare, which were the national standards for health care programs to ensure access and equity in health care services across the country (see Box 6.1).

Box 6.1: A Brief History of Canada's Health Care System

1947 The Saskatchewan Government, led by leader Tommy Douglas, introduces the first provincial hospital insurance program in Canada.

1957 Paul Martin Sr. introduces a national hospital insurance program. Doctors, insurance companies, and big business fight against it.

1960 The Canadian Medical Association opposes all publicly funded health care.

1962 Saskatchewan's NDP government introduces the first public health care program. Doctors walk out, but the strike collapses after 3 weeks.

1965 A Royal Commission headed by Emmett Hall calls for a universal and comprehensive national health insurance program.

1966 Parliament creates a national medicare program with Ottawa paying 50% of provincial health costs.

1977 Trudeau Liberals retreat from 50:50 cost-sharing and replace it with block funding.

1978 Doctors begin extra-billing to raise their incomes.

1979 Canadian Labour Congress convenes the S.O.S. medicare conference to fight extra-billing and joins with community groups to form the Canadian Health Coalition. The Clark Conservative government in Ottawa invites Justice Emmett Hall to chair an inquiry into federal financing of health care and how the provinces use these transfers.

1980 Justice Emmett Hall releases his second Commission Report recommending the abolition of extra-billing and user fees.

1984 Canada Health Act is passed unanimously by Parliament. Extra-billing is banned.

1993 Mulroney government grants 20-year patent protection to brand-name drugs.

1995 Paul Martin Jr. introduces Canada Health and Social Transfer (CHST), causing massive cuts in transfer payments to health and social programs.

1997 National Forum on Health calls for medicare to be expanded to include home care, pharmacare, and a phasing out of fee-for-service for doctors.

1998 Premiers demand say in interpreting the Canada Health Act. Chrétien caves in.

2000 Ralph Klein introduces legislation to allow private hospitals.

2000 Federal Budget offers 2 cents for health care for every dollar of tax cuts, ignoring pleas of Canadians to save medicare.

2002 The Romanow Royal Commission on the Future of Health Care in Canada conducted cross-country public hearings. Final report was tabled in Ottawa on November 28, 2002.

2003 First Ministers' meeting results in a new "Health Accord." Targeted funding in key areas (as prescribed by the Romanow report) shows promise. However, there are no accountability mechanisms and no restrictions on public funding being spent on for-profit health care.

Source: http://www.healthcoalition.ca/History.pdf

■ FEDERALISM: CATALYST FOR INNOVATION?

Federalism is a critical element in the development of health care in Canada (McIntosh, 2004). The institution of federalism has tended to lead to a focus on particular issues while obscuring other key health care issues. Canadian federalism is viewed by some policy analysts as having both constrained and facilitated innovation and opportunities for change (Hutchison, Abelson & Lavis, 2001; Tuohy, 1999).

Federalism divides political authority between federal and regional/sub-national governments (i.e., provinces and territories) and is considered to be the property of constitutions (Brooks, 1996). This means that it is based on state power. Federalism institutionalizes regions by relating them to different governments. The federal and regional governments have constitutional authority to enact laws and collect revenues. In other words, political authority is decentralized. The regionalism that results in the acceptance of a federal constitution is reinforced by the political administrative rivalries between national and regional governments that gave rise to it.[1] Much of this tension between the two levels of government stems from the Canadian Constitution, which sets out the powers and responsibilities of each level of government.

Sections 91 and 92 of the Constitution Act

The Canadian Constitution contributed to, and intensified, the rivalry between the federal and provincial governments by investing responsibility for health care provision in the provincial governments. Neither the federal nor the provincial and territorial governments have exclusive constitutional responsibility for health care (Braen, 2004; Commission on the Future of Health Care in Canada, 2002; Leeson, 2004; Statistics Canada, 2001). The terms set out in sections 91 and 92 of the Constitution Act, 1867, and the various constitutional interpretations of the meaning of these sections provide the core for the federal and provincial governments' claims for a continuing role in health care provision (McIntosh, 2004). While these sections appear to present the exclusive and shared responsibilities of each government, this is not the case. There is some ambiguity, which has contributed to tensions between governments.

McIntosh notes that most of the health and social services that Canadians now consider valid areas of state involvement in actual delivery or regulation were considered to be the responsibility of charitable or religious organizations—that is, private matters in the 19th century (McIntosh, 2004). In the 20th and the 21st centuries, however, the state role evolved into these areas. The courts increasingly determine which level of government is responsible for specific policy initiatives.

In health care, the provinces have primary responsibility for the organization, administration, and delivery of most health care services (Braen, 2004; Leeson, 2004). Section 92(7) of the Constitution Act, 1867 supports the provincial authority over the administration and delivery of health care services, but many constitutional provisions authorize provincial responsibility in this area. The federal government has a role in criminal law, patents, and its often controversial spending power.

The federal government can intervene in health care only through its spending power. It has used this power to set the terms and conditions of medicare. Although since the 1980s it has consistently reduced its transfer payments to the provinces and territories, the federal government retains considerable control over the terms of medicare and also over the provincial governments in the administration of their health insurance plans. Interestingly, it has rarely penalized a province for violating the principles of medicare, although some provinces have routinely allowed extra-billing and the imposition of user fees.

The Charter of Rights and Freedoms as part of the Constitution Act, 1982, exerted a new thrust in public policy debates by enabling individuals and groups to use the courts in efforts to hold governments accountable for policy choices by asserting any of the rights listed in the Charter. The Charter has been used to challenge the state's role in a policy area. In 2005, the Charter provided the basis of a challenge to the Quebec ban on private insurance for medicare-covered services (Rachlis, 2005).

Single-Payer System

Under medicare, the provincial governments are what is termed "single payers" for most medical and hospital services (Rachlis, 2004; Tuohy, 1999; Yalnizyan, 2006). Each province has a single government insurance plan that provides a comprehensive range of medical and hospital services. From the outset as the system developed, there was no provision for private insurance alternatives for these services. Provincial governments were intended to be monopsonists—sole purchasers—of medical and hospital services. Monopsony is an economic term that refers to a state in which demand comes from one source (Tuohy, 1999). If there is only one customer or purchaser for a certain good, that customer has a monopsony in the market for that good or service, or one employer controls or dominates a sector by providing that good or service exclusively. It is similar to a monopoly, but on the demand side, not the supply side.

Since the inception of medicare, various cost-sharing schemes between the two levels of government were devised to ensure the sustainability of the health care system. The financing of provincial health care programs has also been the primary source of tension between the two levels of government as the federal government has reduced its contributions, but continues to dictate to the provinces the terms on which the services are to be delivered. It is considered that the federal spending power has helped to protect the principles of medicare as intended by its founder, Tommy Douglas (see Box 6.2).

Box 6.2: The Five Principles of Medicare

1. *Universality of coverage:* The provinces have to cover 100 percent of their residents for hospital and physicians' services.
2. *Portability of coverage:* The provinces have to cover their residents for care in other provinces at the rates that pertain in other provinces. They are supposed to cover their residents while out of the country, at least at the rates that would have pertained in their home province.
3. *Reasonable accessibility to services:* The provinces are to ensure that services are "reasonably accessible" and that financial charges or other barriers do not impede access. This criterion also requires the provinces to pay reasonable compensation to their health professionals.
4. *Comprehensiveness of services:* The provinces are supposed to cover all "medically necessary" services provided by doctors or within hospitals. This criterion is actually a misnomer because community services (such as home care) are not covered and neither are the services of other providers (except dental services within hospitals—a rare event these days).
5. *Public administration:* The provinces have to administer their health insurance programs either themselves or through a body that is accountable to the provincial government. This criterion is also a bit of a misnomer because it expressly forbids neither for-profit insurers acting on contract with a province nor for-profit providers of services.

Source: Rachlis, M. (2004). *Prescription for excellence: How innovation is saving Canada's health care system*, 37. Toronto: HarperCollins Publishers Ltd.

Cost-Sharing Arrangements

Cost-sharing arrangements have evolved and changed radically since the inception of medicare in Canada. At the outset, the focus was on financing hospital and physician services. Services provided by allied health professionals were covered provided patients had a physician's referral for such services. Over time, a broader range of institutional and community health settings, such as community health centres that combine health and social services, were recognized.

In 1957, the Hospital Insurance and Diagnostic Services Act provided federal-provincial cost-sharing hospital and physician services (Rachlis, 2004; Tuohy, 1999). This act provided a template for future health care programs (Rachlis, 2004). The federal government contributed 50 percent of the costs of these services. The Act required that provincial plans comply with the five principles of medicare: (1) comprehensiveness, (2) accessibility, (3) universality, (4) public administration, and (5) portability.

Medical Care Act

In 1966, the federal government implemented the Medical Care Act, which enshrined the principle of public payment for private medical practice only (Rachlis, 2004; Tuohy, 1999). The Act entrenched private fee-for-service, which became the chief mode of practice organization and physician payment in Canada. The Act was considered a compromise to appease opponents and supporters of medicare. The federal government also promised to continue to pay 50 percent of the costs of provincial programs, provided the provinces complied with the principles of medicare (Rachlis, 2004). Under the terms of the Act, which continue to be in force, physicians send claims for payment to the provincial health insurance plans (Scott, 2001).They are reimbursed on the basis of the fees schedule negotiated by the government and medical association in each province.

When the Medical Care Act came into force, only Ontario refused to comply. All of the other provinces agreed within the first year (Rachlis, 2004). Ontario Premier Robarts preferred a market system similar to that of the US, whereby the government would insure only those who could not afford private care. Prime Minister Trudeau threatened to withhold the transfer from Ontario, forcing Robarts to agree to the federal formula in 1971.

Hutchinson et al. attribute the inclusion of private practice to good fiscal buoyancy/health, positive federal-provincial relations at the time, broad political support for access to health care on the basis of need regardless of income, and physicians' willingness to accept limitations on their entrepreneurial discretion in exchange for professional independence in clinical decision making (Hutchison et al., 2001). A strong economy at the time enabled the government to draw physicians into the program on generous terms, including continued fee-for-service remuneration, clinical autonomy, and control over the location and organization of medical practice. This arrangement placed physicians at the centre of health care at all levels. In short, they became the gatekeepers. It was this promise of power and control that ensured physician support for the system. The legislation did not change the existing structure of health care delivery (see Box 6.3).

Box 6.3: A Summary of Canada's Health Care System

Canada's publicly funded health care system is best described as an interlocking set of ten provincial and three territorial health insurance plans. Known to Canadians as "medicare," the system provides access to universal, comprehensive coverage for medically necessary hospital and physician services. These services are administered and delivered by the provincial and territorial (i.e., state or regional) governments, and are provided free of charge. The provincial and territorial governments fund health care services with assistance from the federal (i.e., national) government.

What Happens First (Primary Health Care Services)

When Canadians need health care, they generally contact a primary health care professional, who could be a family doctor, nurse, nurse practitioner, physiotherapist, pharmacist, etc., often working in a team of health care professionals. Services provided at the first point of contact with the health care system are known as primary health care services and they form the foundation of the health care system.

In general, primary health care serves a dual function. First, it provides direct provision of first-contact health care services. Second, it coordinates patients' health care services to ensure continuity of care and ease of movement across the health care system when more specialized services are needed (e.g., from specialists or in hospitals).

Primary health care services often include prevention and treatment of common diseases and injuries; basic emergency services; referrals to and coordination with other levels of care, such as hospital and specialist care; primary mental health care; palliative and end-of-life care; health promotion; healthy child development; primary maternity care; and rehabilitation services.

Doctors in private practice are generally paid through fee-for-service schedules negotiated between each provincial and territorial government and the medical associations in their respective jurisdictions. Those in other practice settings, such as clinics, community health centres and group practices, are more likely to be paid through an alternative payment scheme, such as salaries or a blended payment (e.g., fee-for-services plus incentives). Nurses and other health professionals are generally paid salaries that are negotiated between their unions and their employers.

When necessary, patients are referred to specialist services (medical specialist, allied health services, hospital admissions, diagnostic tests, prescription drug therapy, etc.).

What Happens Next (Secondary Services)

A patient may be referred for specialized care at a hospital, at a long-term care facility or in the community. The majority of Canadian hospitals are operated by community boards of trustees, voluntary organizations or municipalities. Hospitals are paid through annual, global budgets negotiated with the provincial and territorial ministries of health, or with a regional health authority or board.

Alternatively, health care services may be provided in the home or community (generally short-term care) and in institutions (mostly long-term and chronic care). For the most part, these services are not covered by the Canada Health Act; however, all the provinces and territories provide and pay for certain home care services. Regulation of these programs varies, as does the range of services. Referrals can be made by doctors, hospitals, community agencies, families and potential residents. Needs are assessed and services are coordinated to provide continuity of care and comprehensive care. Care is provided by a range of formal, informal (often family) and volunteer caregivers.

Short-term care, usually specialized nursing care, homemaker services and adult day care, is provided to people who are partially or totally incapacitated. For the most part, health care services provided in long-term institutions are paid for by the provincial and territorial governments, while room and board are paid for by the individual; in some cases these payments are subsidized by the provincial and territorial governments. The federal department of Veterans Affairs Canada provides home care services to certain veterans when such services are not available through their province or territory. As well, the federal government provides home care services to First Nations people living on reserves and to Inuit in certain communities.

Palliative care is delivered in a variety of settings, such as hospitals or long-term care facilities, hospices, in the community and at home. Palliative care for those nearing death includes medical and emotional support, pain and symptom management, help with community services and programs, and bereavement counselling.

Source: www.hc-sc.gc.ca/hcs-sss/pubs/system-regime/2005-hcs-sss/del-pres_e.html#1

Throughout the 1970s and 1980s, both federal and provincial governments were concerned about controlling social spending. With growing inflation at the time, the federal government was uneasy about its spending commitments (Rachlis, 2004). The federal and provincial governments wanted to adjust the funding rules. These concerns led to the passage of the Established Programs Financing Act in 1977.

Established Programs Financing Act (EPF): Shift to Block-Funding

In 1977 the federal government passed the Established Programs Financing Act (EPF). The federal government threatened to act unilaterally unless the provinces agreed to negotiate a block-grant arrangement (Tuohy, 1999). Block grants signified a shift from the cost-sharing arrangements that characterized earlier funding arrangements in health care between the two levels of government. In other words, federal transfers for hospitals, medical care, and post-secondary education were placed in one funding envelope with a commitment to increase funding as the same rate as economic growth (i.e., the gross domestic product, or GDP) (Rachlis, 2004).

Under the EPF, federal transfers to health care—and post-secondary education—consisted of two allocations (Tuohy, 1999):

- A cash transfer was conditional on provincial compliance with the five principles of medicare (i.e., universality, accessibility, comprehensiveness, portability, and non-profit administration) and was determined on the basis of one-half of per capita transfer to a province in 1975–1976. The amount would be determined partially by the rate of increase in GNP and growth in the population in a province, but not at the rate of actual health care costs. In addition, an unconditional transfer was provided in the form of tax points. A tax point or tax room is fiscal compensation in the place of a cash transfer from the federal government to the provincial governments (Madore, 1997). Tax points directly lower the federal income tax rate. For example, when negotiating fiscal arrangements, the federal government would give the provinces the option of opting out of a program and receive an alternative for the federal contribution to a program, often in the form of tax transfers.

  Under the EPF, the tax points were based on the revenues produced by a specific number of percentage points of the amount of income tax of the federal basic tax generated in a province (Tuohy, 1999).
- The impact of the shift to tax points made provinces whose economies grew at less than the GNP financially less well off in the short term. The federal government provided transitional payments to prevent provinces from being made worse off than if the provincial governments had received a cash transfer set at the rate of GNP and population growth. The federal government reduced its income tax rates by 16 percent, and the provinces raised revenues to finance health care and institutions (Rachlis, 2004).

Overall, the shift to block grants heightened tensions between the federal and provincial governments, particularly when the federal government initiated such actions without consultation with the provinces. Ottawa's unilateral action would become the modus operandi when the provinces refused to comply with federal plans. Other concerns in health care also emerged.

In Ontario and some of the other provinces, doctors grew concerned about the decline in their incomes during the late 1970s (Begin, 2007). With the creation of medicare, they were paid for their work; whereas prior to the creation of medicare, about 10 percent of medical bills were not paid (Rachlis, 2004). Yet, by the 1970s, inflation had risen to over 10 percent, such that by 1975, physicians' incomes had begun to fall. To make up the shortfall, some physicians extra-billed patients above the fees set in the fee schedule in their province. The number of Ontario doctors who extra-billed their patients increased from less than 10 percent in 1978 to approximately 20 percent of physicians in the province.

In 1979, the new federal Conservative Minister of Health David Crombie invited Emmett Hall once again to lead an inquiry on the health care system. In his second commission report, one of Hall's key recommendations was for the government to eliminate extra-billing and hospital user fees (Rachlis, 2004). Hall's main contention was that the two practices had led to a two-tiered health care system that jeopardized universal accessibility of health care services.

■ PROTECTING THE FIVE PRINCIPLES OF MEDICARE AND THE WAR ON EXTRA-BILLING

The Canada Health Act of 1984 enshrines the five principles of medicare: (1) universality, (2) uniform terms and conditions, (3) portability, (4) public administration, and (5) comprehensiveness, and specifically banned extra-billing (Rachlis, 2004; Tuohy, 1999). It included a provision that allowed Ottawa to reduce its financial contribution to provinces that permitted physicians to extra-bill their patients as a measure to ensure provincial compliance (Tuohy, 1999). The federal government used this Act to launch its attack on extra-billing, which triggered the 1985 doctors' strike in Ontario. The strike illustrates how Ontario served as a lightning rod for doctors' discontent during the war on extra-billing as the Act contributed to more conflict in Ontario than in any other provinces (Rachlis, 2004; Tuohy, 1999). The relationship between the provincial government and the Ontario Medical Association (OMA) was already particularly confrontational. Added to existing tensions, the election of a Liberal government ended the 40-year Conservative rule in Ontario and also disturbed an accommodation reached by the OMA and the Conservative government.

The actions of the federal Liberal government of the early 1980s should not be construed as expressing an overwhelming commitment to medicare (Tuohy, 1999). Rather, it acted out of concern for its declining popularity. As Tuohy argues, it "seized upon the issue of extra billing as a way of symbolizing its commitment to preserving the universality of the most popular social program" (Tuohy, 1999, 93). It threatened to reduce the federal transfer payment by the amount equal to the estimated amount of extra-billing occurring in an offending province. Interestingly, the federal government hid behind the veil of this commitment while it whittled away at its financial contribution to provincial health care programs (Brooks, 1996; Rachlis, 2004; Tuohy, 1999).

■ CANADA HEALTH AND SOCIAL TRANSFER

The 1995 federal budget replaced the Canada Assistance Plan and the EPF funding for health and post-secondary education with the Canada Health and Social Transfer (CHST). The Canada Assistance Plan (CAP) provided funding for welfare and other provincial social services (Brooks, 1996). The CAP gave federal transfers to provincial welfare programs from 1965–1995 (Banting, 1997). Under the program, the provinces were to provide assistance to all residents in need.

The CHST is a single block transfer that empowers the federal government to freeze and cap transfers to the provinces that both federal Liberal and Conservative governments had done since the early 1980s (Brooks, 1996). This transfer effectively ended cost-shared programs between the federal and provincial governments and signalled a retreat from Ottawa's commitment to national standards, which historically depended on the federal spending power.

Box 6.4: A Brief History of the Health and Social Transfers

2007: Budget restructured the Canada Social Transfer (CST) to provide equal per capita cash support to provinces and territories, effective 2007–08; similar changes to be made to the Canada Health Transfer (CHT) effective 2014–15, when its current legislation is renewed. CST funding has been increased by $687 million in 2007–08 to support the new cash allocation; in 2008–09, it will increase by $800 million for post-secondary education and by $250 million for development of child care spaces. The CST is extended to 2013–14, and will grow by 3% annually as a result of an automatic escalator, effective 2009–10. Federal support for post-secondary education, social programs, and children are notionally earmarked based on provincial spending patterns to make the federal contribution through transfers more transparent. Transition provisions will ensure that no province or territory experiences declines in either its CHT or CST cash relative to what its cash transfers would have been in 2007–08 prior to the implementation of the new equalization program and the move to equal per capita CST cash support.

In addition, Budget 2007 provided provinces and territories with additional funding of $2.4 billion through three third-party trusts to support important initiatives in areas of shared priority: $1.519 billion for clean air and climate change; $300 million for the immunization of girls and women against cancer of the cervix; and $612 million to accelerate the implementation of patient wait times guarantees.

2006, September: Budget provided $3.3 billion through five third-party trusts to help provinces and territories deal with immediate pressures in post-secondary education ($1 billion), affordable housing ($800 million), Northern affordable housing ($300 million), off-reserve Aboriginal housing ($300 million), and public transit capital ($900 million).

2006, May: Budget replaced the ELCC Initiative with the new Universal Child Care Benefit (UCCB), which provides direct support to parents through monthly payments of $100 for every child under the age of 6, effective July 1, 2006. Funding was provided to provinces and territories under the ELCC Initiative for 2005–06 (through a third-party trust) and 2006–07 (directly to provinces and territories) prior to termination of the agreement.

2005, March: Budget introduced a new Early Learning and Child Care (ELCC) Initiative, providing $5 billion over five years (2005–06 to 2009–10) primarily to provinces and territories to support development of a national ELCC framework outlining principles, objectives, and reporting requirements.

2004, September: First Ministers signed the 10-Year Plan to Strengthen Health Care. In support of the Plan, the Government of Canada committed $41.3 billion in additional funding to provinces and territories for health, including $35.3 billion in increases to the CHT through a base adjustment and an annual 6% escalator, $5.5 billion in Wait Times Reduction funding, and $500 million in support of medical equipment.

2004, April: The CHST was restructured and two separate transfers were created, the Canada Health Transfer and the Canada Social Transfer.

2004, March: Budget announced additional funding under the CST for early learning and child care of $75 million in each of 2004–05 and 2005–06; funding would reach $350 million starting in 2007–08.

2004, January: The Government of Canada committed $2 billion through the 2004 CHST supplement for health, nationally allocated equally over 2004–05 and 2005–06.

2003, March: Budget announced $900 million over five years in increased federal support for ELCC. On March 13, 2003, federal and provincial Social Services Ministers reached an agreement on a framework to improve access to ELCC programs and services. In 2003–04, funding was provided through the former Canada Health and Social Transfer (CHST) and in subsequent years through the CST.

2003, February: In support of the February 2003 First Ministers' Accord on Health Care Renewal, Budget confirmed: (1) a two-year extension to 2007–08 of the five-year legislative framework put in place in September 2000 with an additional $1.8 billion; (2) a $2.5 billion CHST supplement, giving provinces the flexibility to draw down funds as they require up to the end of 2005–06; and (3) the restructuring of the CHST to create a separate Canada Health Transfer and a Canada Social Transfer effective April 1, 2004, in order to increase transparency and accountability.

2000, September: First Ministers agreed on an action plan for renewing health care and investing in early childhood development. The Government of Canada committed to invest $21.1 billion of additional CHST cash, including $2.2 billion for early childhood development over five years.

2000, February: Budget announced a $2.5 billion increase for the CHST to help provinces and territories fund post-secondary education and health care. This brought CHST cash to $15.5 billion for each of the years from 2000–01 to 2003–04.

1999: Budget announced increased CHST funding of $11.5 billion over five years, specifically for health care. Changes were made to the allocation formula to move to equal per capita CHST by 2001–02.

1998: CHST legislation put in place a $12.5 billion cash floor beginning in 1997–98 and extending to 2002–03.

1996: Budget announced a five-year CHST funding arrangement (1998–99 to 2002–03) and provided a cash floor of $11 billion per year. For 1996–97 and 1997–98, total CHST was maintained at $26.9 billion and $25.1 billion respectively. Thereafter the transfer was set to grow at GDP–2%; GDP–1.5%; and GDP–1% for the next three years. A new allocation formula was introduced to reflect changes in provincial population growth and to narrow existing funding disparities, moving halfway to equal per capita by 2002–03.

1995: Budget announced that, starting in 1996, EPF and CAP programs would be replaced by a Canada Health and Social Transfer block fund. For 1995–96, EPF growth was set at GNP-3%, and CAP was frozen at 1994–95 levels for all provinces. CHST was set at $26.9 billion for 1996–97 and $25.1 billion for 1997–98. CHST for 1996–97 was allocated among provinces in the same proportion as combined EPF and CAP entitlements for 1995–96.

1994: Budget announced that total CAP and EPF transfers in 1996–97 would be no higher than in 1993–94.

1991: Budget extended the EPF freeze and CAP growth limit, introduced in 1990–91, for three more years to 1994–95.

1990: Growth in CAP transfer for three non-Equalization provinces (Ontario, Alberta, and BC) limited to 5% annually for 1990–91 and 1991–92. The EPF per capita transfer was frozen for 1990–91 and 1991–92 for all provinces.

1989: Budget announced that EPF growth would be further reduced to GNP–3% beginning in 1990–91.

1986: EPF growth was reduced from GNP to GNP–2% indefinitely.

1984: The *Canada Health Act* was enacted. EPF funding was conditional on respect for the five criteria of the *Canada Health Act* (universality, accessibility, portability, comprehensiveness, and public administration) and provisions for withholding funding were introduced.

1983: The post-secondary education portion of EPF was limited to 6% and 5% growth for 1983–84 and 1984–85 under the "6 & 5" anti-inflation program.

1982: GNP per capita escalator would be applied to the total EPF, rather than EPF cash.

1977: Established Programs Financing (EPF) was introduced, with federal funding to be provided in equal parts through a tax transfer and a cash transfer. EPF replaced cost-sharing programs for health and post-secondary education. Provinces received 13.5 percentage points of personal income tax (PIT) and 1 percentage point of corporate income tax (CIT), including some points carried over from the previous post-secondary education program.

The value of the transferred tax points was equalized. The value of the tax points was to grow as economies expanded, and the cash transfer was escalated by the growth rate of per capita GNP. EPF was to be distributed equal per capita over time.

1966: Canada Assistance Plan (CAP) introduced, creating a cost-sharing arrangement for social assistance programs. Conditions attached to federal funding.

Source: Department of Finance, *A brief history of social transfers* (April 29, 2008), www.fin.gc.ca/FEDPROV/hise.html

■ CURRENT ISSUES IN CANADIAN HEALTH CARE

Many issues in health care have arisen in recent years. Chief among them has been the decreasing federal contributions to provincial and territorial health care plans. Brooks and others have argued that the federal position has been to reduce its contribution toward provincial health services while continuing to set conditions on how those services will be delivered (Armstrong & Armstrong, 2003; Brooks, 1996). The reduced federal contribution has thus been the source of much tension between the federal and provincial governments since the early 1980s. The provincial governments have had to shoulder a larger share of health care costs, which increase annually. Thus, declining federal transfers and growing health care costs have contributed to provincial governments opting for various privatization schemes to reduce their health care costs, such as public-private partnership arrangements (P3s) to build hospitals and other social services such as schools and highways. Provinces have also delisted drugs covered by the provincial drug formularies and user fees for a wide range of previously insured services.

■ THE INFLUENCE OF NEO-LIBERALISM

While reduced federal transfers have indeed undermined national standards in health care and other social policy fields, privatization is also driven by an ideological commitment characteristic of increasing neo-liberalism in Canada. Neo-liberalism is a market ideology in which the market is considered to be the most efficient allocator of economic and social resources in a society (Coburn, 2000). Coburn and Teeple trace the rise of neo-liberalism and globalization to the early 1970s during the oil crisis, which prompted many OPEC countries to ratchet back social programs (Teeple, 2000).

Canadian governments have raised alarm bells about the sustainability of medicare in its current form during the 1990s and into the 2000s. The issue of sustainability has fuelled interest in allowing private sector involvement in health care. A key issue is how to pay for the services and programs that promote health, and how to make it politically feasible and attractive (Yalnizyan, 2006). Affordability is expressed in terms of ability to pay. However, governments not only have the responsibility to pay, they also have the capacity to control costs. Government decisions have implications for the public purse and household income, and influence total health care spending in the economy.

■ HEALTH CARE REFORM

Concern about the sustainability of medicare provides an opportunity to explore how it can be reformed to best serve the health care needs of Canadians. As noted elsewhere in this volume, Tommy Douglas and Emmett Hall recommended broadening the programs covered by medicare to include dental care, home care, and other services under medicare. Recent interest has focused on pharmacare to provide coverage of the cost of prescription medications.

The current thrust of the system on diagnoses and curative treatments has increased the cost of health care provision. The system lacks a preventative component. In the view of some critics, prevention would involve addressing the social determinants of health, and in particular reducing the poverty rate among non-elderly families with children to improve their health. Research has established the relationship between income and health (Annals of the New York Academy of Sciences, 1999; Brimblecombe, Dorling & Shaw, 1999; Gordon, Shaw, Dorling & Davey Smith, 1999).

Medicare has many proponents and detractors. The latter seizes upon any perceived failing of the system as evidence of the need to privatize health care. Both sides agree on the need to reform medicare, but there is no consensus on how to proceed. Public opinion polls show that Canadians value the health care system and support reforming it to improve delivery. Few Canadians support privatization as a solution. In addition, some health policy observers have warned that allowing private providers into the health care system would erode medicare in the long term and violate the principle of providing care on the basis of need. They advocate public solutions to addressing problems within the system (Rachlis, 2004; Yalnizyan, 2006).

■ WAIT TIMES

The federal, provincial, and territorial governments continue to wrangle about medicare. They focus their concern on reducing wait times for specialist care. Some provinces such as Alberta, British Columbia, and Ontario have privatized some health services, arguing that private sector involvement will relieve the backlog in the public system. Conservative think tanks, such as the Fraser Institute and the C.D. Howe Institute, have contributed to this view.

A recent health care survey carried out jointly by Statistics Canada and the Centers for Disease Control and Prevention in the United States showed that 31 percent of low-income Americans compared to 23 percent of low-income Canadians reported poorer health (Sanmartin & Ng, 2004). Interestingly, Americans were more likely to report being "very satisfied" with their health care services compared to Canadians, who were more likely to be "somewhat satisfied." How much of this concern is perceived rather than real is questionable.

Studies on health spending in Canada and comparison nations with or without a public health system have shown that the public system is less costly. Table 6.1 shows the health spending for Canada, the United States, the United Kingdom, and Sweden. In all cases, public health care is less costly. Canada's public spending on health care is equated with the single-payer system, which has numerous advantages over a private system (Yalnizyan, 2006). For example, with one centre to receive bills and send out payments, the system reduces administrative duplication. Moreover, approximately 1.8 percent of Canada's provincial and territorial health care costs are directed to the structure responsible for paying physician and hospital claims. In contrast, the US pays three times as much per person for doctors' and hospital services (Yalnizyan, 2006).

The issue of wait times for care has led to discussion among provincial governments to consider an increased role for the private sector in health care or

Table 6.1: Demographic Aspects of Canada and Three Comparison Nations (2005)

	Canada	US	UK	Sweden
GDP per capita (USD)	$34,057	$41,827	$32,896	$32,111
Annual GDP growth in % (1990–2005)	1.8	1.8	2.1	1.7
Share of population > 65 years of age %	13.1	12.4	16.0	17.3
Income inequality—GINI coefficient (2000)	30.1	35.7	32.6	24.3

Source: Organisation for Economic Co-operation and Development 2007. Health Data 2007. Geneva: OECD.

allowing the development of a parallel private system to ease the pressure on the public system. Using public dollars to cover private health care services violates the principles of the Canada Health Act. As noted in the discussion on the terms of the Canada Health Act, provinces that contravene the provisions of the Canada Health Act risk losing some federal health care dollars. The federal government has not acted on these violations. Such a state of affairs leaves the public wondering who will protect medicare and whether it will be there when they or a family member require emergency or long-term care.

■ THE CANADIAN HEALTH SCENE IN INTERNATIONAL PERSPECTIVE

In this section some indicators of Canadian health policy are placed within a comparative perspective. These measures include some demographic data, indicators of the health status of Canadians, and health care system functioning. Canada is examined in relation to the UK, the US, and Sweden. The US provides a comparison with a market-driven approach to health policy, while the UK has a somewhat similar system to Canada, albeit with a separate privately oriented system. Sweden represents a good example of a state-oriented social democratic approach to health policy governance.

Demographics

The US is the wealthiest of these four nations on a per capital gross domestic product basis (Table 6.1). Per capita GDP for the US is $41,827 in US dollars, which is rather more than for the other three comparison nations. In terms of economic growth from the 1990–2005 period, all nations showed rather similar rates of annual change in the GDP. However, striking differences are seen in degree of income inequality as measured by the GINI coefficient, where the US shows the greatest income inequality and Sweden rather less so. Finally, in terms of the percentage of the population over the age of 65 years (a good indicator of the aging of the population) Sweden shows the highest level, and the US the lowest. Canada is near the low end on population aging, yet it is unable to meet the health needs of the population.

Health Status

Life expectancy is the greatest in Sweden and the lowest in the US (Table 6.2). Consistent with this, the US shows the greatest number of premature years of life lost (prior to age 70) and Sweden the lowest. A similar pattern is seen for infant mortality and low birth weight rate. And, not surprisingly, this same pattern holds for obesity rates where Sweden's rate of 10.7 percent is strikingly lower than the 32 percent rate seen in the US.

Table 6.2: Health Status in Canada and Three Comparison Nations (2005)

	Canada	US	UK	Sweden
Life expectancy	80.2	77.8	79.0	80.6
Premature years of life lost/100,000				
Males	4,296	6,418	4,390	3,491
Females	2,669	3,719	2,713	2,141
Infant mortality/1,000	5.3	6.8	5.1	2.4
Low birth weight/100	5.91	8.1	7.5	4.2
Obesity %	18.0	32.2	23.0	10.7

Source: Organisation for Economic Co-operation and Development 2007. Health Data 2007. Geneva: OECD.

Table 6.3: Usage of Health Care System in Canada and Three Comparison Nations (2005)

	Canada	US	UK	Sweden
Physicians/1,000	2.2	2.4	2.4	3.4
Nurses/1,000	10.0	7.9	9.1	10.6
Acute care hospital beds/1,000	2.9	2.7	3.1	2.2
Occupancy rate of acute care beds %	90	67	84	N/A
MRIs/1,000,000	5.5	26.6	5.4	N/A
Hospital discharges/1,000	88	121	245	161
Physician consultations per capita	6.00	3.8	5.1	2.8

Source: Organisation for Economic Co-operation and Development 2007. Health Data 2007. Geneva: OECD.

Usage of the Health Care System

Table 6.3 provides data concerning the health care system. Sweden has the greatest number of physicians available to the population while Canada has among the lowest. While the UK has the greatest number of acute care beds in hospitals, Canada's occupancy rates for these beds are strikingly higher than the other nations. Of interest is the very high number of MRI machines that are available for use in the US. Canada's high occupancy rate for acute care beds is mirrored in its having the highest number of physician consultations. Canada, however, has the lowest rate of hospital discharges than the other nations.

Box 6.5: Health Council of Canada

The Prime Minister and the Premiers accepted the advice of the Kirby Report, *The Health of Canadians—The Federal Role* (October 2002) and the Romanow Commission on the Future of Health Care in Canada (November 2002). Both reports identified the value of an independent council informing Canadians on health care matters while promoting accountability and transparency. Canada's First Ministers established the Council in their 2003 Accord on Health Care Renewal and enhanced its role in the 2004 Ten-Year Plan.

Funded by the Government of Canada, the Council reports to the Canadian public and operates as a non-profit agency. The Council has 26 councillors including representatives of federal, provincial and territorial governments, experts and citizen representatives. Councillors have a broad range of experience bringing perspectives from government, health care management, research and community life from across Canada. The Members of the Council—FPT Health Ministers—are similar to a corporate board of directors, performing a liaison function between the Council and Canada's First Ministers, as well as approving the Council's budget.

The Council will collaborate with Quebec's Council on Health and Well Being.

Supporting the work of the Health Council of Canada is a small secretariat located in Toronto.

Source: Health Council of Canada, www.healthcouncilcanada.ca/en/index. php?option=com_content&task=view&id=2&Itemid=3

Health Expenditures

Total expenditures on health on a per capital basis in equivalent US dollars is presented in Table 6.4. The US spends, on average, $6,401, which is much higher than the comparison nations. Canada spends more than the UK and Sweden on both an absolute dollar basis and also as a percentage of GDP. However, Canada ranks 9th highest among the 30 OECD nations for whom data is available. Of note is that of Canada's $3,326, about 70 percent or $2,400 is publicly financed. Annual growth in spending from 1995–2005 was only 3.2 percent in Canada, which is the lowest among these nations.

Table 6.4: Health Expenditures in Canada and Three Comparison Nations (2005)

	Canada	US	UK	Sweden
Total per capita expenditures (USD)	$3,326	$6,401	$2,724	$2,918
Public per capita expenditures (USD)	$2,400	$2,950	$2,500	$2,600
Total expenditures as % of GDP	9.8	15.3	8.3	9.1
Percentage of expenditures that are public	70	45	87	87
Average annual growth in health expenditures 1995–2005 (%)	3.2	3.6	4.2	3.8
Per capita pharmaceutical expenditures (USD)	$589	$792	N/A	$351
Average annual growth in pharmaceutical expenditures 1995–2005 (%)	5.8	7.1	N/A	3.6
Physician consultations per capita	6.00	3.8	5.1	2.8

Source: Organisation for Economic Co-operation and Development 2007. Health Data 2007. Geneva: OECD.

Per capital spending on pharmaceuticals is highest in the US, but Canada's spending is much higher than seen for Sweden. Similarly, in terms of average growth in costs from 1995–2005, Canada's growth is higher than that for Sweden, but lower than seen in the US.

Public Share of Health Spending

Not surprisingly, only 45 percent of health care spending in the US is public. Canada's rate of 70 percent, while noticeably higher than is the case of the US, is much lower than seen for the UK and Sweden. Indeed, Canada's public coverage is among the lowest of OECD nations.

■ SUMMARY

While wealthier than Sweden, Canada shows much more income inequality. Canada provides a health status profile that, while superior to that seen in the US, falls well behind what is seen in Sweden. This is the case for life expectancy, infant mortality, premature years of life lost, low birth weight rate, and obesity rates.

Canada's health care system spends more than is seen in Sweden on an absolute basis and also as a percentage of GDP. And in Canada, much less of that spending is publicly provided than is the case for Sweden. The growth in health costs, however, in Canada is less than that seen in the other comparison nations. Canada provides less acute care beds in hospital and these show very high occupancy. Finally, Canada has significantly less physicians available and these physicians appear to be very busy as indicated by the average number of consultations.

These findings suggest that Canada's health care system is operating at a higher capacity than is the case in other nations. Despite spending more than Sweden on health care in absolute and percentage of GDP basis than Sweden, health status indicators fall behind those seen in that nation. The sources of these health differences and means by which the health care system can respond to these challenges are taken up in later chapters.

■ CONCLUSIONS

This chapter has described the organization and delivery of health care services in Canada. It has also chronicled the history of public health care and the role of Canadian federalism in shaping it. Medicare is Canada's most valued social program. A comparison of health spending in Canada and comparison nations show that public systems are more cost-efficient than private systems and better serve the health needs of citizens.

Canadian federalism and ongoing federal-provincial conflict have shaped health care in Canada. Federalism, among other dynamics, led to the single-payer system that characterizes Canadian health care. The ongoing conflict between the federal and provincial governments has contributed to discussions about how to sustain the system into the future, not always with a view to strengthening the health care system to ensure its sustainability.

Comparatively Canada provides a health profile that, while superior to the US, falls well behind Sweden. Canada's health care system spends more than does Sweden with rather less to show for it. The system appears to be operating at very high capacity and with fewer physicians, and has more average consultations than three other comparison nations. The sources of these indicators are examined in later chapters.

■ APPENDIX 6.1: A DETAILED HISTORY OF CANADA'S HEALTH CARE SYSTEM

1867	British North America Act passed: federal government responsible for marine hospitals and quarantine; provincial/territorial governments responsible for hospitals, asylums, charities, and charitable institutions.
1897–1919	Federal Department of Agriculture handles federal health responsibilities until Sept. 1, 1919, when first federal Department of Health created.
1920s	Municipal hospital plans established in Manitoba, Saskatchewan, and Alberta.
1921	Royal Commission on Health Insurance, British Columbia.
1936	British Columbia and Alberta pass health insurance legislation, but without an operating program.
1940	Federal Dominion Council of Health created.
1942	Federal Interdepartmental Advisory Committee on Health Insurance created.
1947	Saskatchewan initiates provincial universal public hospital insurance plan, January 1.
1948	National Health Grants Program, federal; provides grants to provinces and territories to support health-related initiatives, including hospital construction, public health, professional training, provincial surveys, and public health research.
1949	British Columbia creates limited provincial hospital insurance plan. Newfoundland joins Canada; has a cottage hospital insurance plan.
1950	Alberta creates limited provincial hospital insurance plan, July 1.
1957	Hospital Insurance and Diagnostic Services Act, federal, proclaimed (Royal Assent) May 1; provides 50/50 cost sharing for provincial and territorial hospital insurance plans, in force July 1, 1958.
1958	Manitoba, Newfoundland, Alberta, and British Columbia create hospital insurance plans with federal cost sharing, July 1. Saskatchewan hospital insurance plan brought in under federal cost sharing, July 1.
1959	Ontario, New Brunswick, and Nova Scotia create hospital insurance plans with federal cost sharing, January 1. Prince Edward Island creates hospital insurance plan with federal cost sharing, October 1.
1960	Northwest Territories creates hospital insurance plan with federal cost sharing, April 1. Yukon creates hospital insurance plan with federal cost sharing, July 1.

1961	Quebec creates hospital insurance plan with federal cost sharing, January 1. Federal government creates Royal Commission on Health Services to study need for health insurance and health services; appoint Emmett M. Hall as Chair.
1962	Saskatchewan creates medical insurance plan for physicians' services, July 1; doctors in province strike for 23 days.
1964	Royal Commission on Health Services, federal, reports; recommends national health care program.
1965	British Columbia creates provincial medical plan.
1966	Canada Assistance Plan (CAP), federal, introduced; provides cost sharing for social services, including health care not covered under hospital plans, for those in need, Royal Assent July, effective April 1. Medical Care Act, federal, proclaimed (Royal Assent), December 19; provides 50/50 cost sharing for provincial/territorial medical insurance plans, in force July 1, 1968.
1968	Saskatchewan and British Columbia create medical insurance plans with federal cost sharing, July 1.
1969	Newfoundland, Nova Scotia, and Manitoba create medical insurance plans with federal cost sharing, April 1. Alberta creates medical insurance plan with federal cost sharing, July 1. Ontario creates medical insurance plan with federal cost sharing, October 1.
1970	Quebec creates medical insurance plan with federal cost sharing, November 1. Prince Edward Island creates medical insurance plan with federal cost sharing, December 1.
1971	New Brunswick creates medical insurance plan with federal cost sharing, January 1. Northwest Territories creates medical insurance plan with federal cost sharing, April 1.
1972	Yukon creates medical insurance plans with federal cost sharing, April 1.
1977	Federal-Provincial Fiscal Arrangements and Established Programs Financing Act (EPF) federal cost-sharing shifts to block funding.
1979	Federal government creates Health Services Review; Emmett M. Hall appointed Special Commissioner to re-evaluate publicly funded health care system.
1980	Health Services Review report released August 29; recommends ending user fees, extra billing, setting national standards.
1981	Provincial/territorial reciprocal billing agreement for in-patient hospital services provided out-of-province/territory.
1982	Federal EPF amended; revenue guarantee removed, funding formula amended.

1983	Royal Commission on Hospital and Nursing Home Costs, Newfoundland, begins April, reports February 1984. Comite d'étude sur la promotion de la santé, Quebec, begins, ends 1984. La Commission d'énquête sur les services de santé et les services sociaux, Quebec, begins January, reports December 1987. Federal Task Force on the Allocation of Health Care Resources begins June, reports 1984.
1984	The Canada Health Act, federal, passes (Royal Assent April 17), combines hospital and medical acts; sets conditions and criteria on portability, accessibility, universality, comprehensiveness, public administration; bans user fees and extra billing. Provincial/territorial reciprocal billing agreement for out-patient hospital services provided out-of province/territory.
1985	Health Services Review Committee, Manitoba, begins, reports November.
1986	Federal transfer payments rate of growth reduced. Health Review Panel, Ontario, begins November, reports June 1987.
1987	Premier's Council on Health Strategy, Ontario, begins, ends in 1991. Royal Commission on Health Care, Nova Scotia, begins August 25, reports December 1989. Advisory Committee on the Utilization of Medical Services, Alberta, begins September, reports September 1989. All provinces and territories in compliance with the Canada Health Act by April 1.
1988	Provincial/territorial governments (except Quebec) sign reciprocal billing agreement for physicians' services provided out-of-province/territory. Commission on Directions in Health Care, Saskatchewan, begins July 1, reports March 1990. Premier's Commission on Future Health Care for Albertans, Alberta, begins December, reports December 1989. Commission on Selected Health Care Programs, New Brunswick, begins November, reports June 1989.
1989–1994	Further reductions in federal transfer payments.
1990	Royal Commission on Health Care and Costs, British Columbia, begins, reports 1991.
1991	National Task Force on Health Information, federal, reports; leads to creation of Canadian Institute of Health Information. Task Force on Health, Prince Edward Island, begins June, reports March 1992.
1994	National Forum on Health, federal, created to discuss health care with Canadians and recommend reforms, begins October, reports 1997.

1995   Federal EPF and CAP merged into block funding under the Canada Health and Social Transfer (CHST), to support health care, post-secondary education, and social services.

1996   Federal CHST transfers begin April 1.

1998   Health Services Review, New Brunswick, begins, reports February 1999.

1999   Social Union Framework Agreement (SUFA) in force; federal, provincial, and territorial governments (except Quebec) agree to collective approach to social policy and program development, including health. Minister's Forum on Health and Social Services, Northwest Territories, begins July, reports January 2000.

2000   First ministers' Communiqué on Health, announced September 11. Commission of Study on Health and Social Services (Clair Commission), Quebec, created June 15, reports December 18. Saskatchewan Commission on Medicare (Fyke Commission), Saskatchewan, begins June 14, reports April 11, 2001. Premier's Advisory Council on Health for Alberta (Mazankowski Council), Alberta, established January 31, reports January 8, 2002. Premier's Health Quality Council, New Brunswick, begins January, reports January 22, 2002.

2001   Standing Senate Committee on Social Affairs, Science, and Technology review (Kirby Committee), federal, begins March 1, publishes recommendations October 2002. Commission on the Future of Health Care in Canada (Romanow Commission), federal, begins April 4, reports November 2002. British Columbia Select Standing Committee on Health (Roddick Committee), begins August, reports December 10. Northwest Territories Action Plan, begins November, reports January 2002. [Health] Consultation Process, Ontario, begins July, results released January 21, 2002. Health Choices—A Public Discussion on the Future of Manitoba's Public Health Care Services, Manitoba, begins January, reports December.

2003   First ministers' Accord on Health Care Renewal, announced February 5.

            Health Council of Canada established to monitor and report on progress of Accord reforms, December 9.

2004   Federal CHST split into two transfers: the Canada Health Transfer (CHT) and the Canada Social Transfer (CST), April 1. First ministers' A 10-Year Plan to Strengthen Health Care, September 16.

Source: http://www.hc-sc.gc.ca/hcs-sss/pubs/system-regime/2005-hcs-sss/time-chron_e.html

■ NOTE

1. See Stephen Brooks's *Canadian democracy: An introduction* (1996) for a full treatment of Canadian federalism and its implications for intergovernmental relations and public policy at the federal and provincial levels.

■ REFERENCES

Annals of the New York Academy of Sciences. (1999). *Socioeconomic status and health in industrial nations: Social, psychological, and biological pathways* (vol. 896). Bethesda: Annals of the New York Academy of Sciences.

Armstrong, H. & Armstrong, P. (2003). *Wasting away: The undermining of Canadian health care.* Toronto: Oxford University Press.

Banting, K. (1997). The social policy divide: The welfare state in Canada and the United States. In K. Banting, G. Hoberg & R. Simeon (Eds.), *Degrees of freedom: Canada and the United States in a changing world,* 267–309. Montreal & Kingston: McGill-Queen's University Press.

Begin, M. (2007). The Canada Health Act: Lessons for today and tomorrow. In B. Campbell & G.P. Marchildon (Eds.), *Medicare: Facts, myths, problems & promise,* 46–49. Toronto: James Lorimer & Company Ltd.

Braen, A. (2004). Health and the distribution of powers in Canada. In T. McIntosh, P.-G. Forest & G.P. Marchildon (Eds.), *The governance of health care in Canada,* 197–232. Toronto: University of Toronto.

Brimblecombe, N., Dorling, D. & Shaw, M. (1999). Where the poor die in a rich city: The case of Oxford. *Health & Place, 5*(4), 287–300.

Brooks, S. (1996). *Canadian democracy: An introduction.* Toronto: Oxford University Press.

Coburn, D. (2000). Income inequality, social cohesion, and the health status of populations: The role of neo-liberalism. *Social Science & Medicine, 51*(1), 135–146.

Commission on the Future of Health Care in Canada. (2002). *Building on values: The future of health care in Canada—Final report.* Saskatoon: Commission on the Future of Health Care in Canada.

Gordon, D., Shaw, M., Dorling, D. & Davey Smith, G. (1999). *Inequalities in health: The evidence presented to the independent inquiry into inequalities in health.* Bristol: The Policy Press.

Health Canada. (2005). *Canada's health care system.* Ottawa: Minister of Health.

Hutchison, B., Abelson, J. & Lavis, J. (2001). Primary care in Canada: So much innovation, so little change. *Health Affairs, 20*(3), 116–131.

Leeson, H. (2004). Constitutional jurisdiction over health and health care services in Canada. In T. McIntosh, P.-G. Forest & G.P. Marchildon (Eds.), *The governance of health care in Canada,* 169–198. Toronto: University of Toronto.

Madore, O. (1997). *The transfer of tax points to provinces under the Canada Health and Social Transfer.* Ottawa: Government of Canada.

McIntosh, T. (2004). Introduction: Restoring trust, rebuilding confidence—The governance of health care and the Romanow Report. In T. McIntosh, Forest, P.G. & G.P. Marchildon (Eds.), *The governance of health care in Canada,* 3–22. Toronto: University of Toronto.

National Coalition on Health Care. (2007). *Facts on health care insurance coverage.* Washington: National Coalition on Health Care. www.nchc.org

Rachlis, M. (2004). *Prescription for excellence: How innovation is saving Canada's health care system.* Toronto: HarperCollins.

Rachlis, M. (2005). *Public solutions to health care wait lists.* Ottawa: Canadian Centre for Policy Alternatives.

Sanmartin, C. & Ng, E. (2004). *Joint Canada/United States Survey of Health, 2002–03.* Ottawa: Statistics Canada.

Scott, C. (2001). *Public and private roles in health care systems.* Buckingham: Open University Press.

Statistics Canada. (2001). *The assets and debts of Canadians: An overview of the results of the Survey of Financial Security.* Retrieved from http://www.statcan.ca:80/english/ freepub/13-595-XIE/9900113-595-XIE.pdf

Teeple, G. (2000). *Globalization and the decline of social reform: Into the twenty-first century.* Aurora: Garamond Press.

Teeple, G. (2006). Foreword. In D. Raphael, T. Bryant & M. Rioux (Eds.), *Staying alive: Critical perspectives on health, illness, and health care,* 1–4. Toronto: Canadian Scholars' Press Inc.

Tuohy, C. (1999). *Accidental logics: The dynamics of change in the health care arena in the United States, Britain, and Canada.* New York: Oxford University Press.

Yalnizyan, A. (2006). *Controlling costs: Canada's single-payer system is costly—but least expensive.* Ottawa: Canadian Centre for Policy Alternatives.

CRITICAL THINKING QUESTIONS

1. How can Canadian federalism contribute constructively to the preservation of medicare in Canada?

2. Why might the medical profession support the preservation of medicare?

3. Why might the medical profession support increased private involvement in the health care system?

4. What possible programs could you envisage as becoming part of the publicly organized health care system?

5. How can the allied health professions (i.e., nursing, physiotherapy, occupational therapy) become engaged in helping to maintain a public health care system?

FURTHER READINGS

Armstrong, H. & Armstrong, P. (2003). *Wasting away: The undermining of Canadian health care.* Toronto: Oxford University Press.

Canada's health care system is often referred to as Canada's best-loved social program. It has been one of the most accessible health care systems in the world and has played a significant role in prolonging the lives of many

Canadians. This book examines how it has come under attack from a variety of sources and the effects these attacks have had on the system.

Canadian Institute for Health Information. (2007). *Health care in Canada 2007*. Ottawa: CIHI.

This report is the eighth in a series of annual reports on Canada's health care system. HCIC 2007 provides a review of key analytic work undertaken at CIHI that highlights CIHI's health care research priorities (access, quality of care, outcomes of care, health human resources, funding/costs/productivity, etc.). Available online at www.cihi.ca

Rachlis, M. (2004). *Prescription for excellence: How innovation is saving Canada's health care system*. Toronto: HarperCollins.

In his latest book, Michael Rachlis argues that the cure for Canada's health delivery system is not more money and not privatization; he says the answer can be found in the system itself. He describes various innovations and best practices across the system that have improved health delivery and enhanced quality for the patients and health professionals. Using an evidence-based storytelling approach, Rachlis argues that innovation will be the key to success, along with maintaining publicly funded support for our hospitals and doctors. Available online at http://www.michaelrachlis.com/product.pfe.php

Raphael, D., Bryant, T. and Rioux, M. (Eds.). (2006). *Staying alive: Critical perspectives on health, illness, and health care*. Toronto: Canadian Scholars' Press Inc.

Staying Alive provides a fresh perspective on the issues surrounding health, health care, and illness. In addition to the traditional approaches of health sciences and the sociology of health, this book shows the impact that human rights issues and political economy have on health. This provocative volume takes up these issues as they occur in Canada and the United States within a wider international context.

RELEVANT WEBSITES

Canada's Health Care System
www.hc-sc.gc.ca/hcs-sss/index_e.html
This government website provides background material and access to a range of sources about Canada's health care system.

Canadian Institute for Health Information
www.cihi.ca
  The Canadian Institute for Health Information (CIHI) provides timely, accurate, and comparable information. Our data and reports inform health policies, support the effective delivery of health services, and raise awareness among Canadians of the factors that contribute to good health.

Commission on the Future of Health Care in Canada
www.hc-sc.gc.ca/english/care/romanow/index1.html
  The Commission on the Future of Health Care in Canada website contains a multitude of commissioned research reports regarding the Canadian health care system. The chair of the commission, Roy Romanow, stated: "The task before us is to draw upon the ingenuity of all Canadians to ensure ... that our health system meets the challenges of the 21st century."

Health Council of Canada
www.healthcouncilcanada.ca/en
  The Health Council of Canada fosters accountability and transparency by assessing progress in improving the quality, effectiveness, and sustainability of the health care system. Through insightful monitoring, public reporting, and facilitating informed discussion, the council shines a light on what helps or hinders health care renewal and the well-being of Canadians.

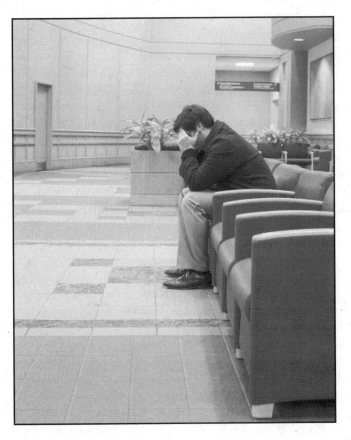

Chapter 7
HEALTH CARE REFORM IN CANADA

■ INTRODUCTION

Since the 1980s, Canadian governments have been preoccupied with issues related to the health care system and how to reform it. The penchant for reform has been driven by concerns that medicare is inefficient and overly costly as it is currently organized. This has fuelled support for allowing a parallel private system to develop to ease pressure on the public system. For example, perceptions of long wait times for specialist care and the non-responsiveness of the health care system to emerging issues have been used to build support for radically overhauling the system. Some critics have proposed privatizing some health care services and allowing private for-profit health care organizations to provide care.

Since 2000, several major reports on health care reform have been released. These include the Mazankowski Report, prepared for the Government of Alberta; the Romanow Royal Commission on Health Care; the Kirby Report from the Canadian Senate; the Fyke Commission on Medicare in Saskatchewan; and the Clair Commission on the Study of Health and Social Services in Quebec (Clair Commission d'étude sur les services de santé et les services sociaux, 2001; Commission on Medicare, 2001; Kirby, 2002; Mazankowski, 2001; Romanow, 2002). Each report proposes a course of action for reforming medicare. Since the Mazankowski, Kirby, and Romanow reports have proven to be the most influential, this chapter examines their key recommendations.

All the authors of the major reports express their commitment to the sustainability of medicare, but differ sharply in their perspectives on medicare and how it can be repaired. Stone's distinction between the polis and the market helps to illuminate the varying concepts of society that inform the orientation of these reports and their recommendations (Stone, 1988). Is the efficient operation of the health care system best accomplished by understanding it to be a communal effort undertaken by society to benefit the community as a whole? Or is it best to allow the health care system's operation to be governed by principles of the marketplace driven by individual interest?

This theoretical distinction helps to raise and answer questions such as: What is the basis for some of the reports recommending privatization and the introduction of user fees for health services? How consistent are these proposed directions with the ethos and principles of medicare as articulated in the Canada Health Act (1984)? And to what extent to these differing reports and their recommendations reflect the various health perspectives and policy theories presented in chapters 2 and 3? Finally, considering the importance of these issues, a key question to be considered is: How well are these issues being addressed in public discussions, if at all?

■ A FRAMEWORK FOR REFORM (MAZANKOWSKI REPORT)

This report was named after Don Mazankowski, who chaired the Premier's Advisory Council on Reform in Alberta. Mazankowski is best known as being minister of finance in Brian Mulroney's Conservative government in Ottawa during the 1980s. His 2001 report calls for fundamental changes in how health care services are delivered and financed to ensure its long-term sustainability (Mazankowski, 2001). Despite an extensive section on the broader determinants of health, most of which was subsequently ignored by the Alberta government (Raphael, 2003), the sections on the health care system have garnered virtually all health policy attention. Mazankowski's primary goal is to "[E]nsure sustainability of the health system for years to come" (Mazankowski, 2001: p. 5).

First off, Mazankowski contends that medicare was never intended to provide the full range of health services, treatments, drugs, and technology. Criticizing the current system as an "unregulated monopoly," Mazankowski advocates a larger role for the private sector in health care and greater choice for consumers. The primary purpose of these recommendations is to stimulate innovation. Specific mechanisms include more direct payments from citizens for health care services, such as user fees, premiums, deductibles, and taxing people for their use of the system. One of his key recommendations was the creation of medical savings accounts (MSAs).

Medical Savings Accounts

MSAs are health accounts formed in conjunction with high-deductible health insurance—that is, the policy pays a significant portion of initial costs—that can be set up by individuals, employers, or governments (Ramsay, 1998, p. 3). As an illustration, employers would set up MSAs for their employees. A portion of these funds would be used to purchase health care for employees. When these funds have been used up, employees would assume full responsibility for paying for their medical care up to a designated cap where catastrophic insurance would then begin.

Mazankowski argues that MSAs would be more cost-efficient than traditional insurance policies. It is claimed that MSAs foster "more prudent" spending of health care dollars without harming the health of individuals (Ramsay, 1998). Rules governing MSA plans could vary with respect to how surplus funds in personal accounts can be used once coverage periods end. In theory, MSAs would reduce demand for services by making individuals financially responsible for their consumption of health services (Shortt, 2002).

Mazankowski argues that MSAs and other co-payment strategies would discourage inappropriate use of health care services, and also "give people more control over their health care spending" (Mazankowski, 2001, p. 17). Mazankowski sees these reforms as increasing choices in health care services, thereby enabling more competition and increased accountability for health care services organization and delivery. He recommends delisting—or removing from public health care system coverage—some services that would now be paid for privately, arguing that "Private innovators could do wonders for our health care system" (Mazankowski, 2001, p. 27).

Further, Mazankowski recommends that private, for-profit health care facilities receive public financing. He also calls for increased development of public-private partnerships (P3s) to build hospitals and provide health care services. A P3 is an arrangement in which a government contracts with the private sector to finance, develop, construct, own, and operate infrastructure and public service (Savas, 2005). The key aspect of P3 arrangements such as those already initiated by Canadian provincial governments is that following the construction of these facilities, such as a new hospital or other public facility, the private corporations that built them would own them and make these facilities available to health care authorities on a lease-back or rental basis.

Regional Health Authorities

Another important aspect of Mazankowski's recommendations is a larger role for regional health authorities (RHAs) in health care. RHAs would work with other health regions to provide health services and also develop service agreements with a range of private or not-for-profit health providers or facilities. These agreements would consider identifying specific areas of specialization.

These collaborations would provide "joint administration," direct contracts with hospitals, and "alternative ownership arrangements and payment mechanisms" (Mazankowski, 2001: p. 50). Authorities would be authorized to raise revenues by charging fees for a range of services that would include instituting co-payments for long-term care and home care, restaurant inspections, environmental assessments, and public health education programs. Acknowledging that RHAs have faced numerous challenges since their inception in Alberta in 1995, Mazankowski believes that his recommendations will address many of these problems (Mazankowski, 2001).

Health Care Guarantee

Mazankowski recommends health care guarantees to reduce wait times for specialists and other specialized health care services (Mazankowski, 2001). Health care guarantees are predetermined wait-time deadlines for various medical procedures. The purpose of these would be to ensure timely access to care. Specifically, if Albertans could not be assured access to needed health services within 90 days, then the RHA where the individual resides would be required to arrange for those services to be provided by either a public or private sector provider. The travel costs of the patient and costs of the service provision would be charged to the region in which the patient resides. The concept of provincial health care guarantees has been endorsed by the federal government as a means of reducing wait times for various medical procedures and treatment (see Box 7.1).

In summary, the key message of the report is that the health care system should be financed less by general taxation and more by direct payments from citizens (Mazankowski, 2001). To further this objective, Mazankowski asserts that such a shift would encourage people to stay healthy such that they would make less use of the health care system. Mazankowski emphasizes that consumers need to be more aware of the cost of providing health care by paying out of pocket for health care

Box 7.1: Why Ontario Keeps Sending Patients South

By Lisa Priest
Globe and Mail

More than 400 Canadians in the full throes of a heart attack or other cardiac emergency have been sent to the United States because no hospital can provide the lifesaving care they require here.

Most of the heart patients who have been sent south since 2003 typically show up in Ontario hospitals, where they are given clot-busting drugs. If those drugs fail to open their clogged arteries, the scramble to locate angioplasty in the United States begins.

"They rushed me over to Detroit, did the whole closing of the tunnel," said Eric Bialkowski, 47, of the heart attack he had on March 14, 2007, in Windsor, Ont. "It was like Disneyworld customer service."

While other provinces have sent patients out of country—British Columbia has sent 75 pregnant women or their babies to Washington State since February, 2007—nowhere is the problem as acute as in Ontario.

At least 188 neurosurgery patients and 421 emergency cardiac patients have been sent to the United States from Ontario since the 2003–2004 fiscal year to Feb. 21 this year. Add to that 25 women with high-risk pregnancies sent south of the border in 2007.

Although Queen's Park says it is ensuring patients receive emergency care when they need it, Progressive Conservative health critic Elizabeth Witmer says it reflects poor planning.

That is particularly the case with neurosurgery, she said, noting that four reports since 2003 have predicted a looming shortage.

"This province and the number of people going outside for care—it's increasing in every area," Ms. Witmer said.

"I definitely believe that it is very bad planning.... We're simply unable to meet the demand, but we don't even know what the demand is."

Tom Closson, the Ontario Hospital Association's president and chief executive officer, said 30 per cent of Ontario's hospital medical beds are currently occupied by patients awaiting more appropriate placements, such as assisted living centres, a nursing home, a rehabilitation facility or even their own homes with proper home-care supports.

That squeezes the system at both ends: Patients in intensive care units whose condition improves cannot get into step-down units, and some emergency patients can't get a bed at all, he said, adding that "everything is jam-packed at the moment."

A method for determining the right mix of beds and health services required in Ontario needs to be developed, he said, noting that that task has not been undertaken on a provincial basis for a decade.

Laurel Ostfield, press secretary to provincial Health Minister George Smitherman, said that in emergencies, where the patient goes becomes a clinical decision.

It is preferable for someone with a heart attack in Windsor to be sent to Detroit, a few kilometres away, rather than on a long ride to London, Ont.

When demand has peaked, government has responded, she said. It struck a neurosurgery expert panel to study the problem and $4.1-million has been provided to stem the tide of US neurosurgery patients.

As well, stand-alone angioplasty services were created in Windsor in May.

Canadian Medical Association president Brian Day said he couldn't speak about the Ontario problem, but noted this country is the last in the Organisation for Economic Co-operation and Development to finance hospitals with global budgets.

Under that model, patients—and often doctors—are sometimes viewed as a financial drain.

"We keep coming back to the same root cause," Dr. Day said in a telephone interview from Ottawa. "The health system is not consumer-focused."

Patients first learn of the problem when they are critically ill.

Jennifer Walmsley went to Headwaters Health Care Centre in Orangeville in October and was diagnosed with a cerebral hemorrhage due to a ruptured aneurysm. That acute-care hospital does not have neurosurgery and no Ontario hospital that does could take her. She was then rushed to a Buffalo hospital.

Headwater's chief of staff, Jeff McKinnon, said three neurosurgery patients have been sent to Buffalo in the past year. Others have gone to Toronto, Mississauga, Hamilton and London.

Radiologist Louise Keevil said Headwaters has an arrangement with neurosurgeons at other Ontario hospitals to send electronic images for their assessment, but "the limiting factor is availability of beds in their hospital."

"The physicians are very accommodating but their hands are tied by availability of service."

Kaukab Usman had a heart attack after a gym workout in Windsor on Dec. 9. She was rushed to hospital and given clot-bursting drugs.

When they failed, she was sent to Henry Ford Hospital in Detroit, where she had angioplasty on one clogged artery and two stents inserted.

"It was a miracle for me to be alive," Ms. Usman said in a telephone interview from Somerset, New Jersey, where she is recuperating.

Aaron Kugelmass, director of the cardiac catheterization laboratory at Henry Ford Hospital, said a system is in place to get these patients the care they need expeditiously.

"We try to make their length of stay in the US as short as possible," said Dr. Kugelmass, associate division chief of cardiology. "If they are stable for discharge, we discharge them to home in Windsor, with clear follow-up plans."

Cross-border emergency health care should become less frequent when Amr Morsi, an interventional cardiologist currently in Orlando, Florida, comes to work at Hôtel-Dieu Grace Hospital in Windsor in April; a second interventional cardiologist is to come on board there by end of year.

When the program is fully functional, Dr. Morsi expects Hôtel-Dieu Grace to be able to do 500 angioplasties a year.

"The idea of starting the program in Windsor is that we will be able to do more of the angioplasty procedures in Windsor without having to send them to Detroit or London," said the Toronto native who did his cardiology training at the University of Toronto.

"It will take some time to decrease the numbers entirely, but that certainly is the long-term plan."

Mr. Bialkowski of Lakeshore, a town east of Windsor, had angioplasty and received four stents. The stents, typically made of self-expanding, stainless steel mesh, were placed at the site of the fully blocked artery to keep it open.

The price to treat him, including a two-day hospital stay in March, 2007, was $40,826.21 (US). With a 35 per cent discount from Henry Ford Hospital, the bill to the Ontario Health Insurance Plan tallied $26,537.03 (US), according to a health ministry document, a copy of which was sent to Mr. Bialkowski.

The father of six, a human resources manager for a manufacturing company based in Windsor, is back at the gym and feels great. It didn't matter where he received the lifesaving care, he said, just so long as he obtained it.

"I guess the Canadian government took care of me," he said.

Source: Globe and Mail (March 1, 2008), A1.

services that they receive. In essence, Mazankowski argues that commercialization schemes through user fees and private sector involvement will foster better quality and timely care.

■ THE HEALTH OF CANADIANS: THE FEDERAL ROLE

Senator Kirby initiated a Senate study of the Canadian health care system at the same time as Romanow began his Royal Commission on behalf of the federal Liberal government of Prime Minister Jean Chrétien. Kirby wrote a number of reports in which he identifies the different roles of the federal government in health and health care, the principles of medicare, and health care financing. The focus here is the sixth report, which presents the final recommendations to reform and renew medicare.

Independent Health Commission

Kirby recommends the creation of an evaluation body or council that would function independently of government to monitor the operation of the health care system. Its primary responsibilities would be to prepare an annual report on the state of the health system and the health of the Canadian population. Such reporting would provide an important impetus to improve health care delivery and health outcomes (Kirby, 2002). This body would consist of one provincial/territorial representative from each of the five major regions in Canada and five representatives from the federal government. The federal government would provide $10 million annually for council operations.

Public versus Private Administration and Delivery of Health Care Services

Kirby argues that it is not important who funds or owns health care services as he believes that the quality would be the same: "The patient and the funder/insurer will be served equally no matter what the corporate ownership of a health care institution might be" (Kirby 2002, p. 39). Kirby asserts that the principle of public administration articulated in the Canada Health Act and other health care legislation refers only to the funding of hospital and physician services, but "*not to the delivery* of those services" (Kirby, 2002, p. 7; italics in source). He asserts there has been widespread misunderstanding about the meaning of publicly funded and administered health insurance, and delivery of health care services. He stresses that under the Canada Health Act, health care services "do not have to be delivered by public agencies" (p. 8).

Cost Efficiency and Medical Savings Accounts

Similar to Mazankowski, Kirby was convinced of the need to make the health care system more effective and efficient (Kirby, 2002). Further, he sees the system, given existing funding levels, as not sustainable. Kirby argues for an infusion of $5 billion annually from the federal government, which he believes is required to reform and renew the health care system.

Also, Kirby also recommends medical savings accounts (MSAs) as a mechanism to prevent inappropriate or overuse of the system (Kirby, 2002). Kirby, too, believes that MSAs will help limit (if not eliminate) unnecessary use of health services, thereby reducing financial pressures on public health care funding. Such accounts will also promote greater efficiency in health care operations (Kirby, 2002).

Health Care Guarantee

Although Kirby acknowledges the lack of reliable data on wait times for particular procedures, Kirby cites "strong" public perception of a waiting list problem as evidence of the need for action (Kirby, 2002). Like Mazankowski, Kirby recommends establishing a national health care guarantee to reduce wait times for health services (Kirby, 2002). Kirby argues that "such a guarantee would serve as a spur to the creation of the necessary standards, criteria and information systems" (p. 113). Kirby argues it will ensure governments provide patients with reasonable access to needed health services in their own or another Canadian province. The guarantee is considered essential to (1) reform the system; (2) restore public confidence in the health care system; and (3) provide evidence of the capacity of government to spend tax dollars responsibly. Further, Kirby argues that not implementing a guarantee will increase the likelihood that the Supreme Court will approve the right of individuals to purchase private-issued insurance to pay for privately delivered health care outside of the public medicare system.

Primary Health Care Reform

Kirby reiterates the need for continuing primary health care reform with emphasis on creating multidisciplinary primary health care teams (Kirby, 2002). He calls for alternatives to fee-for-service arrangements such as capitation (health care providers being paid a set rate for serving a designated population) or some kind of blended approach. He also favours incorporating health promotion and illness-prevention strategies into primary care. Kirby recommends that the federal government provide $50 million annually to help the provinces establish these primary-care groups. All of these arrangements are seen as serving to reduce health care expenditures.

Devolution to Regional Health Authorities

Kirby also favours expanding the role of regional health authorities (RHAs) (Kirby, 2002). Consistent with his interest in introducing mechanisms into the public health care system, Kirby argues for devolving responsibility from senior governments to RHAs to purchase a comprehensive range of health services (Kirby, 2002). RHAs would control finances and select providers on the basis of quality and cost.

Kirby considers that devolution to these authorities would encourage more effective management of health care services. Further, he argues that regionalization will ensure timely provision of health care services (Kirby, 2002). This would occur since regional authorities would be responsible for finding timely care for an individual. If that was not possible, the authority would either have to go to a private health care provider in the local jurisdiction or to a public or private provider in another jurisdiction to provide needed care.

RHAs are also the mechanism by which internal markets would be created. Kirby defines internal markets as "the introduction of market-like mechanisms" into the health care system (Kirby, 2002, 70). Kirby cites internal market reforms that involve devolving responsibilities to regional health agencies as having been implemented successfully in Sweden and the United Kingdom (Kirby, 2002).

Service-Based Funding

The current funding model for hospitals in Canada is global funding. In this model health care service providers apply their funding to provide a range of services. Kirby recommends a shift to service-based funding in which specific areas of activity such as cardiac care or hip replacements are provided with set funding envelopes. Service-based funding would replace all of the current hospital funding methods and include what are called line-by-line budgeting and population-based funding. This means that hospitals would receive funding based on the type and volume of services that they provide (MacDonald, December 2002–January 2003). To this end, Kirby recommends that hospitals develop specializations, such as cardiology care (Kirby, 2002). He argues that service-based funding would reduce costs and make hospitals less dependent on government for financing.

Kirby's report reiterates many of the recommendations found in Mazankowski's health reform report. The key message of both reports is to reduce the perceived dependency of the health care sector upon government financing of health care. Kirby recommends expanding the role of the private sector in health care and introducing a range of market mechanisms to finance the system. He also, however, recognizes the need for stable, though eventually reduced, federal financing.

◼ BUILDING ON VALUES: THE FUTURE OF HEALTH CARE IN CANADA

Prime Minister Jean Chrétien appointed Roy Romanow, former premier of Saskatchewan, to lead a Royal Commission on health care reform (Romanow, 2002). Romanow was to initiate what was called a dialogue with Canadians about the future of the public health care system. Of specific concern was the long-term sustainability of the universally accessible, publicly funded medicare system.

Describing his report as "a roadmap for a collective journey by Canadians to reform and renew their health care system" (p. xxiii), Romanow presents a vision that the health care system is sustainable (Romanow, 2002). His key recommendations focus on retaining a public over private, for-profit service delivery and adding accountability as a principle of medicare in the Canada Health Act. In contrast to the Mazankowski and Kirby reports, he is committed to strengthening the existing public system. In terms of sustainability of the public health care system, Romanow considers the focus on financing and money to be "narrow" and "inadequate." He argues that sustainability "means ensuring that sufficient resources are available over the long term to provide timely access to quality services" (p. 1).

Public versus Private Care

Romanow notes that a key element of his commission's mandate was to make recommendations "to ensure the long-term sustainability of a universally accessible, publicly funded health care system" (Romanow, 2002, p.1). He considers the role that MSAs, various user fees, public-private partnerships, and other market-related mechanisms could play in a reformed health care system. On the basis of the available evidence, including a very large number of commissioned reports, Romanow concludes that all of these have shortcomings with serious implications for the accessibility and quality of health care services.

Not surprising considering the subtitle of his report—"Building on Values"—he calls for a recommitment to the principles of need over income as a guiding principle of medicare. Romanow provides evidence that health care systems are more effective when publicly financed and managed. Health and health care should not be seen as commodities, but rather as essential goods to which all citizens are entitled.

With regard to financial sustainability, Romanow notes that Canada's spending on health care compares favourably with that of other developed countries in the Organisation for Economic Co-operation and Development (OECD) with public health care systems (Romanow, 2002). He recognizes the funding imbalance that has appeared between the federal and provincial governments as a result of steady declines in federal contributions since the 1980s. As a result, the provinces have been required to dedicate increasing proportions of their budgets to health care. He argues that the health care system is under-resourced and requires more federal dollars to maintain sustainability. He recommends "stable and predictable federal funding" in the form of a "cash-only" Canada Health Transfer (Romanow, 2002, p.65).

Health Care Guarantee

Romanow considers the matter of wait times for care and recommends caution in approaching care guarantees (Romanow, 2002). Romanow acknowledges that care guarantees reassure patients and require health authorities, providers, and hospitals to initiate steps to ensure that the health care system can meet time limits established in a guarantee. Yet, he adds that guarantees must be based on an objective assessment of the capacity of the system to provide the required service or treatment within a specific period of time and on the urgency of the condition requiring treatment.

Overall, Romanow is concerned that provincial and territorial health care systems be provided with the flexibility to manage emergency and elective surgical procedures (Romanow, 2002). Care guarantees might introduce rigidity and could direct resources away from life-saving surgery or treatment to meet care guarantees for other health care services.

Direct and Ancillary Health Services

Romanow differentiates between direct and ancillary health services (Romanow, 2002). Ancillary health services are cleaning and food services within hospitals. He recommends public funding of diagnostic and treatment services, but supports contracting out ancillary services to reduce costs and make more resources available for medically necessary services.

Romanow advocates this distinction on the basis that most Canadians seem to accept the provision of ancillary services by for-profit agencies (Romanow, 2002). He adds that many non-profit hospitals currently contract out these services to for-profit corporations. He argues that, based on the available evidence, direct health care services be provided in public and not-for-profit health care facilities since the consequences of private delivery can be life-threatening.

Box 7.2: What Is Missing in the Royal Commission's Final Report?

The Report quite clearly fails to provide a gendered analysis of health care. Plans that fail to take women into account are not only inadequate but also inequitable.

The Report fails to recommend the prohibition of for-profit delivery, even though it presents evidence demonstrating the problems with such delivery.

The Report fails entirely to consider long-term care, chronic care or care for people with disabilities.

The Report fails to discuss reproductive issues and access to these services.

The Report does not apply the lessons on international agreements set out in the final chapter to the other recommendations in the Report, even though they could have a profound impact on them.

What Does the Report Mean for Women?
We applaud the Romanow Commission for demonstrating the sustaining of medicare. A publicly funded system delivered through non-profit services is crucial for all women in Canada. But like other reports on health care reform in the last decade, this Report fails to recognize the significant ways in which health care is an issue for women. Women are 80% of paid health care providers, a similar proportion of those providing unpaid personal care and a majority of those receiving care, especially among the elderly. The sustainability of the system is not just about finances, it is about women's work and women's care. Just as Canada should be a leader in seeing health as a human right, it should also be a leader in promoting gender equality in Canada and globally.

Investing in health care means investing in women. Unless this is understood, planning for care is bound to fail in its objectives.

Source: The National Coordinating Group on Health Care Reform and Women. (2003). *Reading Romanow: The implications of the final report of the Commission on the Future of Health Care in Canada for women*, p. 58. Winnipeg: Centres of Excellence for Women's Health.

Expand Medicare

Romanow recommends expanding the scope of medicare to include home care and palliative home care services to support people in the final six months of their lives (Romanow, 2002). Romanow also recommends developing a program to provide ongoing support to informal caregivers by making them eligible for special benefits under Canada's Employment Insurance program.

Romanow recommends developing a national formulary of prescription medications to ensure consistent coverage of medications in all provinces and territories. The National Drug Agency would work with the provinces and territories to ensure consistent coverage, objective assessments, and cost effectiveness.

Relationship to National Forum on Health Findings

Of all the health reform reports, Romanow's report is most consistent with recommendations made by the National Forum on Health. The National Forum was launched by then Prime Minister Jean Chrétien in 1994 to engage Canadians in a discussion about health care and to recommend innovative ways that the federal government could undertake to improve the health system and the health of the population (National Forum on Health, 1998). The National Forum was set up as an advisory body to the prime minister and the federal minister of health. This body saw its role as considering the long-term and systemic issues associated with health and health care. The National Forum commissioned several papers on systemic issues and produced five volumes on key health issues. It provided several recommendations on how to improve the health care system and the health of the population.

Box 7.3: Recommendations of the National Forum on Health

Among the recommendations of the National Forum were:

- System is sustainable
- Public is preferred over private
- Add accountability to the Canada Health Act principles of public administration, universality, accessibility, portability, and comprehensiveness
- Include home care services
- Improve timely access to services
- Approach health care guarantee with caution; based on principles of fairness, appropriateness, certainty
- Private diagnostic services
- Workers' compensation

■ ANALYSIS OF THE HEALTH REFORM REPORTS

The Mazanowski, Kirby, and Romanow reports reflect the lack of consensus about how to reform medicare. The system has become too large to leave responsibility to the health care professions to manage. Increasing amounts of money are being made available to reform the system, but with little commitment on the part of politicians and government to strengthen the public health care insurance system. They seem unwilling to reform significantly the manner in which services are provided, health care providers are paid, and health care activities are monitored (Rachlis, 2004, 2005).

As a result, the federal and provincial governments tinker at the edges of the system by delisting services and privatizing increasing elements of the system. All of this further reduces the role of government in providing publicly organized and managed health care. Already the Canadian health care system provides significantly less public coverage of health services than do most developed nations

Box 7.4: Preliminary Analysis of the Romanow Report from the Canadian Health Coalition and the Canadian Labour Congress

Overview and Broad Principles

The Romanow Report on the Future of Health Care concluded that there is a consensus among Canadians that medicare is a moral enterprise, not a commercial venture. Canadians believe that equal and timely access to medically necessary health services on the basis of need alone is a right of citizenship. The core values which underpin medicare remain the same: equity, fairness, and solidarity. As a result, Canadians reject diluting the principles of medicare, scrapping national standards, paying privately to get faster care, and treating health care as a business.

In his message to Canadians, Commissioner Romanow said, "I believe it is a far greater perversion of Canadian values to accept a system where money, rather than need, determines who gets access to care." The Report clearly states that Romanow challenged those advocating user fees, medical savings accounts, de-listing public services, greater privatization, and a parallel private system to provide him with evidence that these choices would improve or strengthen the health care system. He clearly said that "The evidence has not been forthcoming." There is no evidence that these solutions will deliver cheaper care or improve access to care. Further, the principles underlying these solutions are directly contradictory to the values of Canadians and the values of medicare.

For those reasons, the Romanow Report rejects a parallel tier of private, for-profit care for the delivery of what he calls direct health care services such as medical, diagnostic, and surgical care. This conclusion is to be applauded. It is based on evidence that for-profit care will harm, not improve, medicare.

However, the Report mistakenly says that a line can be drawn between health services and ancillary services such as laundry, food preparation, cleaning, and maintenance services. These services are said to be appropriate for delivery in the private sector. The labour movement disagrees with this approach. These services are health services and those who provide them are health care workers, and they see themselves as health care workers. These services are pertinent to the health of patients. Good nutrition is critical to people who are sick, and the cleanliness of hospitals is essential to patients, staff, and the public. While the Report has rejected a parallel tier of for-profit care, there does not appear to be a mechanism for ensuring that this does not happen. It does recommend that the Canada Health Act must be clarified to include these services under the Act. The Report needs to be looked at more closely.

Overall, the Romanow Report offers some important steps forward to preserving and expanding medicare for today's and future generations, but it is just a starting point. It has established some fundamental principles which need to be built and expanded upon.

Public-Private Partnerships
The Report rejects the argument that public-private partnerships to design, build and operate health facilities, such as hospitals, will save the public money. Romanow notes that these agreements have been shown to cost more over the longer term, and can have the effect of hospital bed closures and a reduction in nurses and other health staff. Romanow stops short of recommending no public-private partnerships.

Medical Savings Accounts, User Fees and Co-payments, Tax Credits, and Deductibles
Romanow rejects these alternative measures to raise more funding for medicare. In the end, all of these measures violate the core principle of equity and equal access to care based on need for care. These measures promote access based on ability to pay.

MRIs and CT Scans
The Report calls all diagnostic services required to assess a patient's need for health services to come under the conditions of the Canada Health Act, including the prohibitions of user fees, facility fees, and extra-billing. The CHA should be amended to clarify this.

CHST
The Report calls for federal health funding to be taken out of the CHST and put into a new transfer—The Canada Health Transfer. This transfer would be a cash-only transfer and have an escalator clause so that federal funding would keep pace with economic growth and our ability to pay. The CLC has called for this since the CHST was put in place in 1995.

Expansion of the Public System
The Report recommends that the Canada Health Act should be revised to include home care services in priority areas. This would include post-acute home care, including drugs and rehab services, as well as coverage of palliative care in the home during the last six months of life. Also, it would include a program of support for informal caregivers. Home mental health services should immediately come under the CHA. It calls for a Catastrophic Drug Transfer to help provinces with their drug plans. Eventually, the CHA would cover the cost of prescription drugs. It calls for a creation of a National

Drug Agency to control costs and insure the safety of drugs and it also calls for the establishment of a National Drug Formulary to help control costs. Finally, it calls for a review of aspects of the Patent Act. There must be an effective dispute mechanism maintained in the CHA. The dedicated Health Transfer would be directly connected to the principle and conditions in the Act. The Report calls for the development of a Rural and Remote Access Fund to attract and retain health care providers, including opportunities for health professionals in training to gain experience for doctors, nurses and other health providers. The Report states that the current status of injured workers getting preferred access to care violates the principle of equal access to care for all Canadians. The Canada Health Act allows this to take place. This exception needs to be reconsidered.

Accountability

The Report calls for the establishment of a new Canadian Health Covenant which would state Canadian values and would be a guiding force for medicare. A Health Council of Canada would be established to analyze and assess the national health system as a whole. Membership in the Council would include the public, providers, and governments. The Canada Health Act should be revised to include a Sixth Principle of Accountability.

Trade and Health Care

In recognition of the threat to health care from globalization, Romanow sends a clear message to the federal government that current protections for health care in trade agreements must not be weakened. Future expansions and actions must be protected in all future agreements. The right to regulate health care policy should not be subject to claims from foreign companies.

Primary Care Reform

The Primary Care Transfer should drive changes to the primary care system. We need a common national platform for health care reform. Prevention and promotion initiatives would be a part of this. Primary care needs to be delivered in multi-disciplinary teams in a community-based setting. All funding sources for Aboriginal health care should be pooled into a new Aboriginal Health Partnerships Fund. The goal is to improve access to care and provide adequate, stable funding. The system needs to reflect cultural diversity and language barriers to accessing care.

Funding: Making Medicare Sustainable

Civil Society organizations have called for the federal government to increase its share of health funding to 25% of publicly insured health services. The Romanow Report recommends that the federal government move to this standard by 2005–06 with increased funding in each of the next three years. The Report calls for new federal funds to bring the federal share up to 25% of insured health spending provided under current provincial plans. This will require additional investments to be added to the current level of funding. This would mean a new investment of $3.5 billion next year, 2003–04, followed by an additional $5 billion the next year, 2004–05, and a $6.5 billion increase in 2005–06. By 2005–06, these increases will bring the federal cash transfer to $15.3 billion per year. Romanow assumes that this will equal 25% of the public health services insured under provincial health plans. An escalator clause will increase this cash floor according to economic growth. These funding arrangements need to be stable and predictable. These funds would be targeted to specific spending areas over the next two years.

	2003–04/$ billion	2004–05/$ billion
Diagnostic services fund	.75	.75
Rural and remote access	.75	.75
Primary health care	1.0	1.5
Home care	1.0	1.0
Drugs	—	1.0
TOTAL	3.5	5.0

In 2005–06, the federal transfer for that year would rise from $5 billion to $6.5 billion, bringing the total federal cash transfer to $15.3 billion that year.

Source: Ontario Health Coalition, www.web.net/~ohc/docs/nov28-chc.htm

(Organisation for Economic Co-operation and Development, 2005). Thus, central to health care reform is the debate between public versus private financing and delivery of health care services.

Values, Principles, and World Views

Mazankowski's and Kirby's visions of health care are consistent with the market approach defined by Stone (Stone, 1988). Stone describes how the market treats individuals as consumers and how public goods such as health care become commodities. The market is characterized by competition as each individual works to acquire goods and services at the least possible cost. Competition, however, does not ensure quality of the goods and services traded and sold in a market when applied to health care.

Market approaches create inequities in access for vulnerable populations who lack the income to move up in line to receive health care services that they require. If faced with paying health care costs such as user fees, people with low income will simply do without.

Of these reports, only Romanow recognizes these issues and expresses confidence in the overall purpose, function, and form of the public health care system, yet he also identifies areas for improvement. Romanow couches his report in the notion of values and reinforced the notion that medicare expressed a value of equality that Canadians continue to support.

Romanow confirms public confidence in public health care and recommends major new federal investments in the system to ensure its sustainability (Maioni, 2003). Observers wonder, however, if the required cooperation between the two levels of government is feasible, given their tendency toward reducing resources to the system and opting for privatization schemes that result in reducing the role of government in health care.

Box 7.5: New Institutionalism Concepts and the Prospects for Health Care Reform

From a new institutionalism perspective, institutions structure political debate and the solutions that will be considered to address public problems (Hall, 1993; Hall & Taylor, 1996). In health care, federal and provincial institutions impede meaningful reforms of the health care system, particularly in relation to the provision of sufficient funding to ensure its sustainability. The ongoing wrangling between the federal and provincial governments over financing of health care has led to little productive debate on how to change the system with the goal of improving it. The two levels of government can be seen as structuring health care debate and limiting the range of solutions that can be considered to reform the system and improve service delivery and health outcomes. These is also institutional resistance to expand the system not only to provide sufficient resources to core functions of medicare, but also to expand the scope of the system to include dental care, home care, and pharmacare as recommended as early as 1964 by Emmett Hall's report to the federal government.

In contrast to Romanow, Mazankowski and Kirby recommend introducing privatization measures such as user fees for services in order to sustain the system. Opting for private measures or an expanded role for the private sector is an ideological position (Coburn, 2000, 2001; Langille, 2004; Savas,

2005). It prescribes roles and relationships for private institutions and government within a society. The private institutions identified to improve health care represent the market and market-oriented strategies such as user fees, medical savings accounts, and public-private partnerships (Stone, 1988). What happens in these arrangements is that the service or good charged to the private entity in the end belongs to that entity. Critics argue that once these arrangements are in place, it is in the end to bring these goods or services back into the public realm.

All three reports are concerned about the sustainability of medicare, but present very different solutions to ensure its sustainability. Mazankowski recommends user fees and medical savings accounts (MSAs) to reduce inappropriate use. Kirby recommends public over private funding, but also recommends MSAs for reasons similar to Mazankowski's. Romanow unequivocally states that public funding makes the most sense and notes the lack of evidence that privatization will improve the quality of care. These and other aspects of the reports reflect different conceptions of society and how to deliver health care.

Drawing on Stone's distinction between the polis and the market (Romanow, 2002; Stone, 1988), it is clear that the market underlies Mazankowski's and also Kirby's approach to health care reform. Both imply that making the health care system run more like a private business will ensure its sustainability. Both recommend market or private solutions such as medical savings accounts to ensure the sustainability of the system. They both want consumers to be more aware of the cost of health care and to discourage inappropriate or overuse of health care services.

In contrast, Romanow presents the polis in his articulation of the collective responsibility of Canadians to decide how to reform and sustain the health care system. He does not consider health care a commodity to be bought and sold in the market, but rather a public good. He also cites evidence that shows that public health care provides better quality care compared to private health facilities. Romanow also cites the evidence showing that private health care systems are more costly than public health care systems. Romanow's findings and perspective are consistent with the views of the Canadian public.

Underlying all the reports are specific orientations to society and the provision of goods and services. On the one hand, Mazankowski and Kirby emphasize deregulation, user fees, establishing MSAs, and other market mechanisms to reduce costs. They aim to reduce what they perceive as inappropriate use of the health care system. Their recommendations are consistent with Stone's market model, which emphasizes individual responsibility for health.

Box 7.6: Deficit-Reduction Drives Health Care Reform

Much of the concern with reforming medicare has been driven by the focus on deficit reduction by federal and provincial governments since the 1980s. Mendelsohn outlines some of the concerns and perceptions that have shaped the debate about health care (Mendelsohn, 2002). First, the Canadian public hears that the health care system as it is currently organized, i.e., public financing and private provision, is unsustainable. Second, the media and politicians propagate the view that the system is in crisis. Finally, the first two perceptions promote the argument that some form of privatization is the only solution to the ills of the health care system.

In contrast, Canadians are proud of medicare as a made-in-Canada program that differentiates Canada from the United States, and Canada from the United States as a collectivist society concerned about the welfare of all Canadians wherever they may live in the country. Canadians are proud that they share the risk across the population by paying for the system through general revenues to ensure that all have access to health care. In short, health care is a right, not a privilege based on income or ability to pay. In addition, Canadians support the five principles of the Canada Health Act and its core elements. While they perceive that the system has deteriorated since its inception and may need to be updated to reflect changing needs and technology in the health care field, they are concerned about losing medicare, but are willing to accept some modifications to ensure its sustainability into the future.

Mendelsohn notes that Canadians have contradictory views concerning two-tiered medicine. For example, one public opinion poll showed that 33 percent of Canadians were prepared to accept two-tiered medicine, while 73 percent support the option of private facilities if they cannot get timely access in the public system. What is driving these attitudes and perceptions about medicare and health care reform?

Romanow's vision of health care and his preference for a collectivist approach to health care services, if not his view of ancillary service provision, is consistent with the polis, the ultimate political society. Romanow envisions a caring society in which citizens share in the risk of providing care to ensure access to health care for all, regardless of income. These orientations are shaped by ideological commitments to the nature of society and the role of the state versus the market in organizing and distributing societal resources.

In short, the reports reflect two competing world views (Maynard, 2007). These are the collectivist and the libertarian ideologies. The collectivist approach promotes equality as the goal of the behaviour of social institutions. In particular, Kirby's recommendation to shift to service-based funding to hospitals and an expanded role for regional health authorities underscores his desire to deregulate health care services. It also highlights his desire to reduce the role of the state in health care.

Grieshaber-Otto and Sinclair argue that service-based funding represents a fundamental shift in hospital funding (Grieshaber-Otto & Sinclair, 2004). Moreover, they add that Kirby's analysis fails to recognize that hospitals and local health authorities may become less accountable to the public as these institutions become more independent of democratically elected governments. Grieshaber-Otto and Sinclair suggest that Senator Kirby and his Senate colleagues believe that these developments would improve the functioning of the system, thereby validating the policy changes that Kirby and his committee think are necessary (Grieshaber-Otto & Sinclair, 2004).

Kirby's recommendation that governments pay for people to receive treatment in other jurisdictions may not address the fundamental problem of the federal government's underfunding (Grieshaber-Otto & Sinclair, 2004). In essence, the proposed remedy could exacerbate the situation by authorizing additional spending outside the local setting at private market rates. Thus, Grieshaber-Otto and Sinclair and other policy analysts argue that such measures may result in increasing reliance on private, for-profit health entities to provide health care services (Grieshaber-Otto & Sinclair, 2004).

Deregulation and Accountability

Kirby and Mazankowski believe greater competition will lead to more innovation and better quality of care, but cite little evidence to support these claims. They seem unconcerned about the lack of accountability that may result from an expanded private sector role and further deregulation of health care. Mazankowski criticizes medicare as an unregulated monopoly, yet favours further deregulation. It is unclear how further deregulation will improve the quality of services, or how it can maintain public accountability.

Moreover, experiences with deregulation in other jurisdictions suggest the need for caution (Grieshaber-Otto & Sinclair, 2004). Deregulation jeopardizes accountability and obscures lines of authority. For example, the House of Commons Transport Committee in the United Kingdom identified serious flaws in the organization of the privatized railway: "The constant theme throughout our work was the complaint that the current structure of the industry is too fragmented to provide clear lines of responsibility and leadership and a satisfactory basis for improved rail performance" (UK House of Commons Transport Committee,

---

Box 7.7: Canadian Federalism

Maioni argues that unless the federal, provincial, and territorial governments understand shared responsibility for the program, Romanow's solutions to sustain medicare may not be workable (Maioni, 2003). She specifically describes federal-provincial relations as toxic, and therefore not conducive, and potentially detrimental to preserving medicare. She makes an interesting argument about three reforms with respect to money: "more money, money better spent, and accountability for the money" spent on health care (p. 51).

Both Mendelsohn and Maioni identify key dynamics that influence health care and health policy in Canada (Maioni, 2003; Mendelsohn, 2002). Chief among these on the surface is the emphasis on deficit reduction among Canadian governments since the 1980s. This emphasis and that of Mazankowski and Kirby in their reports shows the influence of neo-liberalism, which favours the market as efficient in the allocation and delivery of resources and services in the economy. Teeple and Coburn consider political ideology, particularly neo-liberalism, to be a key driver in policy discussions and as shaping public debates on key issues such as health care.

Sources: Maioni, A. (2003). Romanow—A defence of public health care, but is there a map for the road ahead? *Policy Options, 24*(2), 50–53; Mendelson, M. (2002). Canadians prepared to accept medicare reform in primary care, poll shows. *Policy Options* (November), 27–29.

2004, pp. 5–6). Such fragmentation and blurring of lines of accountability may affect the Canadian health care system should Canadian governments allow further commercialization in health care.

There is need for more consideration of public solutions to remedy the problems of the health care system. Foremost is a need to renew the state's role in health care and recognize the benefits of the single-payer system.

Medical Savings Accounts: Path to Prudent Consumer Use of Health Care Services?

The Fraser Institute, a public policy think tank based in Vancouver, BC, favours an expanded role for the private sector, and the introduction of user fees and MSAs (Ramsay, 1998). Their premise is that MSAs and other user fees will reduce the cost of care, and, in particular, reduce taxes. They argue that American evidence shows that "MSAs are conducive to more prudent health spending without compromising individuals' health…. They have resulted in lower employer and employee costs" (Ramsay, 1998, p. 5). Further, the Fraser Institute suggests that MSAs could lower health expenditures by up to 20 percent (Ramsay, 1998). The rationale for such measures is to make consumers more aware of the cost of health care to reduce their use of health care services.

Research literature on the experience in public systems of Singapore and China, where such plans have been implemented, suggests that the approach does not control costs (Shortt, 2002). MSAs may increase costs. Moreover, MSAs may exacerbate inequalities in publicly funded systems. Low-income individuals are disadvantaged because they will choose to do without health care services if they use up the funds in their MSAs. Such actions may result in fatal consequences for some. They may not have the financial resources to purchase private health care services.

Mazankowski's and Kirby's emphasis on an expanded private sector role in health care raises concerns about meeting the five principles of medicare articulated in the Canada Health Act. As Romanow argues in his report, Canadians remain committed to a publicly funded and administered health care system (Romanow, 2002).

Regionalization of Health

Another important trend in health care reform has been the growing interest in the regionalization of health; that is, the devolution of decision making in health care to local authorities. Regionalization means that responsibility for the delivery of health services is referred to municipal or regional governments. The rationale for regionalization is that local or municipal governments are perceived as best positioned to identify, and are most responsive to, local needs. It is seen as compatible with their mandated responsibility for public health, i.e., sanitation, support to new mothers and families, and population health. Several provincial governments have opted for regionalization based on this rationale not only of local responsiveness, but also to reduce provincial health expenditures.

By the late 1990s, nine of 10 Canadian provinces had devolved health care decision making to local authorities (Lomas, Woods & Veenstra, 1997). Regionalization meant vertical integration of health care services. In other words, vertical integration of health care refers to the entire range of health care services from out-patient to hospital and long-term care services. By the late 1990s, Ontario had not regionalized its health care system, but health care and public health services are organized locally. In 2004, Ontario announced that it will regionalize health services by creating Local Health Integration Networks.

Problems with regionalization related to its design and implementation have been identified. The population health discourse had not translated into mandated programming. Population health and healthy community programs had long been key features of some local public health programs such as the City of Toronto, Peterborough, and other cities across Canada. Concern centred on the potential effect on the public health identity and funding of vertical integration, and that regionalization of public health could result in units that are too small to support local expertise and could impede development and enforcement of province-wide programs. There was also concern that citizen involvement in health care decision making was merely political rhetoric. In addition, critics expressed concern that regionalization would increase rather than reduce costs (Sutcliffe, Deber & Pasut, 1997). Regionalization in the 1990s was clearly different from previous plans to regionalize health care since there was no consensus on whether devolution was good for Canadian health care.

Much of the interest in regionalization stemmed from concerns of the federal and provincial governments with reducing health spending, improving the efficiency of service delivery, equity in service provision, more citizen participation, and more accountability of decision makers (Church & Barker, 1998). In some provinces regionalization had translated into reducing the scope of public health when it should have been amenable to expansion (Sutcliffe, Deber & Pasut, 1997).

Public-Private Partnerships

Another reform adopted by provincial governments are public-private partnerships (P3s). The adoption of P3s is attributable to changes in health care financing, particularly by the federal government. Provincial and territorial governments increasingly consider expanding private sector involvement in health care delivery to reduce their health budgets. Health care costs increase annually. Added to this, reduced federal transfers for health care results in provincial and territorial governments paying more for health care. A P3 is an arrangement in which a government and a private entity—be it a private corporation, individual, or agency—jointly provide a public service or good (Savas, 2005). It refers to a relationship between one government unit and a consortium of private firms to build a highway such as the 407 in Ontario, a hospital, or a school. In other words, a government may contract with a private entity to enable that entity to finance, design, build, own, and operate infrastructure and services that were previously in the public domain. To many health coalitions, P3s signify "privatization by stealth" (National Union of Public and General Employees, 2006). The National Union of Public and General Employees argue that P3s are privatization in secret. There is little opportunity for the public to challenge these arrangements as the best way to provide what are public services.

Savas argues that to consider privatization as merely a call to reduce government is a "serious misunderstanding of the concept" (Savas, 2005, p. 2). In contrast to the authors of *Bad Medicine*, Langille, and others, he argues that "Privatization can be at least as compassionate as the welfare state; properly implemented, it offers even more for the less fortunate among us" (p. 2).

Savas considers three methods of privatization:

1. *Delegation:* The government maintains overall responsibility, but uses the private sector for service delivery, e.g., contracting for services, or outsourcing. Savas says that this can be understood as "partial privatization" because it still requires an active state role while the production or service activity is carried out by the private sector.

2. *Divestment:* The government withdraws its responsibility, and presumably transfers it to the private sector. This is "competitive sourcing." Savas notes that this is the dominant form of privatization in the US and is used by federal, state, and local governments. He describes it as "the most direct form of delegation."

3. *Displacement:* The private sector expands and "displaces" (usurps) a government activity. Savas considers this development to be a "powerful incentive for public agencies."

In contrast to critics of P3s and privatization of health and social services, Savas suggests that P3s are innocuous. Savas fails to demonstrate, however, how low-income and other vulnerable populations would benefit from such arrangements.

The Council of Canadians, the Canadian Centre for Policy Alternatives, and others argue that Canada must approach public-private partnerships and increased commercialization warily and with tremendous caution (Barlow, 2007; Grieshaber-Otto & Sinclair, 2004). Turning over any public good or service to the private sector to deliver for a profit violates the principles of medicare as outlined in the Canada Health Act. A preferable form of private involvement in a public health care system is one in which the private provider is non-profit and is regulated by government statute. This relationship helps to ensure public accountability. For example, hospitals are private, not-for-profit. They are governed by their own board of directors, but are accountable to government for how they spend public dollars to deliver public health care services.

Interestingly, Savas cites Starr's opposition to privatization as an example of ideological and political opposition to P3s: "Privatization undermines the foundation of claims for public purpose and public service…. It shifts power to those who can more readily exercise power in the market. It may also shift income and wealth, depending on the specific form of that policy" (Starr, 1989, pp. 42–44). Starr clearly identifies the movement toward privatization of welfare state programs as a function of structures and interests.

An alternative definition of P3s is provided by Janusz Lewandowski, post-Communist Poland's first minister of privatization, otherwise known as "the Minister of Ownership Transformation." He defined it thus: "The sale of enterprises that no one owns, and whose value no one knows, to people who have money" (Savas, 2005, p. 2). He might have added, "And who will make more as a result of the transaction."

■ CONCLUSIONS

Health care reform in Canada has focused on the financial sustainability of the public health care system. Much of the debate has centred on whether to allow private involvement to ease some of the pressure on the public system.

Health care reform represents a site for governments to reduce public health care spending. The health reform reports of Mazankowski and Kirby welcome increased private sector involvement as a vehicle for innovation in health care. Kirby, however, supports the principle of public financing, but considers that there is little difference whether non-profit or for-profit entities provide health care services. Both Mazankowski and Kirby support medical savings accounts as means to make Canadians aware of the cost of health care, and ostensibly to reduce utilization of health care services.

In contrast, echoing the sentiments of the National Forum on Health, Romanow urges renewing government commitment to medicare around the principles of universality and non-profit delivery of health care services. While he is open to private delivery of what he terms "ancillary services," such as food services, cleaning, and other non-medical care, Romanow acknowledges that he has found no evidence to support a larger private sector role in health care delivery. His main point is the need for stable and secure federal funding to the provinces and territories in order to provide universal and comprehensive health care programs (Maioni, 2003).

The three main reform reports vary in their commitment to allowing private care, reflecting in part the conflict between the polis versus the market concepts of society devised by Stone. The polis signifies a focus on the public interest and the collective in identifying and realizing goals. In contrast, the market consists of viewing society as consisting of individuals who, by competing with each other to promote self-interest, benefit the whole. In health care, as in many other areas, emphasis on the market may distort the operation of public policy and lead to ineffective and inequitable outcomes.

This examination of recent reform proposals in Canada demonstrates this tension between the polis and the market. In health care, the polis reflects the collective desire to provide access to health care to all members of society on the basis of need. In health care, the market represents increasing privatization of health care and the commodification of care. Evidence suggests that such commodification is associated with growing inequities in access to health care and health care outcomes.

■ REFERENCES

Barlow, M. (2007). *Profit is not the cure.* Ottawa: Council of Canadians.

Church, J. & Barker, P. (1998). Regionalization of health services in Canada: A critical perspective. *International Journal of Health Services, 28*(3), 467–486.

Clair Commission d'étude sur les services de santé et les services sociaux. (2001). *Emerging solutions.* Quebec: Government of Quebec.

Coburn, D. (2000). Income inequality, social cohesion, and the health status of populations: The role of neo-liberalism. *Social Science & Medicine,* 51(1), 135–146.

Coburn, D. (2001). Health, health care, and neo-liberalism. In P. Armstrong, H. Armstrong & D. Coburn (Eds.), *Unhealthy times: The political economy of health and care in Canada,* 45–65. Toronto: Oxford University Press.

Commission on Medicare. (2001). *Caring for medicare: Sustaining a quality system.* Regina: Government of Saskatchewan.

Grieshaber-Otto, J. & Sinclair, S. (2004). *Bad medicine: Trade treaties, privatization, and health care reform in Canada.* Ottawa: Canadian Centre for Policy Alternatives.

Hall, P.A. (1993). Policy paradigms, social learning, and the state: The case of economic policy making in Britain. *Comparative Politics,* 25(3), 275–296.

Hall, P.A. & Taylor, R.C.R. (1996). Political science and the three institutoinalisms. *Political Studies XLIV,* 936–957

Kirby, M. J. (2002). *The health of Canadians: The federal role.* Ottawa: Standing Senate Committee on Social Affairs, Science and Technology.

Langille, D. (2004). The political determinants of health. In D. Raphael (Ed.), *Social determinants of health: Canadian Perspectives,* 283–296. Toronto: Canadian Scholars' Press Inc.

Lomas, J., Woods, J. & Veenstra, G. (1997). Devolving authority for health care in Canada's provinces: 1. An introduction to the issues. *Canadian Medical Association Journal,* 156(3), 371–377.

MacDonald, L.I. (December 2002–January 2003). Health care: From reinvesting to reinventing: Interview with Michael Kirby. *Policy Options,* 24(1), 5–9.

Maioni, A. (2003). Romanow—A defence of public health care, but is there a map for the road ahead? *Policy Options, 24*(2), 50–53.

Maynard, A. (2007). How to protect a public health care system. In B. Campbell & G.P. Marchildon (Eds.), *Medicare: Facts, myths, problems, and promise,* 82–86. Toronto: James Lorimer.

Mazankowski, D. (2001). *A framework for reform: Report of the Premier's Advisory Council on Health*. Edmonton: Government of Alberta.

National Forum on Health. (1998). *Building on the legacy. Volume 5: Evidence and information*. Ottawa: National Forum on Health.

National Union of Public and General Employees. (2006). *Public-private partnerships: What they are, why they're a bad idea*. Retrieved from www.nupge.ca

Organisation for Economic Co-operation and Development. (2005). *Health at a glance: OECD indicators 2005*. Paris: Organisation for Economic Co-operation and Development.

Rachlis, M. (2004). *Prescription for excellence: How innovation is saving Canada's health care system*. Toronto: HarperCollins.

Rachlis, M. (2005). *Public solutions to health care wait lists*. Ottawa: Canadian Centre for Policy Alternatives.

Ramsay, C. (1998). *Medical savings accounts: Universal, accessible, portable, and comprehensive health care for Canadians*. Vancouver: The Fraser Institute.

Raphael, D. (2003). Barriers to addressing the determinants of health: Public health units and poverty in Ontario, Canada. *Health Promotion International, 18*, 397–405.

Romanow, R.J. (2002). *Building on values: The future of health care in Canada*. Saskatoon: Commission on the Future of Health Care in Canada.

Savas, E.S. (2005). Privatization and public-private partnerships. Adapted from E.S. Savas, *Privatization in the City: Successes, failures, lessons*. Washington: CQ Press. Online at www.cesmadrid.es/documentos/sem200601_MD02_in.pdf

Shortt, S.E.D. (2002). Medical savings accounts in publicly funded health care systems: Enthusiasm versus evidence. *Canadian Medical Association Journal, 167*(2), 159–162.

Starr, P. (1989). The meaning of privatization. In S.B. Kamerman & A.J. Kahn (Eds.), *Privatization and the welfare state*, 15–48 . Princeton: Princeton University Press.

Stone, D. (1988). *Policy paradox and political reason*. Glenview: Scott, Foresman.

Sutcliffe, P., Deber, R. & Pasut, G. (1997). Public health in Canada: A comparative study of six provinces. *Canadian Journal of Public Health, 88*(4), 246–249.

UK House of Commons Transport Committee. (2004). *The future of the railway*. London: Government of the United Kingdom.

CRITICAL THINKING QUESTIONS

1. What do you think are the main drivers of the call for health care reform in Canada?

2. How can various sectors in Canadian society have their voices heard in health care reform?

3. To what extent do you think Canadians are aware of the various forces driving the health care reform debate?

4. What are your personal views concerning the future of the Canadian health care system?

5. To what extent do you think Canadians are engaged with these issues? Why might this be the case?

FURTHER READINGS

Grieshaber-Otto, J. & Sinclair, S. (2004). *Bad medicine: Trade treaties, privatization, and health care reform in Canada.* Ottawa: Canadian Centre for Policy Alternatives.

This report provides a critical analysis of the three major reports presented above. Available online at: www.policyalternatives.ca/documents/National_Office_Pubs/bad_medicine.pdf -

Kirby, M.J. (2002). *The health of Canadians: The federal role.* (Kirby Report.) Ottawa: Standing Senate Committee on Social Affairs, Science, and Technology.

This is another influential report that has fuelled the call for increasing private sector involvement in the health care system. Available online at: www.parl.gc.ca/37/2/parlbus/commbus/senate/Com-e/soci-e/rep-e/repoct02vol6-e.htm

Mazankowski, D. (2001). *A framework for reform: Report of the Premier's Advisory Council on Health.* Edmonton: Government of Alberta.

This report argues for a range of market-oriented innovations to medicare. Available online at: dsp-psd.pwgsc.gc.ca/Collection-R/LoPBdP/BP/prb0133-e.htm

Romanow, R.J. (2002). *Building on values: The future of health care in Canada.* Saskatoon: Commission on the Future of Health Care in Canada.

Roy Romanow, head of the Commission on the Future of Health Care in Canada, recommended sweeping changes to ensure the long-term sustainability of Canada's health care system. Available online at: www.hc-sc.gc.ca/english/care/romanow/index1.html

RELEVANT WEBSITES

Canadian Centre for Policy Alternatives
www.policyalternatives.ca

The CCPA is an independent, non-profit research organization. It was created to promote research on economic and social policy issues from a progressive perspective.

Canadian Health Coalition
www.healthcoalition.ca
The Canadian Health Coalition is a not-for-profit, non-partisan organization dedicated to protecting and expanding Canada's public health care system for the benefit of all Canadians. The coalition includes organizations representing seniors, women, churches, nurses, health care workers, and anti-poverty activists from across Canada.

Canadian Policy Research Networks
www.cprn.org
The CPRN's mission is to create knowledge and lead public dialogue and debate on social and economic issues important to the well-being of all Canadians. Their goal is to help make Canada a more just, prosperous, and caring society.

Health Council of Canada
www.healthcouncilcanada.ca/en
The Health Council of Canada fosters accountability and transparency by assessing progress in improving the quality, effectiveness, and sustainability of the health care system. Through insightful monitoring, public reporting, and facilitating informed discussion, the council shines a light on what helps or hinders health care renewal and the well-being of Canadians.

National Coordinating Group on Health Care Reform and Women
www.cewh-cesf.ca/healthreform
The group's mandate is to investigate the impact of health care reform on women as providers, decision makers, and users of the health care system. The group's aim is to increase awareness and understanding of the impact of health care reform on women and wish to become involved in the promotion of such activities.

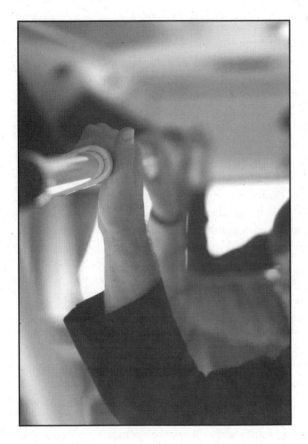

Chapter 8

MARKETS AND HEALTH POLICY

■ INTRODUCTION

Since the 1970s, social and economic changes have dramatically restructured the global economy, specifically the processes of production and investment (Grieshaber-Otto & Sinclair, 2004; Teeple, 2006). In addition, concerns about rising deficits that began in the early 1980s drove both federal and provincial governments to reduce social and health spending (Scarth, 2004). Developed economies such as Canada, the United Kingdom, and the US responded to these changes by adapting their economies and deregulating business activities in several policy areas.

One aspect of this increasing emphasis on economic functioning has seen nations with public health care systems such as Canada and the United Kingdom increasingly looking to the private sector and market mechanisms to deliver health and social services. National governments justify these changes as essential to enhance their competitiveness in the new global economy (Bakker, 1996; Banting, Hoberg & Simeon, 1997). From the perspective of the private sector, health care in particular represents an attractive investment opportunity (Grieshaber-Otto & Sinclair, 2004).

This chapter considers these increasingly important health care markets in Canada. Analysis is also made of the situation in the United Kingdom, where market approaches to health care delivery have become increasingly common. As discussed in Chapter 7, a central and recurring theme in the debate over health care reform in Canada and in the United Kingdom is a call to expand the role of the private sector—or the market—in health care provision. This chapter considers the implications of increasing emphasis on health care markets for both the health care system and for population health.

■ WHAT IS A MARKET?

A market is a complex set of social institutions that enables the exchange of a commodity such as a good (housing) or service (health care) between a seller and buyer (Leys, 2001; Teeple, 2000). The market is thus a mode of exchange that meets the needs of society by buying and selling goods and services as private property or commodities. These goods can be health care services, but also include what are usually termed basic needs such as housing, food, income, education, and recreation, among others.

In the market, the process of distribution is based on competitive supply and demand in the exchange process. The market also comes to represent a means by which labour power and capital, income, and wealth are distributed through processes of production and consumption. Inequalities in such distributions may also give way to differences in political power and influence.

Although often presented as a source of innovation, the effects of markets on societal processes may not always be beneficial or even benign. The market may come to represent significant and powerful economic forces that influence health policy and other public policy arenas. This is especially important since interwoven with markets are politics, ideology, and power (Leys, 2001). Markets have considerable capacity to have influence beyond their purely economic realm into the broader society and the public policy arena.

Consistent with this view, Leys asserts that markets are "highly political" because politics shape market activities as much as do the processes of cost, revenue, and profit margins (Leys, 2001). Understanding the politics of markets and their power to influence many aspects of societal functioning, including health policy development, is integral to understanding their impacts on a society.

■ CHARACTERISTICS OF MARKETS

Leys identifies the characteristics of markets that help explain how they function and influence health care policy (Leys, 2001). This is particularly helpful for understanding the current orientation of governments and others toward market mechanisms to control health care costs.

First, markets are systems consisting of rules and regulations set and enforced by both state and non-state agencies, including market actors through trade associations, informal agreements, and market power such as price maintenance (Leys, 2001). Regulations govern what can be traded, as well as when and where trading can occur. Regulations also influence costs, profit margins, and other aspects of the trading process. Leys suggests that it is at this juncture of shaping regulations that market politics come into play. Despite the assumption that states or governments create regulations, increasing attention is being given to how companies and corporations can adjust the rules to their own advantage. These companies and corporations possess considerable resources to accomplish this.

Second, markets are complex. This is the case since any one market actually consists of a complex of markets that involve transportation, raw and manufactured materials required for product development, insurance, and advertising, among others (Leys, 2001). That is, any one market is embedded directly or indirectly in a broad series of other social relations.

Activities of those who work in markets also participate in other social relations and are shaped by them. Social relations refers to the pattern of relationships between people in a group or organization in which they function (Hale, 1990). Leys suggests that the more important these social relations are, the more changes in a market tend to lead to and accentuate other and larger political issues.

For example, changes in the rules and regulations by which health care services are organized and delivered may influence the ability of certain groups to access and influence health care services. If there is increased emphasis on delivering health care services and these services are turned over to the market, then physicians and other allied health care professionals, such as nurses, may have less ability to influence the course of health policy. And if these newly empowered privately organized service providers have less concern with providing access to marginalized groups, then health consequences for these marginalized groups may emerge.

Increasing market mechanisms for health care delivery may also affect the distribution of income and other economic resources. To make the introduction of market approaches more attractive to citizens, governments may offer tax cuts that will benefit primarily the well-off. Since public health care systems tend to have distributional effects—the well-off pay more for health services in taxes, but tend to use them less—the creation of markets will lead to a transfer of income from lower-income groups to higher-income groups. The health care system then comes to be financed less out of general revenues and more by private sources such as user fees. As discussed elsewhere in this volume, those least able to pay—who also are the most likely to require health services—are especially affected by policy shifts to market approaches.

Third, markets are inherently unstable (Leys, 2001). Their instability reflects the nature of competition. Instability is a function of industry and other market sectors always trying to increase their market share, which is the proportion of industry sales of a good or service that is controlled by an individual company or firm. These processes may be seen as beneficial to market competition, but when provision of basic needs, such as health care services, are included in such processes, this may be problematic.

In addition, Leys argues that market success endows greater power in the market itself possibly at the expense of society as a whole (Leys, 2001). As an example, Leys suggests that global firms can come to take over and control a national market with potential effects of curtailing or discarding certain services. Leys gives an example of Murdoch's News Corporation dominating the national newspaper market in the United Kingdom, but one can imagine health services coming to be dominated by exceptionally powerful private sector health corporations. Competition and resultant side effects of such competition are central to how markets work.

■ THE RATIONALE FOR MARKET COMPETITION

The belief in the competitive market (or health care markets) is based on economic theory, which claims the superiority of markets over government control and regulation of health care. The argument for adopting market approaches to health care services is based on assumptions derived from economic theory (Leys, 2001; Rice, 1997). Some policy analysts and national and provincial policy-makers have come to believe that such markets are the key to reducing health care costs and improving the quality of care.

These beliefs include the following: (1) markets are the source of innovation; (2) deregulation and privatization of health and social services will facilitate such innovation; (3) these activities will allow a reduced role for the state in these policy areas; and (4) efficiencies in cost and operation will result (Coburn, 2001; Leys, 2001; Teeple, 2000). And it is clear that such beliefs are increasingly being put forth in the health policy debate in Canada (see Box 8.1).

The emphasis on the market is supported by political ideologies that are consistent with the central tenets of neo-liberalism and traditional economic theory. These ideologies provide the rationale for emphasizing market processes in several public policy areas, but their effects are especially important when considering health care policy.

The central tenets of neo-liberalism are that a market economy best allocates resources, including income and wealth, in a society (Coburn, 2001). Government policy-makers and elected representatives concerned with health care are especially

---

Box 8.1: University of Toronto Bulletin

Private Health Care Legal But Unprofitable in Canada
Need to Rethink Scope of Public Health Care System Since Some
Growth Areas Not Covered by Canada Health Act
By Sue Toye

March 22, 2001—Contrary to public perception private health care is legal across Canada, however, provincial health insurance legislation, designed to prevent a two-tiered system, makes private practice unprofitable, say U of T researchers.

"The absence of a significant private health care sector is explained by the prohibitions on the subsidy of private practice by public plans," explains law professor Colleen Flood. "These measures prevent physicians from topping up their public sector incomes with private fees. You can' practice privately but you can't get paid by the public health care system."

Flood and doctoral student Tom Archibald surveyed the health insurance legislation of all the provinces in Canada. They found that there is a myriad of regulations that have one objective—to prevent the public sector from subsidizing the private sector, as opposed to rendering privately funded practice illegal. In three provinces—New Brunswick, Newfoundland, Saskatchewan—there are no prohibitions on private insurance from covering medically necessary services that the public health care system provides or restrictions on the fees that could be charged in the private sector. "In these provinces, there are greater economic opportunities for physicians to practice outside the public plan and charge whatever they wish," says Flood. "However, there has not been a surge in private health care in these three provinces because of restrictions on physicians being able to work in both the public and private sectors."

Flood says Canada is still a one-tiered system when providing physician and hospital care. "However, the trouble is there's a lot of growth in other areas that won't be covered by the Canada Health Act such as drugs, gene therapy and home care which receive private financing," she says. "We have to rethink the scope of our public health care system." This study was published in the March issue of the *Canadian Medical Association Journal*.

Source: http://www.news.utoronto.ca/bin1/010322d.asp

---

susceptible to neo-liberal arguments for several reasons. Health care services provided by the state do not generate revenues for the state and consume among the most resources of all public policy areas.

Box 8.2: Cost of Medicare

In a recent report on medicare, the Fraser Institute argues that Canada spends more on health care than other industrialized countries in the Organisation for Economic Co-operation and Development, and provides "inferior" health care compared to those countries without a public health care system (Esmail & Walker, 2005). Further, the institute argues that all of the countries that have fewer years of life lost to disease and lower mortality have private health care systems and user fees at point of access to health care services.

Source: Esmail, N. & Walker, M. (2005). *How good is Canadian health care? 2005 Report: An international comparison of health care systems.* Vancouver: The Fraser Institute.

Neo-liberal arguments become attractive because policy-makers can view health services as a potential site for private investment, which will absolve governments of funding and other responsibilities. By turning to domestic and international private health care agencies to finance and provide health care services, costs and responsibilities can be reduced, yet turning to the private sector leads to the creation of health care markets. Health care then becomes a commodity and not a public service. People become reliant on their incomes to obtain health care services. We are back to the reasons why health care was made into a public affair: to have health services provided on the basis of need, not income!

◼ HEALTH CARE MARKETS

Private financing comes in different forms, but what they all share in common is the creation of health care markets. In addition to medical savings accounts, user fees, and contracting out of services, among others identified in Chapter 7, a government can transfer the financing and delivery of a health care service to the private sector as represented by public-private partnerships (P3s).

As discussed in Chapter 7, a P3 is an arrangement between the public and private sectors to provide a project or service that the public sector has usually delivered (Grieshaber-Otto & Sinclair, 2004; Savas, 2005). There is a continuum of P3 models with considerable variation in the degree to which the private sector is involved. At one end, public assets might be privatized or transferred to the private sector to operate and manage. Other P3 arrangements may involve contracting out services normally provided by public servants to private for-profit firms (Grieshaber-Otto & Sinclair, 2004). Other arrangements may have the private sector operating and managing publicly owned facilities or doing the same for privately owned facilities. Both these directions may be done under short-term, long-term, or indefinite periods. P3 arrangements may also vary in their degree of accountability, government control, or private risk involved.

Box 8.3: Policies for the Market

Tim Rice, a professor in the School of Public Health at the University of California at Los Angeles, identifies the different types of policies espoused by advocates of market mechanisms in health care:

- Providing low-income people with subsidies to allow them to purchase health insurance, rather than paying directly for the services they use.
- Having people pay more money out-of-pocket in order to receive health care services, especially for services whose demand is most responsive to price.
- Requiring people to pay more in premiums to obtain more extensive health insurance coverage.
- Allowing the market to determine the number and distribution of hospitals and what services they provide, and the total number of physicians and their distribution among specialties.
- Deregulating the development and diffusion of medical technologies.
- Eschewing government involvement in determining how much a country spends on health care services.

Provincial governments in Ontario, Alberta, and British Columbia have initiated numerous such arrangements to build schools, highways, and hospitals. In addition, the federal government has publicly stated that these approaches are underutilized in Canada and provide a significant investment in infrastructure to be conducted via public-private partnerships (see Box 8.4). Critics have expressed concerns about the extent to which financial risk remains situated in such arrangements with the public sector, yet any profits accrue to the private sector (Rachlis, 2004). Some argue the primary purpose of P3s is to allow governments to remove expenses from public accounts.

P3s may not only lead to the creation of health markets but may create a web of other markets and commodities such as those in the United States. These markets represent a particular set of social relations that shape how hospitals, doctors, and other health professionals provide care to patients (Armstrong & Armstrong, 2003;

Leys, 2001). These newly created markets include provision of laboratory tests, pharmaceuticals, and ambulatory care, among others.

Box 8.4: Public-Private Partnerships (P3s)

P3s generate "new" money only to the extent that they can generate a revenue stream from a source other than the government that would not otherwise be available to the government. For example, a private hospital operator might be able to generate revenue by offering medical services for sale that are not covered by medicare. Similarly, it may be that Highway 407 was worth more to the successful bidder, 407 International, because it expected to be able to charge higher tolls to highway users than the government would be able to get away with politically. Far from supporting the argument for P3s as a source of "new" money, however, these examples highlight the broader public policy accountability issues raised by P3s. The fact that P3s can, in principle, be used as a way to employ public assets for purposes that the public would not support or to generate revenue at levels that the public would not support is hardly a justification for the concept.

Source: Mackenzie, H. (2004). *Financing Canada's hospitals: Public alternatives to P3s* (p. 5). Ottawa: Canadian Health Coalition. Available online at: www.healthcoalition.ca/3p.pdf

---

In Canada hospitals are private, not-for-profit facilities governed by their own boards of directors, but receive funds from their provincial governments to provide health care services. Although all hospitals remain non-profit in Canada and in the United Kingdom, some hospitals in Canada and the United Kingdom contract out for services such as food provision and cleaning (Armstrong & Armstrong, 2003; Scott, 2001). This has been increasing as governments, by limiting transfers to hospitals, have forced hospital CEOs to make up gaps by contracting out some services to obtain them from the private sector. In the UK, hospital CEOs have reduced the number of registered nursing positions in order to save money. This change lowers the number of nurses available to care for patients on a hospital ward with implications for the quality of patient care in hospitals.

In the United Kingdom, the National Health Service (NHS) had a virtual monopoly on health care, similar to the single-payer system of medicare in Canada (Leys, 2001). In the late 1980s, however, initiatives such as pay-beds in public hospitals, car parking charges, and renting space in hospitals to shops and businesses were introduced to bring in revenues to hospitals (Scott, 2001). Some

Box 8.5: Public Private Partnerships in the United Kingdom

By Dr. Allyson Pollock

The policy of public private partnerships or private finance initiatives (PFIs) as they are called in the UK was a policy dreamed up by the then Conservative government in 1992 to bail out the failing construction industry.... I don't know exactly what models are being proposed for the P3s in Canada, but given that the same management consultants are advising, designing, evaluating, implementing and promoting the policies in Canada as in the UK, it seems likely there will be a remarkable overlap. The decision to rewrite the federal government's capital investment manual is a significant first step to reforming Canada along the UK lines of PPPs.

... PPPs are not a neutral financing mechanism. Neither are they a source of new money or investment. Private finance is debt financing. In other words it is a source of borrowing which has to be repaid—either out of the public purse or by giving the private sector a concession to raise user charges as in toll roads. It is not a neutral financing mechanism as we show in detailed studies of the National Health Services (NHS).

... Using PFI is more expensive for two reasons—the higher cost of borrowing (government borrowing is always cheaper) and the financing cost which can add up to 40% of the total costs of schemes. The financing costs are the rolled up interest that accrues by virtue of long repayment periods and borrowing money in advance. That adds a huge burden to the cost of PFI schemes. In addition PFI results in enormous cost escalation.

... Now coming to the public health concerns. The government can only justify the higher cost of the PFI and PPPs through the value for money analysis. But the real issue for public authorities is how private finance debts are to be repaid. In the UK, National Health Service (NHS) private finance is repaid from the revenue budgets of hospitals. This necessitated a massive change in our accounting systems as for the first time the UK NHS had to pay a charge on capital and this meant creating a stream in the revenue or operating budget to pay for new debt.... The repayment of these very expensive PFIs has put the NHS under enormous pressure. A number of subsidies had to be found. The first was land sales. The second was merging hospitals to release more land and buildings for sale. You might say it was sensible rationalization but it inevitably resulted in major service closure and the diversion of income to pay for the new smaller facility. The third was a diversion of capital grants in budgets intended for public facilities into paying off the debts of the new PFI hospitals.

Source: Excerpt from a presentation made by Dr. Allyson Pollock at a technical briefing on P3s for the Commission on the Future of Health Care in Canada. At the time, Dr. Pollock was head of the Health Policy and Health Services Research Unit at the School of Public Policy, University College London. CUPE. (2002). *Experts tell Romanow commission that public-private partnerships are not the answer*, pp. 1–4. Ottawa: Canadian Union of Public Employees.

Canadian hospitals have implemented similar measures to generate more revenues for hospitals. With increased market-sector involvement, such activities can only increase. Health care should become an important area for investment.

■ IMPACT OF MARKET FORCES AND DEREGULATION ON HEALTH CARE

There is little evidence to support the view that privatized health care provides better quality or is cost-efficient (Evans, 1997; Teeple, 2000). In fact, there is much evidence to support significant government intervention in order to ensure equal access to health care and lower health care costs.

For example, a US study found that user fees at for-profit hospitals contributed to a 20 percent higher risk of death for people with high blood pressure because they were unlikely to see a doctor to get their blood pressure under control (Brook et al., 1983). The same study showed that user fees were as likely to deter appropriate use of health care services as they were to deter inappropriate use of health care services. Similarly, other studies have shown that user fees may deter the poor and elderly from using health care services that they may need (Rachlis & Kushner, 1995).

Another study involving a review and meta-analysis of studies compared mortality rates at private, for-profit hospitals and those of private, not-for-profit hospitals (Devereaux et al., 2002). Findings based on 15 observational studies, including more than 26,000 hospitals and 38 million adult patients, found that private, for-profit hospitals had a small but reliable 2 percent higher risk of death compared to private, not-for-profit hospitals. (Findings were adjusted for a number of possible confounders such as severity of illness, etc.) The authors report that the single available study of infant mortality showed a 10 percent greater risk for for-profit hospitals. These higher mortality rates may be attributable to having fewer and less well-trained staff at private, for-profit hospitals (Rachlis, 2004). The authors concluded that:

> The Canadian health care system is at a crucial juncture with many individuals suggesting that we would be better served by private for-profit health care delivery. Our systematic review raises concerns about the potential negative health outcomes associated with private for-profit hospital care. Canadian policy-makers, the stakeholders who seek to influence them and the public whose health will be affected by their decisions should take this research evidence into account. (Devereaux et al., 2002, p. 1405)

Health care markets may also increase costs. For example, many studies have compared the administration costs of privatized health care compared to public health care systems. Consistently, private health care is associated with higher administration costs (Woolhandler, Campbell & Himmelstein, 2003). Lower administration costs are associated with public health care. .

Box 8.6: Comparison of Health Care Costs in Canada and the United States

In 1999, health administration costs totalled at least $294.3 billion in the United States, or $1,059 per capita, as compared with $307 per capita in Canada. After exclusions, administration accounted for 31.0 percent of health care expenditures in the United States and 16.7 percent of health care expenditures in Canada. Canada's national health insurance program had an overhead of 1.3 percent; the overhead among Canada's private insurers was higher than that in the United States (13.2 percent vs. 11.7 percent). Providers' administrative costs were far lower in Canada.

Between 1969 and 1999, the share of the US health care labor force accounted for by administrative workers grew from 18.2 percent to 27.3 percent. In Canada, it grew from 16.0 percent in 1971 to 19.1 percent in 1996. (Both nations' figures exclude insurance-industry personnel.)

The gap between US and Canadian spending on health care administration has grown to $752 per capita. A large sum might be saved in the United States if administrative costs could be trimmed by implementing a Canadian-style health care system.

Source: Woolhandler, S., Campbell, T. & Himmelstein, D.U. (2003). Costs of health care administration in the United States and Canada. *New England Journal of Medicine, 349*(8), p. 768.

Indeed, considerable evidence shows that the single-payer system is more cost-efficient because there is one place to send all the invoices and from which to receive payment (Yalnizyan, 2006). With a central location for paying and receiving payment, the single-payer system reduces administrative costs by not duplicating administration for different methods of payment. Moreover, as the single supplier and largest buyer of health care services, the government is able to negotiate better prices for products and drugs than may be the case for multiple purchasers.

In support of this argument, the Organisation for Economic Co-operation and Development (OECD) consistently shows that the US, with its market-driven system, spends more on health care than nations with public systems. Table 8.1 shows health spending for member countries of the Organisation for Economic

Co-operation and Development. These reports show that the US spends almost 14 percent of its gross domestic product (GDP) on health compared to, for example, Canada at less than 10 percent.

Table 8.1: Total Health Expenditure as a Share of GDP (2005)

	Public	Total
United States	6.9	15.3
Switzerland	6.9	11.6
France	8.9	11.1
Germany	8.2	10.7
Belgium	7.4	10.3
Portugal	7.4	10.2
Austria	7.7	10.2
Greece	4.3	10.1
Canada	6.9	9.8
Iceland	7.9	9.5
Australia	6.4	9.5
Netherlands	5.5 (2002)	9.2
Sweden	7.7	9.1
Norway	7.6	9.1
Denmark	7.7	9.1
New Zealand	7.0	9.0
United Kingdom	7.2	8.3
Hungary	5.7 (2004)	8.1
OECD average	6.7	9.0

Source: Organisation for Economic Co-operation and Development. (2007). *Health at a glance 2007. OECD indicators.* Paris: Organisation for Economic Co-operation and Development.

Evans argues that that international experience over the last century has shown that increased reliance on the market tends to be "associated with inferior system performance—inequity, inefficiency, high cost, and public dissatisfaction" (Evans, 1997, p. 438). He cites the United States as a key example of allowing market forces to prevail in health care provision. Elsewhere he has criticized the emergence of user fees as "zombies," bad ideas that keep coming back no matter how many times they are buried (Evans, Barer & Stoddart, 1995).

■ DISTINGUISHING BETWEEN ALLOCATION AND DISTRIBUTION IN HEALTH CARE

As stated earlier, the economic theory on which neo-liberalism is based calls for marketization in health care. Anyone who advocates market mechanisms in health care fails to consider whether this is a desirable objective for which governments should strive (Rice, 1997). Rice argues that the much-claimed advantages of competitive markets cannot be fulfilled in health care (Rice, 1997) because economic theory treats allocation and distribution activities of the economy separately. Rice argues further that in health care and in other matters concerned with social welfare, a society must make allocation and distribution decisions simultaneously. These processes cannot be separated.

By way of illustration, Rice presents an example in which a very costly therapy is developed that has been shown to reduce the risk of developing a fatal disease, but its high cost means that only a few people can afford to pay for it (Rice, 1997). This means that it will increase the utility (welfare) of the few who can afford it, but it will probably reduce the utility of the larger group that knows that a life-saving technology is available, but not to them. Thus, reliance on markets may decrease social welfare for the society as a whole. If overall social welfare is to improve, it might therefore be preferable for the government to intervene to ensure that all citizens could have access to the life-saving technology.

Rice and Evans argue that privatization in health care has returned in the health care debate because market mechanisms generate distributional advantages for some powerful interests in societies (Evans, 1997; Rice, 1997). This is how they suggest it happens: First, a more expensive health care system produces higher prices and incomes for providers such as physicians, drug companies, and private insurers. Second, private payment delivers overall system costs on the basis of use or expected use of health care services. If people are charged for services at point of access, then the government contributes less. In effect, income is redistributed from low-income people to high-income people. Also, people with high income can purchase better access or quality for themselves without having to support a publicly funded health care system for those with low-income to ensure they have access to quality health care services. Evans argues that there has thus always been "a natural alliance" of financial interests between service providers and high-income groups. Thus, these interests have a strong incentive to advocate market mechanisms in health care.

In addition, only those who can afford to pay for private care will jump the queue and go to the private system, while those who have low incomes will remain in the public system (Rachlis, 2004). A further concern is that the private system could entice doctors in the public system to private health care with higher incomes and other benefits not provided in the public system (Rachlis, 2005). Allowing a parallel private system to coexist alongside the public system will not be in the best interests of most Canadians, nor will it reduce the wait times in the public system since those waiting for care in the public system cannot afford to consider private care.

■ FACTORS CONTRIBUTING TO MARKETIZATION

Since the postwar period, most industrialized countries have had a mix of public and private economic activity in which a public sphere of economic activity coexists with a private sphere. The mixed economy is derived from a social-democratic conception of the economy that allows for both state and private involvement in public policy spheres such as health care. Leys argues that a flaw in the notion of a mixed economy was a failure to recognize the inherent instability of markets (Leys, 2001). When their survival is threatened, firms in the private sector seek strategies to increase their market and their market share. Firms in the public sector, or Crown corporations, do not contend with this imperative since they are largely prohibited from behaving like private firms. Their mandate is to ensure access to a public good or service, not to increase market share. Leys notes that an important strategy for firms pressured to expand markets is moving into previously non-market spheres such as health care.

The rise in importance of the public sector as a site for investment has been attributed to the decline in manufacturing as a result of international competition (Price, Pollock & Shaoul, 1999). Thus, US and European corporations now see the service sector, including health care services, as an alternative source of profit. To increase the private services sector, however, requires opening up markets in areas in which the state has previously had responsibility for provision. These areas include public services such as health care, education, and housing. By opening up the sector as a market, it allows domestic and foreign corporate entities to create private clinics or other for-profit health services. Thus begins the process of commodifying services that were once deemed public services to be a matter of right to citizens of a country.

■ COMMODIFICATION AND DECOMMODIFICATION

While Chapter 10 elaborates on the concepts of commodification and decommodification, these concepts have relevance for understanding health care market issues. Esping-Andersen devised the concepts of decommodification and commodification to determine the extent to which individuals must depend on their market-derived incomes to obtain specific goods and services such as health care (Esping-Andersen, 1990). Decommodification refers to a state in which individuals are not reliant on their incomes to obtain a service such as health care. In other words, health care is a public service provided on the basis of need, as it is in Canada.

Commodification means that individuals are reliant on their incomes and the market to obtain a service such as health care. In the US, for most Americans to have health insurance, they must be employed, and the employer must provide health benefits. Some American employers do not provide health insurance for their employees. This means that many Americans must purchase their own health insurance. As a result, many Americans may do without health care because they are either not employed, have employers who do not provide health benefits, or are unable to afford either insurance or care. The US health care system is embedded in the US market economy.

Increasing numbers of studies are finding growing dissatisfaction among providers, as well as consumers, with the health care market approach in the US. A recent interview study of local health care leaders in the US found that most doubted the capacity of market-based reforms to improve the efficiency and quality of US health care (Nichols, Ginsburg, Berenson, Christianson & Hurley, 2004). Many of the respondents appeared to reluctantly accept that government intervention may be necessary to improve care:

> What is palpable across the 12 communities we studied is the recognition that private market forces are limited in their ability to achieve social objectives in health care services, and a growing sense that a broader conversation about what to do next should begin soon. (Nichols et al., 2004, p. 20)

In the Canadian context, allowing market forces into health care could very well violate the principles of medicare as specified in the Canada Health Act. In addition, as discussed in previous chapters, directing public revenues to private entities may not violate the letter but perhaps the spirit of medicare, particularly with regard to universality and public financing and administration of the health care system. All citizens, regardless of where they live in Canada, have a right to health care on the basis of need. Some argue this calls for health care services to have public financing *and* public administration (see Box 8.7).

Box 8.7: Ontario Health Tax

No Easy Cure for Health Tax
By Thomas Walkom
Toronto Star

Dalton McGuinty says that, if re-elected, his Liberals would keep their irritating health tax because there is no other choice. "We need every penny," he said on Thursday.

At one level, the Ontario premier is correct. Health care costs are rising faster than the rate of inflation. If Ontarians want any kind of meaningful comprehensive health insurance, they must be prepared to pay for it—either out-of-pocket (which the US experience shows to be more expensive) or through their taxes. There is no such thing as a free lunch.

However, McGuinty did not mention his government's mixed record in curbing these accelerating health costs. While it is true that we have to pay for the health care we want, it is not true that in all cases we have to pay so much.

In particular, we do not have to pay as much for drugs, which today represent the fastest-growing element of health costs. The McGuinty Liberals understand this. Last year, Health Minister George Smitherman proposed a series of mild legislative reforms designed to encourage Ontarians to use cheaper generic versions of expensive brand name drugs.

Smitherman also wanted the government's Ontario Drug Benefit Plan—the largest purchaser of pharmaceuticals in the country—to negotiate better deals with drug firms.

The idea in both cases was to scale back the spiralling $3.5 billion annual cost of the provincial drug plan for welfare recipients and seniors.

But when Smitherman unveiled his plan, the big drug companies went ballistic. One, GlaxoSmithKline, warned it might pull its branch plants out of Ontario unless the government relented.

Within weeks, the Liberals quietly reversed themselves. Most of Smitherman's controversial drug reforms were either watered down or scrapped.

In other areas of cost containment, the government has been almost as timid. Its decision to set up so-called local health integration networks is good in theory. These networks could provide a rational administrative framework for the complex and often competing array of hospitals, nursing homes, and other institutions that make up the Ontario health system.

But the McGuinty Liberals have been hesitant to offend the big power blocs (doctors, nurses, hospitals). So it is not yet clear whether this new system will be any more useful than the largely ineffective array of powerless district health councils it replaced.

Instead, this government, like those before it, has focused on scrimping in areas where it faces the least political resistance—like providing diapers for incontinent residents of nursing homes. As the *Star*'s Moira Welsh revealed this summer, the government's $1.20 a day allowance is so skimpy that some nursing homes make their elderly residents sit in urine-soaked diapers for hours in order to save pennies.

None of this is to suggest there is a costless answer to the health puzzle. True, it might make more sense to fund diapers for the elderly rather than the already hefty profits of Big Pharma. But even if we eliminated the provincial drug benefit program entirely, we would still be spending roughly $16.5 billion a year on health care (by comparison, the McGuinty health tax rakes in only $2.6 billion).

One way or the other, we have to pay for the services we want.

The opposition says McGuinty broke his no-new-taxes promise when he instituted his so-called health premium. The opposition is right. But if he hadn't done that he would have faced great pressure to break his no-cuts promise—which would have been worse.

Source: The Toronto Star (September 9, 2007), A6.

■ IMPACT OF PRIVATE HEALTH CARE MARKETS ON POPULATION HEALTH

The creation of health care markets is consistent with an individualized approach to health care as discussed in Chapter 2. In tandem with increasing commodification of health care services is an emphasis on individualized approaches to health in which the individual must preserve her or his own health by making proper lifestyle choices, such as having a diet of fruits and vegetables, moderate alcohol consumption, and regular physical activity.

In addition, as stated elsewhere, one of the primary concerns about creating private health care markets is that they reduce access to health care, particularly for vulnerable populations such as those with low income or those who are living in poverty. Such developments could accentuate unequal health outcomes.

Market approaches also have the potential to heighten inequalities in living conditions that are known to determine health. As background, during the 1980s, class-related health differences in health outcomes in the UK were reported in the famous Black Report and revisited in *The Health Divide* (Townsend, Davidson & Whitehead, 1992). Research—since replicated numerous times—has shown that social class is strongly related to health status (Coburn, 2000). That is, people with lower social class, occupational status, or income and wealth, have poorer health status compared to those higher up on the class, occupational, or income ladder. This relationship is one of the most robust findings in the health and social sciences (Davey Smith, 2003; Gordon, Shaw, Dorling & Davey Smith, 1999; Raphael, 2008).

While it has been argued that all countries show socio-economic differences in health status, income and wealth gaps among Canadians have been widening since the 1980s (Yalnizyan, 2000). Much of these growing social inequalities have been attributed to Canadian governments withdrawing from numerous programs that provide Canadians with income and employment security (Scarth, 2004; Stanford, 2004). These developments have been marked by the increasing influence of the market sector in Canadian society. And evidence from the United Kingdom indicates that such increases are good predictors of growing health inequalities (Shaw, Dorling, Gordon & Davey Smith, 1999).

In Canada, research into health inequalities has focused on how life expectancy and the incidence of various chronic diseases, such as heart disease and diabetes, as measures of population health differ among population groups. For example, life expectancy for men who reside in the poorest of Montreal's health districts is 13 years less than for men residing in the richest districts of Montreal (Agence de la santé et des services sociaux de Montréal, 2007). Much of this is explained by the fact that approximately half of the population in the poorest health districts in Montreal have incomes below Statistics Canada's low income cut-off (LICOs). Wilkins has documented profound differences in mortality rates from a variety of afflictions as a function of average neighbourhood income (Wilkins, Berthelot & Ng, 2002).

This is little doubt that increasing the role of the market in Canadian society tends to be related to growing social and health inequalities (Raphael, 2000). The available data concerning this conclusion is, to date, mixed. Wilkins documents that income-related differences in mortality due to diabetes, suicide, and deaths from mental illness are increasing while differences in heart disease are declining (Wilkins et al., 2002).

Neo-liberalism has been shown to foster higher income inequality (Coburn, 2000; Kaplan, Pamuk, Lynch, Cohen & Balfour, 1996; Lynch, 2000). This is so because neo-liberal policies weaken the welfare state by reducing the state's role in health and social services. Most industrial countries and many developing nations have introduced neo-liberal policies that result in reduced social welfare and increased private sector involvement in social welfare provision.

The welfare state, of which health care is a key component, is a mode of redistribution whereby higher-income groups pay higher taxes in order for low-income groups to have access to health services of which they tend to need more. As stated earlier in this chapter, weakening the welfare state results in redistributing income from low-income groups to high-income groups. It also means that there are lower revenues available to the state to spend on health care. This results in lower health spending.

Another way to think about the issue of markets and health is to consider the health status of nations whose political economies are dominated by the marketplace rather than the state. Esping-Andersen argued that liberal political economies, such as Canada, the US, and the United Kingdom, are more receptive to market influence on public policy, while social democratic nations such as Norway, Denmark, and Sweden have greater state intervention in service provision. Do these nations differ in health status?

Navarro and Shi (2001) examined predictors of low infant mortality and higher life expectancy in a comparison of OECD countries from 1945–1980. Infant mortality has been identified as an important indicator of the general health status of a nation. Life expectancy is also an indicator of overall well-being in a population. The study found that countries with a social democratic tradition not only had more comprehensive health care systems, but were more likely to have lower infant mortality rates and longer life expectancy. Liberal nations such as Canada showed opposite trends.

More specifically, infant mortality in Sweden improved from 16.6 per 1,000 in 1960 to 4.0 per 1,000 in 1996. In contrast, infant mortality in the United States was 26 per 1,000 in 1960 and fell to 7.8 per 1,000 in 1996. Canada's rate went from 27.3 per 1,000 to 6.0 per 1,000. These relationships are consistent with other international comparisons. Increased market influence is associated with increases in social and health inequalities. Ultimately Canadians have to decide whether they wish to have markets dominate the organization and allocation of health care services and other health-related public policies. As will be discussed in Chapter 9, the form that welfare states assume in different countries reflects both different political ideologies and different class structures.

■ IMPLICATIONS FOR HEALTH POLICY DEVELOPMENT

The dominance of neo-liberalism in Canada and other industrialized countries has restructured domestic policies, which has implications for health policy and health provision. Its strength as the dominant political ideology reflects the influence of particular interests that stand to benefit from the shift to market-driven financing and delivery mechanisms. This can undermine the influence of other civil society actors that wish to preserve and improve medicare. It means that some perspectives may be shut out of the policy-development process. Indeed, governments sometimes undermine or ignore the voices that challenge the dominant perspective (Rochon & Mazmanian, 1993). The restructuring may undermine the ability of national governments to set domestic policy and weaken democratic processes (Teeple, 2000). In fact, the commitment to market principles and practice exemplified in neo-liberalism is opposed to those of democracy. It has been argued that this is because the market and democracy constitute two different approaches to resource allocation. The market signifies the social distribution of goods and services through an exchange between buyer and seller (Teeple, 2000). Democracy refers to a form of political organization in which citizens have a role in political decision making. There is concern that neo-liberalism undermines citizen participation and the democratic process. The requirements of economic globalization (to be examined in Chapter 11) invest greater power in transnational corporations at the expense of civil society.

■ CONCLUSIONS

The creation of health care markets is the desired outcome of those advocating increased privatizing of health care services. The creation of health care markets is driven by political ideology commitments to market-driven policies buttressed by the economic interests of particular sectors. The establishment of these markets has implications both for access to health care for Canadians and for the allocation of political, economic, and social resources among the population. The intellectual support for such developments, neo-liberalism, is based on economic theory that stresses the micro-economics of the individual, whereby self-advancement and self-interest are seen as the driving force in human motivation.

The growth of health care markets has special implications for access to health care for specific groups in Canada. As such, the advent of health care markets would shift care from being an entitlement as a right of citizenship to a commodity. And those who are the most disadvantaged—and therefore the most likely to need such services—would suffer the greatest consequences from such a shift.

Health care markets may increase costs and have been associated with generally inferior care as compared to care provided by public systems. Studies have found greater mortality rates in private, for-profit hospitals. This may be due to use of less-experienced staff, and reduced staff complements. Greater use of market approaches may also increase the burden on individual households to provide health care for family members (Armstrong & Armstrong, 2003). This burden tends to fall on women, who are usually the primary care providers in their families.

The creation of health care markets is not an isolated development, but is tied to government responses to the requirements of economic globalization. Later chapters explore how these forces shape health-related public policy as well as national politics (Leys, 2001; Teeple, 2000). Indeed, some critics argue that globalization interferes with and undermines national governments' capacity to set domestic policy and, in particular, to continue to provide public health care.

Recent international agreements that set forth the terms of trade between nations impose obligations on national governments. These terms may require changes to health care in Canada. Health care is a government monopoly since provincial governments are the sole suppliers of health care services. Some of the private alternatives recommended by Mazankowski and Kirby could violate the terms of international trade treaties to which Canada is signatory (Grieshaber-Otto & Sinclair, 2004). In addition, Canada's treaty commitments could make it difficult to reverse commercializing reforms initiated by several provincial governments in future.

■ REFERENCES

Agence de la santé et des services sociaux de Montreal. (2007). *Atlas santé Montreal.* Montreal: Carrefour montrealais d'information sociosanitaire.

Armstrong, H. & Armstrong, P. (2003). *Wasting away: The undermining of Canadian health care.* Toronto: Oxford University Press.

Bakker, I. (1996). Introduction: The gendered foundations of restructuring in Canada. In I. Bakker (Ed.), *Rethinking restructuring: Gender and change in Canada,* 3–25. Toronto: University of Toronto Press.

Banting, K., Hoberg, G. & Simeon, R. (Eds.). (1997). *Degrees of freedom: Canada and the United States in a changing world.* Montreal & Kingston: McGill-Queen's University Press.

Brook, R.H., Ware, J.E., Rogers, W.H., Keeler, E.B., Davies, A.R., Donald, C.A. et al. (1983). Does free care improve adults' health? *New England Journal of Medicine, 309,* 1426–1434.

Coburn, D. (2000). Income inequality, social cohesion, and the health status of populations: The role of neo-liberalism. *Social Science & Medicine, 51*(1), 135–146.

Coburn, D. (2001). Health, health care, and neo-liberalism. In P. Armstrong, H. Armstrong & D. Coburn (Eds.), *Unhealthy times: The political economy of health and care in Canada,* 45–65. Toronto: Oxford University Press.

Davey Smith, G. (Ed.). (2003). *Inequalities in health: Life course perspectives.* Bristol: Policy Press.

Devereaux, P.J., Choi, P.T.L., Lacchetti, C., Weaver, B., Schunemann, H.J., Haines, T. et al. (2002). A systematic review and meta-analysis of studies comparing mortality rates of private for-profit and private not-for-profit hospitals. *Canadian Medical Asociation Journal, 166*(11), 1399–1406.

Esmail, N. & Walker, M. (2005). *How good is Canadian healthcare? 2005 Report: An international comparison of healthcare systems.* Vancouver: The Fraser Institute.

Esping-Andersen, G. (1990). *The three worlds of welfare capitalism.* Princeton: Princeton University Press.

Evans, R.G. (1997). Going for the gold: The redistributive agenda behind market-based health care reform. *Journal of Health Politics, Policy, and Law, 22*(2), 427–465.

Evans, R.G., Barer, M.L. & Stoddart, G.L. (1995). User fees for health care: Why a bad idea keeps coming back. *Canadian Journal on Aging, 360*(8), 360–390.

Gordon, D., Shaw, M., Dorling., D. & Davey Smith, G. (1999). *Inequalities in health: The evidence presented to the Independent Inquiry into Inequalities in Health.* Bristol: The Policy Press.

Grieshaber-Otto, J. & Sinclair, S. (2004). *Bad medicine: Trade treaties, privatization, and health care reform in Canada.* Ottawa: Canadian Centre for Policy Alternatives.

Hale, S.M. (1990). *Controversies in sociology: A Canadian introduction.* Toronto: Copp Clark Pitman Ltd.

Kaplan, G.A., Pamuk, E.R., Lynch, J.W., Cohen, J.W. & Balfour, J.L. (1996). Income inequality and mortality in the United States. *British Medical Journal, 312:7037,* 999–1003.

Leys, C. (2001). *Market-driven politics.* London: Verso.

Lynch, J. (2000). Income inequality and health: Expanding the debate. *Social Science & Medicine, 51,* 1001–1005.

Navarro, V. & Shi, L. (2001). The political context of social inequalities and health. *International Journal of Health Services, 31*(1), 1–21.

Nichols, L.M., Ginsburg, P.B., Berenson, R.A., Christianson, J. & Hurley, R.E. (2004). Are market forces strong enough to deliver efficient health care systems? Confidence is waning. *Health Affairs, 23*(2), 8–21.

Price, D., Pollock, A.M. & Shaoul, J. (1999). How the World Trade Organisation is shaping domestic policies in health care. *The Lancet, 354,* 1889–1892.

Rachlis, M. (2004). *Prescription for excellence: How innovation is saving Canada's health care system.* Toronto: HarperCollins.

Rachlis, M. (2005). *Public solutions to health care wait lists.* Ottawa: Canadian Centre for Policy Alternatives.

Rachlis, M. & Kushner, C. (1995). *Strong medicine: How to save Canada's health care system.* Toronto: HarperCollins.

Raphael, D. (2000). Health effects of new right policies. *Policy Options, 21:8,* 57–58.

Raphael, D. (Ed.). (2008). *Social determinants of health: Canadian perspectives* (2nd ed.). Toronto: Canadian Scholars' Press Inc.

Rice, T. (1997). Can markets give us the health system we want? *Journal of Health Politics, Policy, and Law, 22*(2), 383–426.

Rochon, T.R. & Mazmanian, D.A. (1993). Social movements and the policy process. *Annals of the American Academy of Political and Social Sciences, 528,* 75–87.

Savas, E.S. (2005). Privatization and public-private partnerships. Adapted from *Privatization in the city: Successes, failures, lessons.* Washington: CQ Press. Online at: www.cesmadrid. es/documentos/Sem200601_MD02_IN.pdf

Scarth, T. (Ed.). (2004). *Hell and high water: An assessment of Paul Martin's record and implications for the future.* Ottawa: Canadian Centre for Policy Alternatives.

Scott, C. (2001). *Public and private roles in health care systems.* Buckingham: Open University Press.

Shaw, M., Dorling, D., Gordon, D. & Smith, G.D. (1999). *The widening gap: Health inequalities and policy in Britain.* Bristol: The Policy Press.

Stanford, J. (2004). Paul Martin, the deficit, and the debt: Taking another look. In T. Scarth (Ed.), *Hell and high water: An assessment of Paul Martin's record and implications for the future,* 31–54. Ottawa: Canadian Centre for Policy Alternatives.

Teeple, G. (2000). *Globalization and the decline of social reform: Into the twenty-first century.* Aurora: Garamond Press.

Teeple, G. (2006). Foreword. In D. Raphael, T. Bryant & M. Rioux (Eds.), *Staying alive: Critical perspectives on health, illness, and health care,* 1–4. Toronto: Canadian Scholars' Press Inc.

Townsend, P., Davidson, N. & Whitehead, M. (Eds.). (1992). *Inequalities in health: The Black Report and the health divide.* New York: Penguin.

Wilkins, R., Berthelot, J.-M. & Ng, E. (2002). Trends in mortality by neighbourhood income in urban Canada from 1971 to 1996. *Health Reports (Stats Can), 13*(Supplement), 1–28.

Woolhandler, S., Campbell, T. & Himmelstein, D.U. (2003). Costs of health care administration in the United States and Canada. *New England Journal of Medicine, 349*(8), 768–775.

Yalnizyan, A. (2000). *Canada's great divide: The politics of the growing gap between the rich and poor in the 1990s.* Toronto: Centre for Social Justice Foundation for Research and Education.

Yalnizyan, A. (2006). *Controlling costs: Canada's single-payer system is costly—but least expensive.* Ottawa: Canadian Centre for Policy Alternatives.

CRITICAL THINKING QUESTIONS

1. What is it about health care that does not make it a typical commodity?
2. What are some of the forces that are in favour of privatizing health care in Canada?
3. Why might the public be led to believe that markets in health care would improve the functioning of the health care system?
4. Why are governments apparently so willing to consider market solutions to health care problems?
5. What would be the result of bringing a market approach to health policy in general and to health care in particular?

FURTHER READINGS

Barer, M.L., Evans, R.G., Hertzman, C. & Johri, M. (1998). *Lies, damned lies, and health care zombies: Discredited ideas that will not die.* HPI Discussion Paper 10. Houston: The University of Texas-Houston Health Science Center.

This report discusses how ideas related to the value of markets in health care are discredited yet refuse to die. Available online at: www.chspr.ubc.ca/node/407

Esping-Andersen, G. (1990). *The three worlds of welfare capitalism.* Princeton: Princeton University Press.

Few discussions in modern social science have occupied as much attention as the changing nature of welfare states in Western societies. Gosta Esping-Andersen, one of the foremost contributors to current debates on this issue, provides a new analysis of the character and role of welfare states in the functioning of contemporary advanced Western societies.

Leys, C. (2001). *Market-driven politics.* London: Verso.

This book provides an original analysis of the key processes of commodification of public services, the conversion of public-service workforces into employees motivated to generate profit, and the role of the state in absorbing risk.

Macarov, D. (2003). *What the market does to people: Privatization, globalization, and poverty.* Atlanta: Clarity Press.

The book examines privatization and globalization as the most recent and widespread causes of poverty and looks at the divisive impact of the market-driven economy on medical services, education, and social welfare. It illustrates international, national, and local efforts to reduce or eliminate poverty, and considers the prospects for a drastic reduction in worldwide poverty in the future.

Navarro, V. (2007). *Neo-liberalism, globalization, and inequalities: Consequences for health and quality of life.* Amityville: Baywood Publishing Company, Inc.

This book assembles a series of articles that challenge neo-liberal ideology. Written by well-known scholars, these articles question each of the tenets of neo-liberal doctrine, showing how the policies guided by this ideology have adversely affected human development in the countries where they have been implemented.

RELEVANT WEBSITES

Canadian Centre for Policy Alternatives
www.policyalternatives.ca

The Canadian Centre for Policy Alternatives produces many reports on health policy and incomes in Canada.

The Canadian Health Services Research Foundation
www.chsrf.ca/home_e.php

The CHSRF supports the evidence-informed management of Canada's health care system by facilitating knowledge transfer and exchange, bridging the gap between research and health care management and policy. See especially their "Myth-busters" and "Evidence Booster" sections at: www.chsrf.ca/mythbusters/index_e.php

National Coalition for Health Care in the United States
www.nchc.org/facts/coverage.shtml

This provides information and insights on the state of health care in the United States, and regular reports on the impact of a privatized health care system.

UBC Centre for Health Services and Policy Research
www.chspr.ubc.ca/about

The UBC Centre for Health Services and Policy Research stimulates scientific inquiry into population health and into ways in which health services can best be organized, funded, and delivered. The centre's researchers and staff carry out a diverse program of research and development designed to deliver data, tools, and analysis useful to understand and renew health care, and improve the health of Canadians.

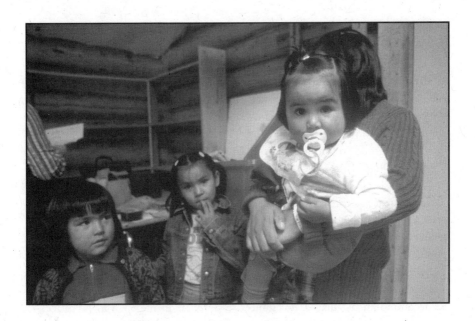

Chapter 9

HEALTH POLICY IN BROADER PERSPECTIVE: WELFARE STATES AND PUBLIC POLICY

■ INTRODUCTION

The form that health care policy and health-related public policy take in Canada is part of what has been termed the advanced welfare state (Myles, 1998). The advanced welfare state was a significant development in most developed political economies following the Second World War. The source of the welfare state in Canada as we know it today is to be found in the insecurities and experiences of Canadians during the Depression and the Second World War (Teeple, 2000). In policy studies, the welfare state refers to a set of social reforms—such as public pensions, public health care, employment insurance, and social assistance—implemented by governments to provide citizens with various supports and benefits. These reforms are important since such policies have been shown to be important predictors of the overall health of a population (Raphael, 2007c).

Rather than seeing the advent of the advanced welfare state as being a reasoned governmental response to perceived citizen need, it has been argued that in Canada it was actually a governmental concession to the significant and sustained calls for reforms by citizens and the labour movement (Teeple, 2000). The welfare state has been defined as "a capitalist society in which the state has intervened in the form of social policies, programs, standards, and regulations in order to mitigate class conflict and to provide for, answer, or accommodate certain social needs for which the capitalist mode of production in itself has no solution or makes no provision" (Teeple, 2000, p. 15).

Whatever the reason, as a result working families and individuals won some security against the unbridled operations of the economic system. A key guiding principle behind the welfare state is that provision of public programs and services is an entitlement of citizenship rather than commodities, which require purchase by earned income. These various programs and supports enabled people to maintain a decent standard of living that was not totally dependent on their ability to earn market income. In essence, many programs and supports come to be decommodified—that is, not subject to purchase in the open marketplace—a key concept in understanding the form and function of the welfare state in nations such as Canada.

In Canada, the welfare state also redistributes economic resources from high-income earners to low-income earners. As one example, the health care system is funded by general revenues received from citizen taxes (Teeple, 2006). High-income earners pay greater taxes in both absolute (dollar amounts) and relative (tax rates) amounts (Murphy, Roberts & Wolfson, 2007). Higher income earners, however, are less likely to become ill and make use of the health care system (Raphael, 2007b). Thus, the public health care system is a very effective means of assuring the provision of health care to citizens as well as economic redistribution. Whether this latter goal was an intention of its creation may be uncertain, but it clearly serves these dual purposes.

Canada has developed a more generous welfare state as compared to that of the United States, but evidence indicates that it shows greater similarity to the US version in being what is called a liberal welfare state than it does with the more developed and generous European standard (Saint-Arnaud & Bernard, 2003). In Europe two alternatives to the liberal welfare state emerged during the late 19th and 20th centuries: the conservative and the social democratic (Esping-Andersen, 1990, 1999).

Esping-Andersen identifies clusters of social democratic (Sweden, Norway, Denmark, Finland); conservative (France, Belgium, Germany, Italy); and liberal economies (Canada, Ireland, United States, United Kingdom, Australia) that differ in their kind and degree of social provision (Esping-Andersen, 1990). And these differences have been shown to be related to both the comprehensiveness of their health care system as well as the health of their populations (Coburn, 2006; Navarro & Shi, 2001).

Yet in every case, economic globalization has exerted powerful pressures on the state, which has resulted in some weakening of the welfare state in most industrial countries (Banting, 1997a; Teeple, 2000). In both Canada and the United States— both already with relatively undeveloped liberal welfare states—this has especially been the case. This chapter examines the nature of the Canadian welfare state. It considers how the three political economy typologies of the welfare state theorized by Gosta Esping-Andersen helps to make sense of how Canada develops and enacts health care and health-related public policy. The health-related consequences for the Canadian population of this public policy approach are also considered.

■ HISTORY OF THE WELFARE STATE

The welfare state refers to state intervention in the provision of supports and services that include education, social services such as employment insurance and training, public pensions, social assistance, and health care (Banting, 1997b). In addition to providing citizens with various kinds of security, the creation of the welfare state also served as a vehicle to promote resource distribution and promote class harmony (Teeple, 2000).

The modern welfare state as it evolved in Canada and other developed nations is sometimes called the Keynesian welfare state (KWS), named after the economist John Maynard Keynes (Townsend, 1993). The main point of his work was that the state should intervene in the workings of the market economy in order to support societal functioning and citizen well-being (see Box 9.1).

Box 9.1: The Keynesian Welfare State

The modern welfare state is often referred to as the Keynesian welfare state (KWS), the name deriving in part from the economist John Maynard Keynes. The principal assumption in his work was the existence of a national economy in which, he argued, the state could intervene to influence levels of investment and domestic income and thereby partially regulate unemployment through national "demand management" policies. Such intervention represented a certain socialization of the costs of production (with state credits, guarantees, grants, and concessions) and of working-class reproduction (through public works and forms of income support), as part of a political compromise with the working classes in an attempt to moderate the business cycle (to prevent a repeat of the unrest of the 1930s), to help rebuild the war-destroyed economies of Europe (to ensure the reconstruction of capitalism), and to contain or diminish a growing interest in socialism due to the experience of the 1930s and the devastation of the war. In an open letter to Roosevelt about the New Deal, Keynes wrote: "If you fail, rational change will be gravely prejudiced throughout the world, leaving orthodoxy and revolution to fight it out." Donald Winch argues that Keynesian policies were "an effective weapon for use against the Marxists on the one hand and the defenders of old style capitalism on the other; a real third alternative, the absence of which before the General Theory had driven many into the Communist camp."

Source: Teeple, G. (2000). *Globalization and the decline of social reform: Into the twenty-first century* (p. 9). Aurora: Garamond Press.

The experiences of the Depression and the two world wars increased the working class's demands for more security and protection from the down-cycles of the business cycle and the market's deleterious effects upon personal well-being. Many citizens had come to believe that the dominance of the market economy had demonstrated that it benefited one class—owners of business and the wealthy—at the expense of the majority. The emerging welfare state emerged as a political compromise worked out by the state between the market sector and the working class to reconcile the negative effects of the business cycle, especially in its most extreme form such as the Depression of the 1930s (see Box 9.2).

Box 9.2: The Business Cycle

Definition
Business cycles are periodic swings in an economy's pace of demand and production activity. These cycles are characterized by alternating phases of growth and stagnation. A period in which real GDP is rising steadily is called an economic expansion, and a period in which it is falling steadily is called a recession. The early stage of an expansion, following a recession, is called an economic recovery. Although these cycles are part of the natural ebb and flow of economic activity, their length is difficult to predict.

How Does It Affect Canadians?
Business cycles have a direct impact on Canadians. Periods of economic boom bring jobs, growth, and economic prosperity. Slowdowns in the economy, on the other hand, hurt businesses and put people out of work.

Examples
The most serious economic contraction experienced in Canada in the last century was the Great Depression in the early 1930s. Canada has also had two serious recessions in more recent years—in 1982 and in the early 1990s. In the late 1990s and early 2000s, Canada experienced a period of healthy economic expansion and prosperity.

Source: Government of Canada (2008). *Economic concepts: The business cycle.* Available online at: http://www.canadianeconomy.gc.ca/english/economy/business_cycle.html

The post-Second World War welfare state was also intended to help rebuild the war-damaged economies of Europe. By doing so, it repaired and preserved the capitalist economic system and restrained growing socialist activity that first arose during the Depression and continued to grow during the Second World War (Teeple, 2000). Thus, these social and economic reforms were meant to ameliorate the inequalities and insecurity created by the market economy, and at the same time preserve the market economic system that produced these insecurities.

The development of the welfare state—its specific social reforms and means of implementing these—differed among nations in time and circumstance. For example, Sweden, an exemplar of the social democratic approach, began to build its welfare state during the 1930s (Esping-Andersen, 1985). The German welfare state, an exemplar of the conservative approach, began as early as the 1870s. The liberal welfare state—always undeveloped as compared to social democratic and conservative nations—showed its greatest development during the post-Second World War period. It was only during this period that Canada, the US, and the UK began to implement universal publicly organized health care.

■ THEORIES OF THE WELFARE STATE

Various theoretical frameworks on the welfare state have been developed to understand the characteristics of different welfare states and the influences that shaped their development. Typologies arrange national welfare states into categories or clusters on the basis of one or more characteristics. A limitation of typologies is that they may mask important differences between nations that at first appear to be in the same category (Olsen, 2002).

One such typology is dichotomous. The dichotomous typology contrasts between residual welfare states and institutional welfare states (Olsen, 2002). The residual welfare states are less developed and provide a smaller range of social welfare measures. These include less generous benefits and lower income replacement rates upon job loss or acquiring a disability. Overall, levels of social expenditures are lower as compared to welfare states characterized as institutional.

Residual states target benefits at the less well off in a society. Eligibility criteria are very stringent and there are usually a multitude of rules and obligations that include means testing (Olsen, 2002). Once benefits are approved, there are waiting periods before these are provided and these benefits are then provided for short entitlement periods. There is little state commitment to reducing poverty.

In contrast, an institutional welfare state does not treat public welfare programs as last resorts to be in place for emergencies or situations of urgent need (Olsen, 2002). Institutional state welfare benefits and services are seen as citizen-entitled social protections and social investments. The general approach is one of promoting well-being and preventing problems rather than providing services and supports on a reactive or remedial basis. Benefits and services are more comprehensive, covering a wider range of contingencies, and are more generous, of higher quality, and more easily accessed than benefits in a residual welfare system. The institutional approach sees the allowing of the free market to allocate resources to be an inferior means of addressing many types of social need.

Olsen identifies a limitation with the binary residual-institutional approach as it can lump very different kinds of welfare states into the same category (Olsen, 2002). For example, the residual welfare states of southern Europe—Greece, Italy, Portugal, and Spain—differ from the English-speaking residual welfare states—Canada, the US, the UK, and Ireland. The binary typology has limited application, but it does provide a starting point for comparing different types of welfare states.

Box 9.3: Dichotomous Welfare State Typology: Residual versus Institutional

The first widely adopted typologies constructed to detail and classify the social policy orientation of various nations were often dichotomous, distinguishing between two major ideal types of welfare provision: a *residual* welfare state and a more comprehensive *institutional* welfare state. Building on the quantitative concerns highlighted by the leader-laggard approach, the residual-institutional typology was designed to place greater emphasis on some of the more qualitative dimensions of welfare states.

... *Residual* welfare states are less comprehensive; they have a much narrower range of social welfare measures and cover far fewer social contingencies than institutional welfare states. They also provide more modest benefit levels and income replacement rates and, consequently, are characterized by considerably lower levels of social expenditure. And since residual welfare state programs are targeted at the poor or less well off, far fewer people are eligible for benefits. Allocating benefits largely on the basis of demonstrated need, these programs typically maintain other stringent eligibility conditions, rules, and obligations, including relatively long qualifying and waiting periods before benefits may be accessed, short periods of benefit entitlement, and a variety of grounds for disqualifying benefit recipients. Not surprisingly, there is also a very high social stigma attached to many of the benefits provided by residual welfare states. Best represented by the United States, the residual welfare state is premised on the notion that the market (and, to a lesser extent, the family) is the "natural" and best means for meeting the needs of citizens. Public measures are considered to be only supplementary, serving primarily as temporary substitutes when private welfare channels break down or are otherwise unavailable.

The *institutional* welfare state model, in contrast, does not treat public welfare programs primarily as a last resort to be activated during periods of emergency and urgent need (interruptions in earnings due to illness or unemployment, for example). Rather, they are embraced as an important first line of social protection, often emphasizing prevention rather than simply reactive or remedial measures. The free market, in turn, is considered to be a largely inferior way of addressing certain types of basic human needs. The character of institutional welfare states also stands in stark contrast to those categorized as residual; benefits and services cover a wider range of contingencies, are more generous and of a higher quality, and are more easily accessed.

Source: Olsen, G. (2002). *The politics of the welfare state* (pp. 69–70). Toronto: Oxford University Press.

■ ESPING-ANDERSEN: THREE WORLDS OF WELFARE CAPITALISM

Esping-Andersen's three welfare state typology has been widely applied and also the subject of much critique (Bambra, 2004; Esping-Andersen, 1990), yet it seems to have withstood the test of time and has contributed to a substantial body of research on welfare states (Saint-Arnaud & Bernard, 2003). It also sheds light on why and how health care and health-related policies developed in Canada and how such policies can be influenced. Esping-Andersen considers whether the welfare state is best understood by analyzing a nation's social policies or by examining the institutional forces that shape these collections of a nation's social policies. Supporting the later approach, he argues that welfare state regimes are actually a complex of interrelated legal and organizational characteristics. In essence, the term "welfare state" in industrial capitalist societies signifies the set of features by which major institutions define social citizenship and provide welfare provision. The major institutions of the market economy, the state, and the family have unique interconnections that can take different forms (von Kempski, 1972).

At the time of his initial development of the three ideal welfare state types, Esping-Andersen recognized that while societies he included in the welfare state typology did not comprise a large number of cases, they did distinguish themselves into three distinct groups (Esping-Andersen, 1990). The distinguishing feature of these nations was their identification with three specific traditions of political mobilization and political philosophy: conservatism, liberalism, and socialism. These features were linked, he argued, to particular aspects of their contemporary social policy approach as well as their broader political and economic features (Arts & Gelissen, 2001). The form that welfare states assume in different countries is shaped by economic interests and political ideology.

The result of this work was Esping-Andersen's *Three Worlds of Welfare Capitalism* (Esping-Andersen, 1990). His three welfare state typology—liberal, conservative, and social democratic—classified nations on the basis of their established patterns of welfare provision. These patterns—based on the interrelationships of the state, the market, and the family—specified the mix each nation provided of public sector, private sector, and civil sector social programs. Canada is squarely identified as a liberal welfare state.

Table 9.1: Members of Each Esping-Andersen Welfare State Type

Liberal	Conservative	Social Democratic
Australia	Austria	Denmark
Canada	Belgium	Finland
Ireland	France	Norway
New Zealand	Germany	Sweden
UK	Italy	
USA	Japan	
	Netherlands	
	Switzerland	

Source: Adapted from Esping-Andersen, G. (1990). *The three worlds of welfare capitalism* (p. 52). Princeton: Princeton University Press.

Liberal Welfare States

The liberal welfare state is the most undeveloped form. It provides modest universal transfers and social-insurance plans to citizens, which is usually done with some form of means or income testing to determine eligibility (Esping-Andersen, 1990). As a result, social assistance is usually provided only to the least well-off. This type of regime provides basic social safety nets, minimal relief for individuals who are unable to compete successfully in the marketplace, and few benefits or programs as a right of citizenship or national residency. It is clearly a residual approach to social welfare based on the belief that when welfare benefits are too generous, recipients will prefer to depend on these benefits rather than seek out employment for earned income. For Esping-Andersen, the liberal welfare state is exemplified by Australia, Canada, Ireland, New Zealand, the United States, and the United Kingdom.

The term "liberal" signifies its historical roots in 19th-century political economy, which embodies principles of a laissez-faire orientation associated with the early industrializing capitalist nations. "Liberal" does not refer to the North American usage as being somewhat more progressive than those who call themselves conservative. It can be argued that the conservative nations in Esping-Andersen's typology (see Table 9.1) are actually more progressive in their provision of social security than liberal nations. Liberal nations are also rather more likely to take up policies considered to represent current neo-liberal thought: emphasis on the marketplace as the arbiter of the distribution of resources among the population.

While even liberal welfare states redistribute economic resources from the well-off to the less well-off in a society through progressive income taxes and the operation of public health care systems, the extent of this redistribution is rather less as compared to other welfare state types (Navarro & Shi, 2001). Consistent with this, benefit levels tend to be low. The chief objective of this form of redistribution is to help address the needs of the least well-off, but there is little effort to compensate the disadvantaged for their past experiences or protect them from future hardships. Benefits are best seen as being of last resort, similar to the residual concept of the dichotomous typology.

Conservative Welfare States

Conservative regimes are characterized by either paternalist and sometimes authoritarian approaches that historically have had strong ties with the Church (Esping-Andersen, 1990). Examples of these are Germany, France, Netherlands, Belgium, Spain, and Italy. Esping-Andersen considers these nations as "corporatist" because of their "statist" and "organicist" traits. In other words, conservative welfare states are structured to maintain and reproduce the existing differences in status, income, and wealth among social classes and sectors. There is rather little commitment to creating an egalitarian society.

Conservative welfare regimes use a range of separate but state-mandated and state-directed social insurance programs for members of different sectors of the economy. These are financed primarily by employers and workers. The benefit levels provided vary by sector, with higher-paid employees receiving more generous payments. Conservative welfare states stress social insurance as opposed to social assistance or universal measures. They redistribute income over the life cycle of a single individual or family to ensure that support is available in old age, sickness, or during periods of unemployment.

The conservative welfare state is characterized as retaining status differences between social classes, but doing so with less emphasis on the market and commodification as the provider of welfare. The church has a prominent role in shaping the conservative or corporatist welfare regime with emphasis on the family and promoting the traditional nuclear family. The emphasis is on the family providing social welfare. The state provides when the family has exhausted its own resources for taking care of family members. Family benefits promote traditional motherhood.

The conservative regime is also a corporatist welfare state (Esping-Andersen, 1990). In this sense, conservative relates to classical conservatism, which highlights community, authority, hierarchy, and tradition, together with a disposition to resist change and preserve traditions and societal values. Christian norms and traditional family roles are more central than the market.

Social Democratic Welfare States

Social democratic regimes have broad and extensive programs that provide economic and other forms of security to its citizens. For example, many social insurance programs are compulsory in the workplace, which, when combined with traditionally high employment levels, provide a very developed welfare state. Access to programs and benefit levels are based on a record of contributions made by employers and employees. Even when such contributions have not been made, benefits tend to be comprehensive. Coverage is strikingly more developed than those provided by liberal regimes.

The social democratic welfare state regime comprises nations that emphasize universalism and decommodification of social rights. In other words, the state provides universal rather than targeted social welfare. The social democratic welfare states strive for far-reaching objectives closer to optimal conditions rather than providing the basic minimum characteristic of the liberal welfare states. The orientation of social democratic welfare regimes toward social problems is preventative. An important part of the approach is to promote equality and eliminate poverty through more equal distribution of economic resources, including income.

In social democratic regimes, full employment is a key priority and active labour policies focused on employment training are extensive (Esping-Andersen, 1990). In contrast, liberal regimes such as Canada and the US have rather less commitment to active labour policies, the result of which is that workers with high education are more likely to take educational and training opportunities than those with less education (Myers & de Broucker, 2006). Liberal regimes have more insecure employment that provides few or no benefits.

The key feature then of social democratic regimes is provision of basic citizen entitlements such as access to a well-paying job, comprehensive health care, safe working environments, and secure retirements. Pensions are usually tied to inflation to keep older citizens well above the poverty line (Esping-Andersen, 1990). Social democratic regimes also tend to have strong active labour market policies that promote training and retraining programs for workers. Such regimes are similar to institutional welfare states that see citizen welfare as both social rights and social investment.

■ DECOMMODIFICATION AND STRATIFICATION

Esping-Andersen's typology is based to a large part on the degree of decommodification and social stratification within a society (Arts & Gelissen, 2001; Esping-Andersen, 1990).

Commodification and Decommodification

Commodification refers to the degree to which citizens are dependent on the market and earned incomes for the provision of goods and services. Decommodification refers to the degree to which citizens are not dependent on their market incomes to obtain these goods and services. When a service is decommodified, it is provided as a matter of right (Esping-Andersen, 1990). In other words, services such as education, child care, employment training, and health care as examples are provided by the state in a "public economy" that coexists alongside the private capitalist market. These are powerful concepts that illuminate the role of the state versus the market in social welfare provision. These concepts and how they play out in a nation have strong implications for the development of health-related public policies in addition to traditional health care services.

Stratification

In his treatise on the welfare state, Esping-Andersen defined the welfare state as a "system of stratification": "Welfare states are key institutions in the structuring of class and the social order" (Esping-Andersen, 1990, p. 55). This refers to welfare states' capacity to reinforce or reduce existing patterns of inequality within a country. This occurs through the shaping of kind and degree of social solidarity, class divisions, and status differences. For example, the liberal welfare state maintains and reinforces existing patterns of inequality since there is rather little state intervention in the workings of the marketplace. There is little institutional or ideological commitment, for example, to reduce or eliminate poverty. This contrasts with the social democratic regime, which has a deep commitment to reducing inequality and poverty. Similarly, the conservative regime is committed to preserving the family and "socializ[ing] the costs of family-hood" by supporting families prior to using up all of their own resources. This is not an approach conducive to reducing inequality, though it does reduce the rough edges associated with being on the lower end of the status hierarchy.

Health care and health-related policies and their impacts therefore reflect differing national political ideologies: liberal, social democratic, or conservative. By highlighting political ideology, the typology provides means for understanding both national trajectories in health policy, but also the impacts of the resurgence of neo-liberalism as a political ideology on some, but not all, welfare regimes. For example, it has been argued that liberal welfare regimes, already market-oriented, are more susceptible to the influence of neo-liberalism and globalization on their policymaking (Raphael, 2003). And, as has been noted, health care policy is one area of increased market sector interest.

■ USEFULNESS OF THE ESPING-ANDERSEN WELFARE TYPOLOGY

Since the publication of *The Three Worlds of Welfare Capitalism*, debates have raged over: (1) the accuracy of the Esping-Andersen's typology; (2) its sensitivity to issues of gender and diversity; and (3) the impact of economic globalization on the quality of these different forms of the welfare state (Kasza, 2002).

On the role of gender, Esping-Andersen responded to these concerns in his 1999 volume, *Social Foundations of Post-industrial Economies* (Esping-Andersen, 1999) by exploring the issues of female employment and child care among the three welfare types. In her detailed examination of the relationship between decommodification and defamilialization, Bambra identified much overlap between these concepts, concluding that much of the critique of Esping-Andersen as being gender-blind was unfounded (Bambra, 2004).

Esping-Andersen generally focuses on the nature of income and other related financial supports as an indicator of welfare state form and did not relate the welfare state to health care, a critical component of the welfare state. In many social democratic nations, health care developed as an integral component of the welfare state. In liberal nations such as the UK, national governments created a public health care system before developing the other service components of the welfare state.

■ WELFARE STATES AND HEALTH-RELATED PUBLIC POLICIES

Raphael (2007a) recently compiled information on how Canada stacks up against other developed nations in terms of supports and benefits. His analysis sheds much light on where Canada stands as a member of the liberal welfare state club.

■ SOCIETAL COMMITMENTS TO CITIZENS AND GOVERNMENTAL SPENDING

A key aspect of health-related public policy is degree of support for citizens. The Organisation for Economic Co-operation and Development (OECD) calculates the percentage of each country's gross domestic product (GDP) that is transferred to citizens. Transfers refer to governments taking fiscal resources generated by the market economy and distributing them to the population as services, monetary supports, or investments in social infrastructure. Such infrastructure includes education, employment training, social assistance or welfare payments, family supports, pensions, health and social services, and other benefits.

Nations may choose to transfer relatively small amounts, allowing the marketplace to decide how economic resources are distributed. Or, a nation may choose to intervene to control the marketplace and give itself decision-making authority concerning these allocations. As it turns out, the nations that transfer a greater proportion of resources are more likely to have less income inequality, lower poverty rates, and generally better health status among the population compared to those countries that transfer less (see Box 9.4).

Box 9.4: Taxes and Services

Cost of cutting taxes not worth the savings
Elaine Power and Jamie Swift
Toronto Star

Two of the major political parties in the upcoming election are promising tax cuts to "put more money in taxpayers' pockets."

"Great," we think. Who wouldn't want more money in their pockets, especially as the post-holiday credit-card bills arrive?

There are two important questions we need to consider before jumping to the conclusion that tax cuts are a good thing: (a) will tax cuts really put more money in our pockets? and (b) what are the costs of those tax cuts?

The first problem is that tax cuts at the federal level mean, in part, reduced income transfers to the provinces, which then download the problem to municipalities.

We've already lived through a decade of decreased federal funding to the provinces, compounded by provincial tax cuts and downloading of services. So Ontario's city governments must make tough decisions: Raise taxes. Cut services. Impose user fees for services that were once free. Or all of the above.

It's a new version of the old "trickle-down" theory of economics. Some people, especially the more affluent, may end up with more money because of Ottawa's tax cuts. But it is not a sure thing.

More important are the costs of tax cuts.

What doesn't get funded—or is inadequately funded—because "we can't afford it"? Tax cuts affect programs that Canadians value: education, health care, public health, the environment, income support programs, and so on. They erode "public goods" such as clean air and water that are impossible to produce for profit.

Tax cuts already have a proven track record: The Walkerton water disaster. An ongoing crisis in health-care funding. Aboriginals living in Third World conditions. Inadequate funding for education. A growing gap between the rich and the poor. Reduced help for marginalized groups like "high- risk" youth and victims of domestic abuse. One in six children living in poverty, and double that rate for Indian, immigrant and visible minority children. A deplorable lack of affordable housing.

The simple fact is that tax cuts undermine the government's ability to act. And this is exactly what the tax cutters intend. Tax cuts are an integral component of a particular ideological position, often called neo-liberalism, which argues—without supporting evidence—that the market can always provide goods and services better than government.

But can the market provide health care for all?

Evidence from the American experience suggests not. Can the market provide affordable housing for the alarming number of workers who do not earn a living wage? Evidence from the past 10 years of tax-cutting in Ottawa and Queen's Park, combined with a retreat from social housing programs, suggests not.

Downloading onto municipal governments also underpins the neo-liberal worldview. Our cities have the least fiscal capacity and are least able to regulate a market dominated by a small number of ever more powerful corporations.

Canadians are not overtaxed. The Organisation for Economic Co-operation and Development ranks Canada among the lowest taxed industrialized nations: 21st among 30 industrialized nations, and fifth among the seven largest.

We wove our social safety net after World War II, when Canadians saw themselves as nation-builders. In the wake of the events of the 1930s and 1940s, we had a collective sense that no one should ever again have to suffer the humiliations of unemployment and poverty experienced during the Great Depression.

Canadians believed then—as we do now—that we could look after each other and work together to achieve whatever national goals we set for ourselves. We could build a better future for all Canadians. We still can.

Taxes are the price we pay for a decent, caring, and civilized society.

When a candidate promises you tax cuts, ask him or her what the real cost will be. Instead of gazing down at the bottom line, let's start asking ourselves what kind of Canada we want to build together. And let's demand that our politicians work for the public good.

Elaine Power teaches in Queen's School of Physical and Health Education and Jamie Swift teaches in Queen's School of Business.

Source: Toronto Star (January 19, 2006), A17.

Among the developed nations of the OECD, the average public expenditures in 2001 was 21 percent of gross domestic product (GDP) (Organisation for Economic Co-operation and Development, 2007). There is great variation among countries with Scandinavian nations such as Denmark (spending 29.2 percent of GDP) and Sweden (spending 28.9 percent of GDP) being the highest public spenders. Canada ranks 24th of 30 wealthy industrialized nations and spends just 17.8 percent of GDP on public expenditures. The only nations that allocate a smaller percentage of GDP to public expenditure are Japan (16.9 percent), the US (14.8 percent), Ireland (13.8 percent), Turkey (13.2 percent), Mexico (11.8 percent), and Korea (6.1 percent). Other wealthy developed nations spending relatively more—in addition to Denmark and Sweden—are France (28.9 percent), Germany (27.4 percent), Belgium (27.2 percent), Austria (26 percent), and Finland (24.8 percent).

How do these differences in spending translate into specific policy areas? Figures 9.1a–9.1d shows how Canada compares to a number of OECD nations in transfer of resources to its citizenry as indicated by the percentage of GDP allocated to public expenditures on health, old age, incapacity-related benefits, and families.

Canada has among the highest public expenditures on health care with Germany, Iceland, Sweden, France, and Denmark spending more. But public spending on health care in Canada represents only about 70 percent of total health spending, which is among the lowest of OECD nations (Organisation for Economic Co-operation and Development, 2005). The US ranks relatively low on public health care spending as even more of its spending comes from private sources than is the case in Canada.

It is in the other areas of benefits and supports to citizens—that is, health-related policy—that Canada provides limited support compared to other developed economies. In fact, among OECD member countries, Canada has among the lowest spending for seniors, primarily pensions. Contributing 4.8 percent of GDP for seniors' pensions makes Canada 26th of 29 developed economies. Canada also is among the lowest spenders on incapacity or disability-related issues, allocating less than 1 percent of its GDP. It ranks 27th of 29 modern industrialized nations. Canada also ranks very low on family benefits at 25th of 29 of these developed economies.

Figure 9.1a: Public Expenditure on Health as % of GDP, 2001

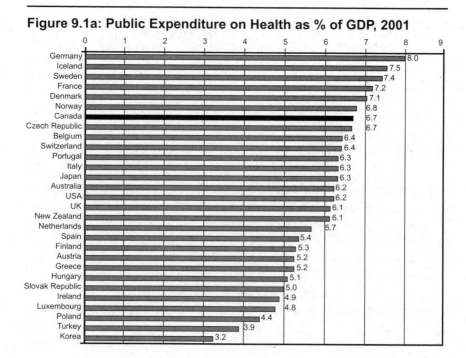

Figure 9.1b: Public Expenditure on Old Age as % of GDP, 2001

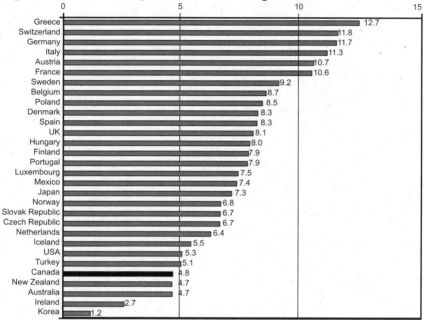

Figure 9.1c: Public Expenditure on Incapacity-Related Benefits as % of GDP, 2001

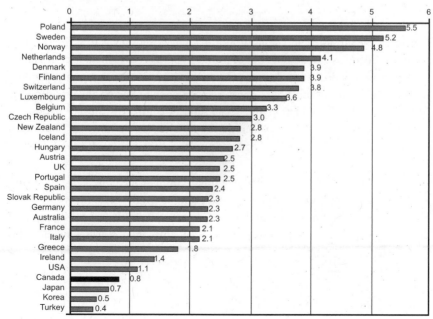

Figure 9.1d: Public Expenditure on Family as % of GDP, 2001

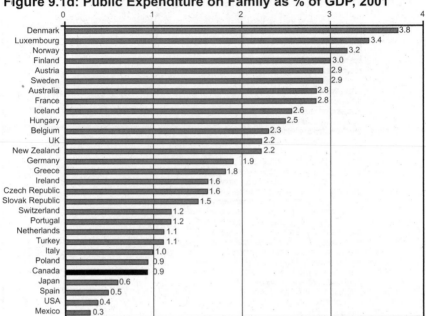

Source: Organisation for Economic Co-operation and Development. (2004). Social expenditure database, www.oecd.org/els/social/expenditure

Income support to other age-groups in the population comprises family benefits, wage subsidies, and child support paid by governments to help keep low-income individuals and families out of poverty. Social services include counselling, employment supports, and other community services. Consistent with its spending in other social and health policy areas, Canada is quite low on income supports to the working-age population and social services compared to other nations. It spends 2.8 percent of GDP on income supports to the working age population (rank 27th of 30), and spends 2.2 percent on social services (rank 8th of 30) (see Box 9.5).

Active labour policy is another area of government spending concerned with support for training and other policies that promote employment for workers that have lost their jobs through restructuring. Canada contributes just 1.14 percent of GDP to such policies, which gives it a ranking of 15th of 22 developed nations for which data was available.

> ### Box 9.5: Hurricane Katrina Reflects the Lack of Social Infrastructure in the United States
>
> Inequalities in the US have long been associated with race. Hurricane Katrina exemplified racial inequalities and the lack of public supports for people who lost everything they owned and were too poor to leave New Orleans before the storm hit.
>
> "Racial disparities are leading indicators of trouble, and just like canaries gasping for air, the marginalized are signaling that this democracy is in trouble because injustices are reproducing themselves and structural arrangements are benefiting a few at the expense of the many. Without a doubt, the greatest burdens in this country are shouldered by poor people of color, but they are not the only ones who are suffering. The uneven way we fund schools harms white students as well as students of color. The way our institutions perpetuate and increase wealth disparities has shrunk the middle class. Slashing social safety net programs in the name of increasing personal responsibility has added millions of people to the ranks of the working poor. Consequently, we can use the Katrina crisis as a launching pad not only for investigating the way we think and talk about race in this country, but also for developing a new discourse on race and class that highlights how the public and private are related, how democracy and structural arrangements that produce disparate outcomes are incompatible, and why institutional inequality concerns us all. In this way, our discussion about race can become transformative; instead of dividing people, it can bring them closer together in a collective reimagining of a just society" (p. 68).
>
> *Source:* Powell, J.A., Kwame Jeffries, H., Newhart, D.W. & Stiens, E. (2006). Towards a transformative view of race: The crisis and opportunity of Katrina. In C. Hartman & G.D. Squires (Eds.), *There is no such thing as a natural disaster: Race, class, and Hurricane Katrina*, 59–84. New York: Routledge.

◼ IMPLICATIONS FOR PUBLIC POLICY AND HEALTH

How do public policy commitments affect differing living conditions that are known to be key determinants of health? Some of the issues examined here are resources available to the unemployed, the level of social assistance benefits, minimum wages, and pension benefits. These can mean the difference between having income and employment security and good health, and living in poverty and having poor health.

Unemployment Benefits

Figure 9.2 shows the percentage benefit replacement for individuals—at the average production worker level—unemployed over a five-year period. For most Canadians, benefits available over a five-year period would be employment insurance (EI), which expires after one year of benefits. At that point, a family with liquid assets would need to spend these in order to be eligible for social assistance benefits. Therefore, for non-destitute families, EI provides only 20 percent replacement income over this period, which ranks Canada 23rd among 28 industrialized nations in its benefit level. Even if families did qualify for social assistance, the benefit percentage is equivalent to only 50 percent of average income. Canada ranks 22nd of 28 nations.

Figure 9.2: Average Percentage of Net Replacement Rates over 60 Months of Unemployment, for Four Family Types and Two Earnings Levels without and with Social Assistance, 2002

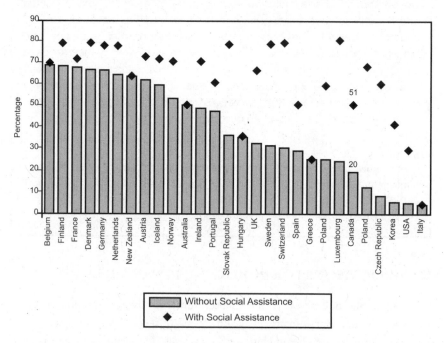

Source: Organisation for Economic Co-operation and Development. (2005). *Society at a glance: OECD social indicators 2005 edition* (p. 43). Paris: OECD.

Social Assistance or Welfare

The OECD considers social assistance and welfare support as "benefits of last resort." On average, a married couple with two children receives social assistance benefits at 37 percent of median average income. In international comparisons, Canada places 17th of 23 OECD nations in its provision of social assistance. This means that 15 other nations provide more generous income support than Canada does. Moreover, social assistance in Canada is targeted to low-income or destitute families and individuals who must be means or income tested to demonstrate their need for such support.

Figure 9.3: Average Net Incomes of Social Assistance Recipients as Percentage of Median Equivalent Household Income, Married Couple with Two Children, 2001

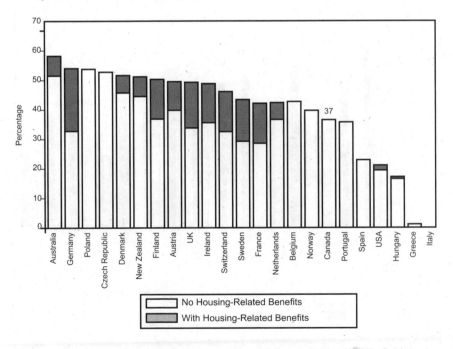

Source: Organisation for Economic Co-operation and Development. (2005). *Society at a glance: OECD social indicators 2005 edition* (p. 45). Paris: OECD.

Minimum Wages

In comparison to other advanced nations, Canada provides among the lowest minimum wages. Figure 9.4 provides data that show how Canada compares with other nations on minimum wages. Here, we are concerned with minimum wages that are provided at a level that enables people to obtain what they require in order to maintain their health.

A Canadian family with two children and one full-time minimum wage earner places the family at 47 percent of the median household income. This falls below what is usually considered the poverty line at 50 percent of median poverty level. A two-parent family with two children and both parents employed full-time at

Figure 9.4: Net Incomes at Statutory Minimum Wages, Married Couple with Two Children as Percentage of Median Household Income, 2001

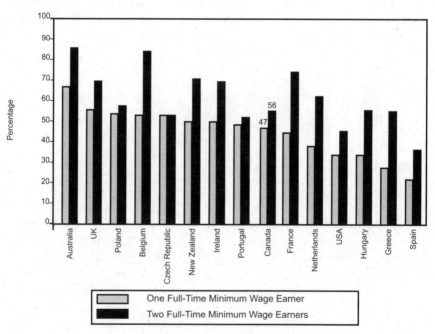

Source: Organisation for Economic Co-operation and Development. (2005). *Society at a glance: OECD social indicators 2005 edition* (p. 45). Paris: OECD.

minimum wages receives 56 percent of median income. This family is therefore identified as a low-wage earning family. Of 15 developed industrialized countries, Canada ranks 9th for lone-parent working families and 10th among 15 such nations for two-parent working families.

Pensions

The Canada Pension Plan (CPP) is an income benefit program paid to retired individuals who have contributed to the plan during their working lives. The OECD compares data on the value of pension benefits provided by each nation in relation to the gross earnings of an average production worker (Organisation for Economic Co-operation and Development, 2005). For a worker earning 50 percent of an average production worker, the CPP offers a rate of 89 percent of earnings. For Canadian residents earning the average production worker's income, the rate is 57 percent. In international comparisons, Canada's rates for average-waged workers are quite low, ranking Canada 22nd of 30 wealthy industrialized nations. For very low-paid workers, Canada ranks 12th among 30 wealthy industrialized nations.

Support for People with Disabilities

On support for people with disabilities, Canada allocates less than 1 percent of GDP toward disability benefits (Organisation for Economic Co-operation and Development, 2003). This means that Canada ranks 17th among 20 industrialized nations.

■ IMPLICATIONS FOR HEALTH POLICY AND THE CANADIAN WELFARE STATE

Canada's approach to health-related public policy appears to be rather undeveloped as compared to other nations, which include both social democratic as well as conservative welfare states. These findings become understandable when Canada is recognized as being a liberal welfare state where the primary governmental ideological inspiration is one of minimizing government intervention (Saint-Arnaud & Bernard, 2003). The implications of this for developing and implementing health and health-related public policy is that there are formidable ideological and societal barriers to such action. The means by which these barriers can be overcome may involve the same processes discussed in terms of maintaining the public health care system in Canada: building political and social movements in support of health.

■ WELFARE STATES AND HEALTH OUTCOMES

The relationship between welfare state regime and health outcomes can be succinctly summarized: Population health is usually better in social democratic nations and worse in liberal nations. Navarro and Shi related the welfare state typology to health policy and health outcomes (Navarro & Shi, 2001). Specifically, they looked at the social democratic, Christian democratic/conservative, liberal, and the formerly fascist regimes of Europe and compared their health and social spending patterns and the impact on population health status in four main areas: (1) the primary determinants of income inequalities; (2) the levels of public expenditures and health care benefits coverage; (3) public support of services for families; and (4) infant mortality as a measure of population health status for the period 1946–1990. They found that political traditions that were committed to the redistribution of economic and social resources and full-employment policies, such as the social democratic parties, tended to be more successful in enhancing population health status. Table 9.2 shows public expenditures on health as a percent of gross domestic product from their study.

Between 1960 and 1990, social democratic regimes had the largest public expenditures on health care, followed by the Christian democratic regimes. In contrast, the liberal Anglo-Saxon regimes tended to have the lowest expenditures in this area.

Table 9.2 shows that the social democratic regimes also had the highest coverage of most of their population for medical care. Christian democratic political economies had similarly high health care coverage of most of their populations. Among the liberal Anglo-Saxon political economies, the United Kingdom provided 100 percent medical coverage to all of its population for all of the years examined. Canada provided 71 percent health care benefits coverage in 1960, and 100 percent coverage for the other years examined in their analysis. In the US, less than half of its population had health care benefits coverage for all the years examined in the analysis. Navarro and Shi showed that these investments in health reduced the poverty rate in social democratic and Christian democratic countries, whereas the poverty rates in liberal Anglo-Saxon political economies were two to three times higher than those for the social democratic and Christian democratic regimes, particularly in the United States, followed by the United Kingdom and Canada. In addition, social democratic countries also tend to have the lowest infant mortality rates for the period 1960–1996 (Navarro & Shi, 2001). These findings have been replicated in more recent analyses (Coburn, 2006; Navarro et al., 2004).

Table 9.2: Public Expenditures on Health, 1960–1990, Percent of GDP

	1960	1970	1980	1990
Social democratic political economies				
Austria	3.0	3.4	5.3	5.3
Sweden	3.2	6.1	8.7	7.9
Denmark	3.2	5.2	7.7	7.1
Norway	2.3	4.1	5.9	6.5
Finland	2.1	4.2	5.1	6.5
Mean	2.8	4.6	6.5	6.7
Christian democratic political economies				
Belgium	2.3	5.0	5.5	6.9
Germany	3.2	4.6	7.0	6.7
Netherlands	1.3	5.0	5.9	6.1
France	2.4	4.3	6.0	6.6
Italy	3.0	4.5	5.6	6.3
Switzerland	1.9	3.1	4.6	5.7
Mean	2.4	4.4	5.8	6.4
Liberal Anglo-Saxon political economies				
United Kingdom	3.3	3.9	5.0	5.1
Ireland	2.9	4.3	7.1	4.9
United States	1.3	2.7	3.9	5.1
Canada	2.3	5.0	5.5	6.9
Mean	2.4	3.9	5.3	5.5
Former fascist dictatorships				
Spain	—	2.4	4.4	5.7
Portugal	—	—	—	—
Greece	—	—	3.1	3.5
Mean	—	2.4	3.8	4.6

Source: Navarro, V. & Shi, L. (2001). The political context of social inequalities and health. *International Journal of Health Services, 31*(1), 1–21.

■ POLITICAL IDEOLOGY AS AN INFLUENCE

Political ideology and its manifestation in public policy then is a key influence on health care expenditures, health-related public policies, and population health outcomes. Esping-Andersen's typology is therefore relevant to understanding how health policy is made and implemented in Canada. Given that Canada has a public health care insurance system, is it appropriate for Canada to be lumped in with the United States in the liberal cluster? It would appear initially not, but the similarities of Canadian public policies on a range of health-related public policy approaches does appear to support this placement (Bernard & Saint-Arnaud, 2004). This has especially been the case as differences between the two countries may have narrowed as a result of closer integration of the Canadian and US economies during the 1980s and into the 1990s as a result of free trade treaties, specifically the Free Trade Agreement (FTA) and the North American Free Trade Agreement (NAFTA).

In spite of trade agreements linking the two political economies, the US has a private health care system, while Canada still has a public system to which all citizens have access on the basis of need, not income. Although about 30 percent of health care costs in Canada are not covered by the public system—a very high figure in international comparison—and there is increasing privatization of parts of the Canadian health care system, Canada still scores higher than the US in terms of access for low-income populations (Sanmartin & Ng, 2004).

And while low-income populations in both countries are more likely to report poor or fair health than the high-income populations, a greater percentage of low-income Americans (31 percent) do so compared to low-income Canadians (23 percent) who reported poor or fair health. In addition, the primary reasons for unmet health care needs differ between nations. In Canada, wait times for care have become the most frequently given reason, whereas in the United States, it is cost or lack of health insurance that deters Americans from seeking health care services they need.

And while income and health inequalities have been growing in Canada, Canada continues to emerge as more egalitarian compared to the United States in terms of redistributive health and social policies (Siddiqi & Hertzman, 2007). Whether these specific differences between the Canadian and US health care systems and health-related public policies will maintain these different profiles remains uncertain.

■ THE WELFARE STATE IN DECLINE

Chapter 1 noted how Canada and other Western developed political economies have reduced health and social spending in response to global economic pressures.

This has been done, it is stated, to enhance national competitiveness in the global economy. Studies indicated that less-developed welfare states have effects upon health as illustrated by higher infant mortality rates and shorter life expectancies (Navarro et al., 2004). In other words, the more governments invest in social and economic resource redistribution, the better population health outcomes tend to be. In addition, liberal—also Anglo-Saxon—economies appear to be more susceptible to the policy influencing effects of neo-liberalism and globalization (Hemrijck, 2002). Why has neo-liberalism penetrated the Anglo liberal economies but not to the same degree in social democratic or conservative regimes? In short, why are some welfare states more resilient than others?

As with other issues, many explanations have been posited to account for such globalization-resistant resiliency. Swank argues that the reason for this is because the same class and political institutions that mediated and shaped welfare states in the age of expansion now shape domestic responses to internationalization (Swank, 1992, 1998). He thus concludes:

> Where institutions of collective interest representation—social corporatism and inclusive electoral institutions—are strong, where authority is concentrated, and where the welfare state is based on the principle of universalism, the effects of international capital mobility are absent, or they are positive in the sense that they suggest economic and political interests opposed to neo-Liberal reforms ... have been successful in defending the welfare state. (Swank, 1998, p. 44)

In contrast where political institutions fragment interest representation and political authority, as in the Anglo-American democracies, the ability of investment capital to move from place to place exerts downward pressure on social provision.

A related explanation is to consider the political organization of society and specifically the electoral process. In *Fighting Poverty in the US and Europe*, Alesina and Glaeser (2004) address this very issue with regard to differences in the size of the welfare state. While they agree with Swank that institutions and political ideology are important influences, they add that the European wars of the 19th and 20th centuries fuelled a variety of grievances among the working classes that provided fertile ground for socialist and communist parties to build support.

In response to these organized movements, many European nations instituted some form of proportional representation in which the percentage of legislative seats is determined on the basis of the percentage of votes that a political party receives in an election. This means that smaller—and usually not dominant—political parties can gain influence in policymaking to a much greater extent than is the case in first-past-the-post systems that are typical of liberal political economies. Left or social democratic parties have been able to use this mechanism to further their goals of more comprehensive welfare states such that the presence of proportional representation is an excellent predictor of size and depth of welfare states.

Canada does not have proportional representation, but has had periods of minority federal governments where the left party (the CCF and later the NDP) have held the balance of power. It was during these times, especially during the 1960s, that progressive changes such as public pensions and Canada's health care system were established. In Canada, the establishment of proportional representation would enable smaller political parties like the New Democratic Party and the Green Party to gain more seats and more influence on the political system and on public policy outcomes. The arguments for proportional representation raise interesting issues with respect to the welfare state. This is an area rich for further research into its value in furthering the welfare state and the development of health care and health-related public policy.

◼ CONCLUSIONS

This chapter has examined the form and function of the welfare state. It examined how and why Canada fits into Esping-Andersen's liberal welfare state group. Being a liberal welfare state has shaped the Canadian approach to health and social programs. And how Canada approaches these issues has implications for population health. More developed welfare states show increased public health and social expenditures and better population health.

Social democratic regimes have the highest investment in health and social spending and the best population health outcomes, while liberal welfare states have the lowest spending and worse outcomes. In addition, Canada's spending in these areas has declined since the 1980s. Already at a disadvantage, the Canadian response to the economic pressure associated with increasing economic globalization has further weakened the Canadian welfare state.

Much of this has to do with Canada already being a liberal welfare state. In addition, the absence of proportional representation also makes it more difficult for left-leaning political parties, such as the NDP and the Green Party, to influence public policy. The liberal political economies appear to be more susceptible to neo-liberal-influenced responses to the demands of economic globalization, an issue further addressed in the next chapter.

■ REFERENCES

Alesina, A. & Glaeser, E.L. (2004). *Fighting poverty in the US and Europe: A world of difference.* Toronto: Oxford University Press.

Arts, W. & Gelissen, J. (2001). Welfare states, solidarity, and justice principles: Does the type really matter? *ACTA Sociologica, 44*, 283–299.

Bambra, C. (2004). The worlds of welfare: Illusory and gender blind? *Social Policy and Society, 3*(3), 201–211.

Banting, K. (1997). The social policy divide: The welfare state in Canada and the United States. In K. Banting, G. Hoberg & R. Simeon (Eds.), *Degrees of freedom: Canada and the United States in a changing world*, (267–309). Montreal & Kingston: McGill-Queen's University Press.

Bernard, P. & Saint-Arnaud, S. (2004). *More of the same: The position of the four largest Canadian provinces in the world of welfare regimes.* Ottawa: Canadian Policy Research Networks.

Coburn, D. (2006). Health and health care: A political economy perspective. In D. Raphael, T. Bryant & M. Rioux (Eds.), *Staying alive: Critical perspectives on health, illness, and health care* (pp. 59–84). Toronto: Canadian Scholars' Press Inc.

Esping-Andersen, G. (1985). *Politics against markets: The social democratic road to power.* Princeton: Princeton University Press.

Esping-Andersen, G. (1990). *The three worlds of welfare capitalism.* Princeton: Princeton University Press.

Esping-Andersen, G. (1999). *Social foundations of post-industrial economies.* New York: Oxford University Press.

Hemrijck, A. (2002). The self-tranformation of the European model. In G. Esping-Andersen (Ed.), *Why we need a new welfare state* (pp. 173–214). Oxford: Oxford University Press.

Kasza, G. (2002). The illusion of welfare regimes. *Journal of Social Policy, 31*(2), 271–287.

Murphy, B., Roberts, P. & Wolfson, M. (2007). High-income Canadians. *Perspectives on Labour and Income, 8*, 1–13.

Myers, K. & de Broucker, P. (2006). *Too many left behind: Canada's adult education and training system.* Ottawa: Canadian Policy Research Networks.

Myles, J. (1998). How to design a "liberal" welfare state: A comparison of Canada and the United States. *Social Policy and Administration, 32*(4), 341–364.

Navarro, V., Borrell, C., Benach, J., Muntaner, C., Quiroga, A., Rodrigues-Sanz, M. et al. (2004). The importance of the political and the social in explaining mortality differentials among the countries of the OECD, 1950–1998. In V. Navarro (Ed.), *The political and social contexts of health*, 11–86. Amityville: Baywood Press.

Navarro, V. & Shi, L. (2001). The political context of social inequalities and health. *International Journal of Health Services, 31*(1), 1–21.

Olsen, G. (2002). *The politics of the welfare state.* Toronto: Oxford University Press.

Organisation for Economic Co-operation and Development. (2005). *Health at a glance: OECD indicators 2005.* Paris: Organisation for Economic Co-operation and Development.

Organisation for Economic Co-operation and Development. (2007). *Society at a glance: OECD social indicators 2007 edition.* Paris: Organization for Economic Cooperation and Development.

Raphael, D. (2003). Addressing the social determinants of health in Canada: Bridging the gap between research findings and public policy. *Policy Options, 24*(3), 35–40.

Raphael, D. (2007a). Canadian public policy and poverty in international perspective. In D. Raphael (Ed.), *Poverty and policy in Canada: Implications for health and quality of life,* 335–364. Toronto: Canadian Scholars' Press Inc.

Raphael, D. (2007b). Interactions with the health and service sector. In D. Raphael (Ed.), *Poverty and policy in Canada: Implications for health and quality of life,* 173–199. Toronto: Canadian Scholars' Press Inc.

Raphael, D. (Ed.). (2007c). *Social determinants of health: Canadian perspectives* (2nd ed.). Toronto: Canadian Scholars' Press Inc.

Saint-Arnaud, S. & Bernard, P. (2003). Convergence or resilience? A hierarchical cluster analysis of the welfare regimes in advanced countries. *Current Sociology, 51*(5), 499–527.

Sanmartin, C. & Ng, E. (2004). *Joint Canada/United States survey of health, 2002–03.* Ottawa: Statistics Canada.

Siddiqi, A. & Hertzman, C. (2007). Towards an epidemiological understanding of the effects of long-term institutional changes on population health: A case study of Canada versus the USA. *Social Science & Medicine, 64*(3), 589–603.

Swank, D. (1992). Politics and the structural dependence of the state in democratic capitalist nations. *American Political Science Review, 86*(1), 38–54.

Swank, D. (1998). *Global capital, democracy, and the welfare state: Why political institutions are so important in shaping the domestic response to internationalization.* Berkeley: Centre for German and European Studies, University of California at Berkeley.

Teeple, G. (2000). *Globalization and the decline of social reform: Into the twenty-first century.* Aurora: Garamond Press.

Teeple, G. (2006). Foreword. In D. Raphael, T. Bryant & M. Rioux (Eds.), *Staying alive: Critical perspectives on health, illness, and health care,* 1–4. Toronto: Canadian Scholars' Press Inc.

Townsend, P. (1993). *The international analysis of poverty.* Milton Keynes: Harvester Wheatsheaf.

von Kempski, J. (1972). Zur Logik der Ordungsbegriffe, besonders in den Sozialwissenschaften. In H. Albert (Ed.), *Theorie und Realitat. Ausgewahlte Aufsatze zur Wissenschaftslehre der Sozialwissenschaften,* 115–138. Tubingen: J.C.B. Mohr (Paul Siebeck).

CRITICAL THINKING QUESTIONS

1. What was your reaction upon finding that Canada is considered a liberal welfare state?

2. To what extent should business interests dictate health policy in Canada?

3. Should the Canadian approach to provisions of citizen benefits and supports be reoriented to be more like those seen in European nations? What would be the arguments in favour of this? What arguments could be used to oppose this shift?

4. What public policies would need to be changed to improve the economic security of Canadians, thereby improving their health and quality of life?

5. What are some of the barriers to having Canadians become aware of the importance of public policies addressing economic and social security as determinants of health and quality of life?

FURTHER READINGS

Bambra, C. (2007). Going beyond the three worlds of welfare capitalism: Regime theory and public health research. *Journal of Epidemiology and Community Health 61*(12), 1098–1102.

In this analysis, Bambra reviews the original Esping-Andersen typology of welfare states and provides the range of related conceptualizations. Most of these find Canada to be a firm exemplar of a liberal welfare state.

Banting, K., Hoberg, G. et al. (Eds.). (1997). *Degrees of freedom: Canada and the United States in a changing world.* Montreal & Kingston: McGill-Queen's University Press.

A comparative study of Canadian and American responses to the changing international economy and to changing patterns of social diversity in domestic society, *Degrees of Freedom* traces the impact of these pressures on the economic and social structure, culture, political institutions, and policy regimes of the two countries.

Eikemo, T. & Bambra, C. (2008). The welfare state: A glossary for public health. *Journal of Epidemiology and Community Health, 62*, 3–6.

This article provides background information on welfare states for those working in the health field.

Esping-Andersen, G. (1990). *The three worlds of welfare capitalism.* Princeton: Princeton University Press.
Esping-Andersen, G. (1999). *Social foundations of postindustrial economies.* Toronto: Oxford University Press.

These two books provide a typology of Western welfare states that takes into account a range of social policies and links these with variations in the historical development of Western countries. The author describes how profound differences that exist among liberal (e.g., the US, Canada, the UK), conservative (e.g., Germany, France, Italy), and social democratic (e.g., Sweden, Norway, Denmark) political economies translate into widely differing lived experiences among citizens of these nations.

Organisation for Economic Co-operation and Development. (2007). *Health at a glance: OECD indicators 2007*. Paris: Organisation for Economic Co-operation and Development.

Organisation for Economic Co-operation and Development. (2007). *Society at a glance: OECD social indicators 2007 Edition*. Paris: Organisation for Economic Co-operation and Development.

These reports provide a wealth of data that puts Canadian social and health indicators within an international perspective.

RELEVANT WEBSITES

Clare Bambra's website at the University of Durham, UK
www.dur.ac.uk/school.health/staff/?username=dhs0cb1

Dr. Bambra's research focuses on public policy and health inequalities; work and health; comparative social policy, politics, and health; and urban regeneration and health. She has many articles listed on welfare states and social and health indicators.

Innocenti Research Centre (IRC)
www.unicef-icdc.org

The IRC works to strengthen the capacity of UNICEF and its co-operating institutions to respond to the evolving needs of children and to develop a new global ethic for children. It promotes the effective implementation of the Convention on the Rights of the Child in both developing and industrialized countries, thereby reaffirming the universality of children's rights and of UNICEF's mandate.

Organisation for Economic Co-operation and Development
www.oecd.org

This site provides a wealth of reports, publications, and statistics about every aspect of society in modern industrialized states. Many of its contents are free or available electronically through a university's library.

Public Policy at The Robert Gordon University
www2.rgu.ac.uk/publicpolicy

An introduction to social policy. This module on social policy examines social welfare and its relationship to politics and society. It focuses on the social services and the welfare state.

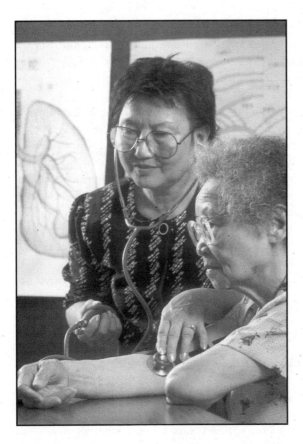

Chapter 10

CANADIAN FEDERALISM, THE CANADIAN SOCIAL UNION, AND HEALTH POLICY

■ INTRODUCTION

Canadian federalism has been both a support and impediment with regard to the development of health policy in Canada (Prince, 2003). On one hand, it initially provided a vehicle for the federal government to use its spending power to finance health and social programs. On the other hand, federalism has come to be a continuing source of conflict between the two levels of government as provincial governments demand more and more federal dollars to support health and social programs. Until recently, it seemed that federalism could not be restored to the state of co-operation between the two levels of government that was seen during the 1950s and 1960s when the Canadian welfare state as we know it came about (Noel, St-Hilaire & Fortin, 2003).

The era of co-operative federalism in which the two levels of governments participated in cost-sharing of many health care and health-related public policy programs came to an apparent end in the 1980s (Cameron & Simeon, 2002). By 1980, increasing concern with reducing budget deficits led to health care and various social programs becoming the targets of governmental restructuring and retrenchment. Rather than seeing budget deficits as resulting from policies that shrank revenues, the culprits were seen as being health care and other program spending (Banting, 1997). The "politics of fiscal deficits" not only began to shape intergovernmental relations but also public perceptions as to the causes and solutions to the growing public sector deficits.

In recent years the federal and provincial governments have hammered out different agreements in an attempt to renew the spirit of co-operation in social provision that had prevailed during the creation of the welfare state. The Social Union Framework Agreement (SUFA) was the product of such negotiations in 1999. It was followed by the health accords of 2000, 2003, and 2004. These agreements represent a collaborative federalism in which the federal and provincial governments work together in these policy areas (Noel et al., 2003). This chapter examines SUFA and the health accords of 2000, 2003, and 2004, and considers their impact on the development and implementation of health policy in Canada. The chapter also considers the prospect for continued collaborations among the federal and provincial/territorial governments in these efforts.

■ A BRIEF HISTORY OF CANADIAN FEDERALISM

Prince (2003) and others have identified three primary periods of Canadian federalism: (1) co-operative federalism, (2) executive federalism, and (3) collaborative federalism. Although largely descriptive categories, these periods as designated can help to locate different intergovernmental initiatives in health and social policy.

Co-operative Federalism: 1950s to the early 1960s

The first period is the 1950s to the early 1960s, which is characterized as co-operative federalism. This was the stage in which the two levels of government cost-shared social programs to ensure universal access to these programs. There was general recognition and acceptance by both governments of their obligations for social provision. For many, this was the golden age of the Canadian welfare state that saw the creation of the Canadian health care system and the general growth of social programs and services.

Executive Federalism: Mid-1960s to the 1990s

The second phase from the mid-1960s to the 1990s is described as executive federalism, a term coined by Doug Smiley (Smiley, 1980). Smiley argued that during this period Canada drifted away from what he termed "classical federalism," in which each order of government carried out the responsibilities assigned to it by the Constitution. Smiley defined executive federalism "as the relations between elected and appointed officials of the two levels of government in federal-provincial interactions and among the executives of the provinces in interprovincial interactions" (p. 91). Smiley argued that the institutions and processes of executive federalism began to become more oriented toward conflict rather than consensus.

Box 10.1: The Social Union Framework Agreement

The "social union" initiative is the umbrella under which governments will concentrate their efforts to renew and modernize Canadian social policy. It focuses on the pan-Canadian dimension of health and social policy systems; the linkages between the social and economic unions; and the recognition that reform is best achieved in partnership among provinces, territories, and the government of Canada. The primary objective of the social union initiative is to reform and renew Canada's system of social services and to reassure Canadians that their pan-Canadian social programs are strong and secure. In working to build a strong social union, the government of Canada and the provinces and territories have reached a broad consensus that the first priorities should be children in poverty and people with disabilities.

First ministers created the Federal-Provincial-Territorial Council on Social Policy Renewal in 1996. The purpose of the council was to guide the social union initiative. The council monitors activities on overarching social policy issues and, as well, coordinates and supports "sectoral" councils that examine cross-sectoral issues such as supporting children and people with disabilities. The council includes representation from nine provinces, three territories, and the government of Canada, and is co-chaired by Diane Finley, minister of Human Resources and Social Development Canada, and Chester Gillian, minister of Health and Social Services, Prince Edward Island.

Source: http://www.socialunion.ca/menu_e.html

Collaborative Federalism: Mid-1990s into 2000s

Finally, the current era of federalism reflects recognition by both levels of government of a crisis in Canadian federalism to the point of being almost dysfunctional. Simeon and Willis describe a "widespread sense of policy and institutional failure" (Simeon & Willis, 1997, p. 150). It is essentially driven by an agenda of reparation (Prince, 2003). This reparation has occurred in the face of demands by the provinces and territories for stable, predictable, and sufficient funding of social transfers and programs. The reinstatement of previously frozen and reduced federal funding was apparent in the restored federal funding levels in the Health Accord of 2003 under the Canada Health and Social Transfer, and is also evident in the transfers to the provinces for programs for people with disabilities.

■ IMPLICATIONS OF RECENT DEVELOPMENTS FOR HEALTH POLICY

Related to these phases of Canadian federalism are the actual policy processes that took place. Prince specifies four principal phases of recent national policy change and spending from the 1980s through the 1990s (Prince, 2003). Prince's phases refer to public policy orientations rather than focusing on the nature of intergovernmental relations. There is an attempt to make sense of the types of policies that emerged at each phase.

1980–1984: Maintaining Governmental Roles

The period 1980–1984 saw the maintenance of the important role that governments played in social provision even in the light of economic shocks taking place as globalization began to take hold (Myles, 1998).

1984–1988: Restraining Social Program Costs

However, governmental commitments to the maintenance of health and social programs began to weaken during the mid-1980s. Upon election of his party to power in Ottawa in 1984, Conservative Prime Minister Brian Mulroney initiated a number of actions that increased provincial spending requirements for health and other programs. Mulroney froze federal transfers to the provincial governments for health care and post-secondary education (Banting, 1997). In the health care field, this development represented the first retreat by the federal government in meeting its obligations to health care under the Canada Health Act.

This phase also marked the beginning of the rise of global economic pressures on nation-states that culminated in the free trade era. The 1988 election became a referendum on free trade, which the Conservatives won in spite of significant opposition to free trade during the lead-up to the election. In 1989, Canada and the US signed the Free Trade Agreement.

Much of the opposition to free trade agreements centred on their potential threat to medicare and other social programs. The belief was that the requirements for open investment contained in these agreements made it difficult for nations to pass laws that protect publicly provided health care and other services from being open to private investment and potential takeover. As such, these agreements could be seen as threatening the ability of governments to set domestic policy. National sovereignty in numerous policy areas could be weakened. These issues are taken up in the following chapter.

1988–1997: Restructuring the Role of Government

From 1988–1997, the federal government—both Conservative and Liberal—began to restructure the role of government in social provision. This was associated with significant curtailing of federal—and in some cases provincial—health care and other program spending. The term "restructuring" can be seen as a euphemism for significantly reduced governmental social spending.

By the time the Free Trade Agreement came into effect in 1989, then Prime Minister Mulroney reduced federal transfers to the provinces, forcing them to bear a greater proportion of health and other social program costs. The federal government spared few social programs. For example, in 1995, the new federal Liberal government of Jean Chrétien replaced the Established Programs Financing Act (EPF) (1977) with the Canada Health and Social Transfer (CHST) (Brooks & Miljan, 2003). Under the CHST, the federal government began to retreat from its commitment to match provincial spending on health. From then on, the federal contribution to health would be based on the previous year's level of provincial spending, adjusted to take into account change in a province's gross provincial product. As a result, Ottawa's share of public health care spending fell steadily.

Also, prior to the CHST, provinces had been provided with separate funding envelopes for health care, social services, and post-secondary education. Under the CHST, only one funding envelope was provided such that provinces came to decide how CHST monies would be allocated. Since health care was seen as the main priority by most provincial governments, funds were made available for this budget area at the expense of the other funding areas. This led to profound reductions in many provinces to social assistance funding, which adversely affected the less well-off.

1997 to the Present: Repairing the Social Union

By 1997, governments of all stripes began to recognize that the social infrastructure was deteriorating and that there was a need to reinvest in social programs. Hence, the federal, provincial, and territorial governments decided to redefine the social union. Prince notes that the social union is a broad term that refers to three separate issues (Prince, 2003).

Box 10.2: The Social Union Framework (SUFA) and the Social Union

Prince distinguishes between SUFA and the social union (Prince, 2003). SUFA is one agreement. Prince defines the social union as referring to three different issues. The first is a sequence of processes and structures instigated by the annual premiers' conference in 1995, and thereafter by the Provincial/Territorial Council on Social Policy Renewal. The second is the policy decisions and intergovernmental relations such as action plans, budget allocations, and program changes that emerged. And the third is perspectives on federalism and social policy. Prince argues that this latter stage also exemplifies the belief systems about the appropriate roles of and relationships between states, the economy, families, and communities. In short, the social union "refers to the long-term ideas and infrastructure of Canadian social policy" (Prince, 2003, p. 126).

Source: Prince, M.J. (2003). SUFA: Sea change or mere ripple for Canadian social policy? In S. Fortin, A. Noel & F. St-Hilaire (Eds.), *Forging the Canadian social union: SUFA and beyond*, 122–156. Montreal: Institute for Research on Public Policy.

■ THE SOCIAL UNION FRAMEWORK INITIATIVE AND AGREEMENT (SUFA)

The "social union" initiative refers to government efforts to renew and modernize Canadian social policy. It aims to strengthen the role of government vis-à-vis social provision as entitlements to citizens. The focus is on national health and social policy systems, the linkages between the social and economic unions, and the recognition that reform is best managed co-operatively among the provincial, territorial, and the federal governments (see Box 10.3). The concept of a social union is that a unified nation shares a set of norms, standards, and objectives concerning the basic elements of social citizenship (Cameron & Simeon, 2002).

Box 10.3: The Purpose of SUFA

Alain Noel and others at the Institute for Research on Public Policy argue that the purpose of the Social Union Framework formulated in 1999, and the health accords that followed in 2000 and 2003, was to provide the basis for more constructive and co-operative intergovernmental relationships, or more collaborative/co-operative federalism in social policy (Noel, St-Hilaire & Fortin, 2003). SUFA was intended to provide common guiding principles and a code of conduct for interactions between the federal, provincial, and territorial governments in health care, post-secondary education, training, social assistance, and social services. Its objectives were to:

- help governments work together to address the needs of Canadians;
- establish adequate, stable, and sustainable funding for social programs;
- undertake efforts to avoid administrative overlap and duplication;
- mediate and resolve intergovernmental disputes, and improve public accountability and transparency.

Source: Noel, A., St-Hilaire, F. & Fortin, S. (2003). Learning from the SUFA experience. In S. Fortin, A. Noel & F. St-Hilaire (Eds.), *Forging the Canadian social union: SUFA and beyond*, 1–29. Montreal: Institute for Public Policy Research.

Prior to the signing of SUFA, the federal government used the 1995 budget to bring down the federal deficit primarily through spending reductions (Facal, 2005). It reviewed its spending programs in its own areas of jurisdiction, but also radically reduced its transfer payments to the provinces. With its introduction of the Canada Health and Social Transfer (CHST), actual federal funding cuts of $6 billion occurred over a two-year period. These cuts took place in health care, social services, and post-secondary education. In addition to its lofty stated aims, SUFA was also an attempt to placate the provincial and territorial governments by sketching out controls over federal actions.

The SUFA itself is a non-constitutional yet formal agreement intended to clarify the roles of the two levels of government in public policy (Fortin, Noel & St-Hilaire, 2003). The federal, provincial, and territorial governments (with the exception of Quebec) signed the document in February 1999. SUFA was intended to renew the social union and make explicit the obligations and commitments of the two levels of government in the health, social services, post-secondary education, social assistance, and training policy domains.

In practice, SUFA was an attempt to specify the means by which the federal government could exercise—yet be under some provincial control—its power in public policy areas that the Canadian Constitution identifies as exclusive provincial jurisdiction (Cameron & Simeon, 2002; Facal, 2005). The agreement prohibits the unilateral use by the federal government of its spending power.

The first ministers stated that the SUFA provided a template for fostering more constructive and co-operative relations between the federal, provincial, and territorial governments in health and social provision (Fortin et al., 2003). First ministers are the heads of the federal and provincial and territorial governments; that is, the prime minister and the premiers of the provinces and territories. One of the first sets of agreements to emerge from SUFA has been concerned with health care. Concerns have been raised about the elitist nature of SUFA (see Box 10.4).

Box 10.4: Concerns with the SUFA

Policy analysts have criticized the document as an exemplar of "elite accommodation" (Cameron & Simeon, 2002). Others argue that SUFA fails to define social union and to resolve the disputes that brought it into being (Noel et al., 2003). In short, it is considered little more than rhetoric on paper. Another concern was that Quebec had not signed on to the agreement. Quebec had not participated actively in interprovincial meetings from 1995 to mid-1998 (Facal, 2005). The Quebec government refused to endorse SUFA because the other provinces did not appear ready to support its demand for recognition of the unconditional right to opt out with full financial compensation from the federal government for any province prepared to assume full responsibility in areas of exclusive provincial jurisdiction. A similar rationale led to the development of the health accords of 2000 and 2003.

Sources: Cameron, D. & Simeon, R. (2002). Intergovernmental relations in Canada: The emergence of collaborative federalism. *Publius: The Journal of Federalism* 32(2), 49–71; Noel, A., St-Hilaire, F. & Fortin, S. (2003). Learning from the SUFA experience. In S. Fortin, A. Noel & F. St-Hilaire (Eds.), *Forging the Canadian social union: SUFA and beyond*, 1–29. Montreal: Institute for Public Policy Research; Facal, J. (2005). *Social policy and intergovernmental relations in Canada: Understanding the failure of SUFA from a Quebec perspective*. Public Policy Paper 32. Regina: University of Regina.

■ THE HEALTH ACCORDS OF 2000, 2003, AND 2004

The first focus of federal and provincial governments meetings under SUFA was to consider health care issues. As a result of these meetings, the federal health minister and his provincial and territorial counterparts produced two health accords in 2000 and 2003.

The Health Accord of 2000

The health accord of 2000 increased federal transfer payments to provinces and territories for health care and other programs through the Canada Health and Social Transfers by $21.1 billion over five years (Noel et al., 2003). The short title for the first Health Accord Agreement was the Accord on Health Care Renewal. This sum also included $2.2 billion for early childhood development within the CHST. The health care-related funds entailed:

- $1 billion over two years to the provinces and territories to shore up necessary diagnostic and treatment equipment;
- $800 million to provinces and territories for innovation and reforms in primary care;
- $500 million to Canada Health Infoway to help expedite the adoption of modern information technologies in order to ensure better health care.

The Canada Health Infoway is an independent, non-profit agency with a membership comprising 14 federal, provincial, and territorial deputy ministers of health (Canada Health Infoway, 2007). Its mandate is to facilitate the use of electronic health information systems and electronic health records across Canada.

Some considered the accord of 2000 to be a pre-election stopgap initiated by the federal government to defuse the health care issue (Fortin et al., 2003). While transfer payment increases announced at the same time were considerable—at $21.1 billion over five years—they have not to date had a significant impact on health services (Fortin et al., 2003).

Health Accord 2003

Three years later in 2003, the first ministers returned to the bargaining table to negotiate a new health accord, which followed the release of the reports on health reform by Senator Michael Kirby and Roy Romanow (Noel et al., 2003). This accord provided more federal funding for primary health care, home care, and catastrophic drug coverage. This accord was clearly a response to the recommendations of the Kirby and Romanow reports on health care reform. The accord also created an independent Health Council of Canada. The membership would consist of health care experts, representatives from both levels of government, and the public with the goal of monitoring and reporting on health care and broader population health issues.

Like the previous health accord of 2000, the health accord increased federal funding. The first ministers established an "enhanced accountability framework" (Canada Department of Finance, 2007). Under the framework, the first ministers committed to providing comprehensive and regular reports to the public based on comparable indicators pertaining to health status, health outcomes, and quality of services. Governments agreed to establish the Health Council, as recommended by Romanow, to monitor and provide annual public reports on the implementation of the accord.

The accord was also intended to improve wait times for care, access to home and community care, as well as provide catastrophic drug coverage. These provisions were consistent with Kirby's recommendations, so the 2003 accord may have been seen as a way of satisfying some requirements of the federal reports on health care reform. The 2003 health accord was intended, like the SUFA before it, to bring about "more constructive and cooperative federalism" (Noel, St-Hilaire and Fortin, 2003, 1). Following its implementation, however, the premiers expressed their dismay about what they considered to be less than adequate levels of federal funding.

Health Accord 2004

The first ministers met again in 2004 and added to the commitments made in the 2003 Health Accord (Health Canada, 2006). The Health Accord of 2004—also known as the 10-Year Plan to Strengthen Health Care—promises to sustain and renew the health care system, and assures long-term funding to achieve these goals. The 2004 accord also promises to reduce wait times for care and improve access with a focus on cancer care and heart treatments, diagnostic imaging, joint replacements and sight restoration. The federal investments of $41 billion over 10 years specified in the 2004 accord enables governments to plan ahead with the assurance of enhanced federal funding. The first ministers also committed to regular reports on the performance of the health care system to the Canadian public.

The concern remains whether these commitments of renewal and improved funding levels are merely words on paper. The next sections consider the impacts of the 2000, 2003, and 2004 health accords in particular, and the SUFA in general.

■ EVALUATION OF THE IMPACT OF SUFA AND THE HEALTH ACCORDS

SUFA and the 2000, 2003, and 2004 health accords are intended to foster more co-operative relations between the two levels of government in the health and social policy fields (Noel et al., 2003). To date, it is unclear what impact any of these agreements have had on health and social service provision by either level of government.

While SUFA provided the federal and provincial governments some room to manoeuvre in their health reform efforts, it has provided little fostering of political debate over two critical issues on the health policy agenda (Maioni, 2000). These are: Who should be allowed to set the rules in health care? What should the rules be? Perhaps the most critical issue is what role the federal government should play in the health care sector with respect to setting the rules.

And concerning these rules, a primary question, which appears to be a focus of provincial concern: What should be the boundaries between the public sector and private markets in provincial health care systems? A key issue underlying both these questions is whether private markets should have a role in health care delivery at all (see Box 10.5).

Although both federal and provincial governments have welcomed a private sector role, some have argued that involvement of the private sector runs counter to the spirit, if not the provisions, of the Canada Health Act (Rachlis, 2004). Others argue that private sector financing and delivery of health care services jeopardizes the sustainability of public health care itself (Canadian Health Coalition, 2008). Rather than address the problems of the public health care system, private sector involvement may worsen the situation.

Box 10.5: Privatized Medical Care No Cure for Waiting Lists
By Colleen M. Flood and Meghan McMahon
Toronto Star

A constitutional challenge to Ontario legislation that prohibits the purchase of private health insurance for medically necessary health care services (dubbed the "Ontario Chaoulli") was announced on Sept. 5.

It's another call for increased privatization, based on the misinformed notion that an expanded role for private insurance will remedy wait times in Canada.

Just last month, the outgoing president of the Canadian Medical Association, Dr. Colin McMillan, put forward Medicare Plus, the CMA's solution for sustaining our health care system. It proposed expanding the role for private insurance and private payment, and allowing physicians to work for the public system and treat private patients, too.

After a stream of backlash from the Canadian Healthcare Association, the Registered Nurses Association of Ontario, Canadian Doctors for Medicare, and others, the CMA responded by saying that it is time to examine the nature of the public versus private health care debate.

Indeed it is. Will the CMA's recommendations make Medicare better? The evidence says no.

Currently, Canadian regulations prevent doctors who are paid by public Medicare from also providing medically necessary care for private payment.

But doctors can "opt out" of the public system and "go private" (except in Ontario).

Why do we have this regulation? Because if we didn't, doctors would naturally want to spend much more of their time than they presently do treating private patients—as these patients often have easier conditions to treat and they (or their insurer) will pay more.

A doctor, like any normal person, will be attracted to working for more and doing less—who can blame them? So it is not surprising that some members of the CMA like the idea of Medicare Plus.

But from the public's perspective, and from the perspective of most patients, it's a bad idea. If you are a patient wealthy enough to pay privately or you have private insurance, then you may fare better under Medicare Plus. But lines for treatment in the public hospitals will grow longer and longer.

The CMA's recommendation also ignores the simple fact that, in the absence of an increase in the number of doctors (where will we get them from?), the introduction of a parallel private system must mean that the doctors we do have will be distributed between both public and private patients.

Private patients will pay more to have their medical needs met on a preferential basis, leaving public patients on ever-growing waiting lists. Evidence suggests that allowing doctors to practise in the public and private sectors will not, as Medicare Plus states, "improve access for the entire population."

Other countries that allow doctors to work on an unregulated basis in the public and private sectors—like New Zealand, the UK, and Ireland—currently have, or have had, chronic problems with long waiting lists.

The evidence doesn't seem to indicate that having parallel private health insurance or "Medicare Plus" has cured waiting lists in these countries. Where waiting lists have been wrestled down—as in the UK—it has been through a huge infusion of public money and improvements in the management of public hospitals. The cure has not come from more private money or private insurance.

And countries like France that appear to have a large private sector actually heavily regulate doctors who work privately—including the price they can charge and the amount of time they can spend treating private patients. So what looks on the surface to be "private" is not really: it's quasi-public because of such heavy regulation.

So we could follow the European route—and heavily regulate doctors who "go private"—or we can stick with the cleaner and simpler approach of requiring doctors who are paid by public Medicare to be paid only by Medicare but still allow doctors to "go private" if they are prepared to work completely within the private payment sector.

But we have to recognize that even with European-style regulation we would be embracing the idea that it's fine for folks with more money to jump queues and get preferential treatment from doctors.

This is in direct opposition to the principle of equity that has historically guided the Canadian Medicare system, which was created in part to eliminate distinctions between the rich and poor in access to medically necessary health-care.

Canada's healthcare system needs reform—but reform based on the best available evidence and guided by Canadian values. On the issue of waiting times, for example, the Institute of Health Services and Policy Research—part of the Canadian Institutes of Health Research—funded research that helped establish the first-ever national benchmarks for waiting times in December 2005. CIHR-IHSPR is committed to providing evidence-based solutions that will improve the health care system. Let us not make the mistake of misusing the wealth of evidence that strongly supports a public health-care system like Canadian medicare.

Source: The Toronto Star (September 18, 2007), AA8

■ SUFA, HEALTH CARE, AND HEALTH-RELATED PUBLIC POLICY

Some question the "privileged" position of health care in the debate on the SUFA (McIntosh, 2000). Specifically, McIntosh cautions that other aspects of the social union—much of it concerned with health-related public policy—could be abandoned in the process. Further, he argues that labour market policies are especially important in that they lie at the centre of social and economic policies, which "makes their overall direction a crucial component of a re-created social union" (p. 48).

Yet, McIntosh agrees that the "crisis" in the health system is real and requires the attention of policy analysts and governments. But labour market policy is also about health and clearly constitutes an important health-related public policy area. As an important social determinant of health employment (Jackson, 2004; Tremblay, 2004), McIntosh notes that secure attachment to the labour market in "well-paid, meaningful employment" is critical to human health and well-being (p. 48).

Indeed, McIntosh highlights the obsession of Canadian politicians with health care and the failure to consider promoting human health and well-being as a critical health policy outcome. He also notes the lack of an overarching vision for labour market policy or any other public policy and little consideration of potential consequences of continuing in such a manner.

The federal, provincial, and territorial governments renewed the Social Union Framework Agreement in 2002, but even then it was apparent that it was becoming peripheral to the actual functions and ongoing negotiations taking place in intergovernmental relations. The document said much about building for the future, but as Pat and Hugh Armstrong and others have argued, it does nothing to prevent further erosion of health care (Armstrong & Armstrong, 2003). The health accords lack enforcement mechanisms. They are statements of commitment, but provide little direction for governmental action.

■ IMPLICATIONS OF THE NEGLECT OF SUFA

The Social Union Framework Agreement was intended to assure the Canadian public of the willingness and ability of Canadian governments to co-operate. Gibbins (2003), of the Canada West Foundation, argues that SUFA was perceived by some as representing a fundamental transformation of the Canadian federal system that would usher in an "unprecedented level of cooperation, formality and civility to intergovernmental relations" (Gibbins, 2003, 31). It had also assured increased citizen participation in the previously exclusive world of intergovernmental relations. Others noted that SUFA excluded Quebec, which was seen as a major flaw, but the health accord struck in the fall of 2000 at least brought Quebec into the SUFA framework in health care.

Lazar argues that SUFA is primarily about process rather than outcomes (Lazar, 2000). It is primarily concerned with how governments should relate to one another and to citizens in making social policy. It says rather less about developing new social policy commitments (Lazar, 2000). The SUFA calls for joint federal-provincial planning and coordination in social policy, more citizen and stakeholder participation in decision making, and increased accountability and transparency. Lazar concludes that SUFA is potentially "a major departure in Canadian social policy and in the management of the federation" (Lazar, 2000, 11). He notes that it is difficult to assess its impact because most of its activities have occurred behind closed doors. In short, the process has not increased transparency or increased citizen involvement, a key component of the agreement.

SUFA has failed to change the politics of social policy or health reform (Maioni, 2000). The warring between the two levels of government continues. This is particularly so since the federal government has tended to focus on particular health care issues such as wait times, which seems to exacerbate tensions between the federal and provincial governments. The intent was to renew collaborative federalism that had characterized the 1950s and 1960s when the two levels of government cost-shared social and health programs. There was a commitment to ensure that all citizens had access to necessary health care and social programs.

Governments were cognizant of their obligations to ensure universal access to social programs.

What is also significant is that none of the health accords even refers to the Social Union Framework (Noel et al., 2003). It is therefore questionable how much impact the SUFA has had on the health accords. The agreements outline commitments to public accountability, transparency, and joint planning specified in the Social Union Framework. What they appear to have excluded were agreement on key issues such as the level of the federal financial commitment to health care and the appropriate level to ensure sustainable funding, and how the provinces are to report on how they spend this contribution. At least, the 2004 health accord enhanced the mandate and scope of the new Health Council. In the end, the documents spout much rhetoric, but no action or commitment on the part of any governments to health care and its sustainability into the future.

In addition, the Social Union Framework Agreement and the health accords provide promises with respect to health care, such as upholding the principles enshrined in the Canada Health Act. They do not specify, however, how these principles will be ensured. Nor do they address the issues of privatization and increased commercialization of health care that commentators such as the Canadian Centre for Policy Alternatives, various provincial governments, and others consider to be key issues.

The federal government has a role to play in preventing the further commercialization of health care. As Maioni argues, the agreement neither addresses nor offers means to address the continuing dispute over who should set the rules in the health sector, or what rules should govern the Canadian health care system (Maioni, 2000).

■ ABSENCE OF QUEBEC

What is notable is Quebec's absence from the SUFA. The federal and provincial governments, with the exception of Quebec, affirmed federal spending in areas of provincial jurisdiction and specified the rules for intergovernmental relations in social policy. Trying to make sense of Quebec's absence, Noel asks, "If the situation is so one-sided, why did all provincial and territorial governments except Quebec accept the agreement?"(Noel, 2001 58–59). Quebec may have objected to the affirming of the federal spending power and, by extension, its authority in exclusive provincial jurisdiction. At first ministers' meetings, Quebec asserted its right to opt out of national programs and receive federal compensation.

Noel suggests that SUFA brought together a process that was already underway, which he attributes to federal fiscal and social policies (Noel, 2001). He adds that initiatives on the Social Union by the provinces and territories did not emanate from a wish to collaborate on social policy. Rather, they emanated from a desire on the part of these governments to rail against the CHST and the reduced federal cash transfers that it brought. This does not mean that the provinces and territories are more socially progressive and enlightened than the federal government. On the contrary, the provinces and territories wanted limits on the federal spending power that would be consistent with the decreasing value and reliability of federal transfers. Noel suggests that the Quebec government, under then Premier Lucien Bouchard, united with the other provinces after the federal government implemented the National Child Benefit. In the end, the provinces and territories acted to protect themselves. This provided yet another opportunity for Quebec also to oppose federally imposed requirements.

Noel concludes that a more constructive stance for the provinces and territories would be to change the course of events by taking advantage of the SUFA review and renewal process to re-establish a common position and advocate simple but forceful demands (Noel et al., 2003). These would be demanding increases in social transfers and repairing the fiscal imbalance. In the same vein, they could also attempt to insert an enforcement mechanism in the form of a statement of principle in SUFA for "adequate, affordable, stable and sustainable funding for social programs" (p. 3).

SUFA has failed to protect social programs such as medicare from further commercialization. The framework and health accords reflect governments' general tendency to develop social policy in a vacuum. The processes that led to SUFA and the health accords of 2000, 2003, and 2004 reflect unwillingness by both levels of government to address the key issues, to arrive at an agreement on what contributes to health, how it can be maintained, and the role of governments in promoting the health and well-being of the population.

Moreover, these processes are almost entirely concerned with health care to the exclusion of other key issues that are known to contribute to health such as labour market policy, housing, income, and other issues. Fundamentally, governments lack vision to do what is necessary to improve and maintain the health of the population. There are many ways to improve, as demonstrated by the actions and policies of governments in western Europe, where public spending on health and social programs far exceeds the commitments of Canadian governments. The penchant of Canadian governments to commercialize health care reflects a drift toward an American model of social provision.

■ THE HARPER GOVERNMENT

There is little evidence that the minority government in Ottawa under Stephen Harper can provide a more constructive approach to those of previous federal governments. For example, the Harper government promises 6 percent more toward health care than its previous financial contributions in 2006 and 2007. Federal Health Minister Tony Clement considers that this is evidence that Ottawa is prepared to cover most of the increases in health spending. In response, the minister expects that the provinces will develop wait time targets in five priority health care categories by the end of this year. In short, the Harper government is unlikely to deliver any new resources or policies compared to those of previous Liberal administrations in Ottawa.

Public policy organizations, such as the Canadian Centre for Policy Alternatives (CCPA), monitor federal and provincial public policy issues and propose alternative public policies to address key health and social policy issues. They specifically oppose commercialization strategies in health and social provision to address the problems of the health care system.

For example, in an editorial prepared for the Canadian Centre for Policy Alternatives, Colleen Fuller argues that "private health care is not the solution" (Fuller, 2000, p. 1). She cites research that shows for-profit hospitals are 3–11 percent more costly than not-for-profit hospitals. Fuller adds that the shift of services from the hospital to the community was in the right direction, but notes that "if people cannot get services in their communities on the same terms and conditions they get them in the hospital, they are going to head for a growing line-up for a hospital bed. This is how user fees act as a barrier to access, and this is how people respond" (Fuller, 2000, p. 1). Fuller concludes that the first ministers should have agreed to interpret the Canada Health Act more generously and progressively than they did. She means that they should clearly define home care, long-term care, and out-patient rehabilitation as services covered by the no-user-fee rules of the legislation.

As far as increasing accountability as raised in the health accords and in the Social Union Framework Agreement, the Canada Health Act requires regular provincial reporting on their health care spending. The Act states very clearly that if provinces fail to report to the federal health minister how they are complying with national standards, they will not receive any federal money. Fuller argues that reporting is essential to ensure that the principles of the CHA are enforced, and that user fees are not erecting a barrier to access (Fuller, 2000). The absence of enforcement mechanisms to ensure the compliance of all parties to the terms of SUFA and the health accords shows these documents are merely platitudes to preserving medicare. It reflects a lack of political leadership to do what is necessary to improve the health of the population and preserve an important social program that defines Canada.

The accords and other measures are well intentioned in attempting to reaffirm the commitments of the federal and provincial governments in social and health provision. Without commitments backed up by action by both governments, these agreements are merely words to show the Canadian public that governments are still thinking about health care.

■ CONCLUSIONS

The SUFA and health accords of 2000, 2003, and 2004 can be understood as efforts to renew a collaborative federalism between the two levels of government. Both the federal and provincial governments recognized the demise in cordial relations and general decline in social provision. Although these agreements to date have shown little impact in improving relations between governments, they have initiated an important national discussion about the appropriate role of government in social provision.

These agreements may signify more in terms of altering and perhaps improving intergovernmental relations and process to assure the Canadian public that the two levels of government are communicating. Fundamentally, the agreements do not articulate a clear vision with respect to what both levels of government wish to achieve in health and social policy. The primacy of health care in the agreements may lead to excluding other fundamental public policy issues that are germane to health, such as income and employment security, housing security and labour policy, as McIntosh suggests. Discussion has failed to move much beyond health care and the appropriate roles of the federal and provincial governments in health policy, and in these public policy areas that research has shown are more critical to health than health care.

■ REFERENCES

Armstrong, H. & Armstrong, P. (2003). *Wasting away: The undermining of Canadian health care*. Toronto: Oxford University Press.

Banting, K. (1997). The social policy divide: The welfare state in Canada and the United States. In K. Banting, G. Hoberg & R. Simeon (Eds.), *Degrees of freedom: Canada and the United States in a changing world*, 267–309. Montreal & Kingston: McGill-Queen's University Press.

Brooks, S. & Miljan, L. (2003). *Public policy in Canada: An introduction*. Toronto: Oxford University Press.

Cameron, D. & Simeon, R. (2002). Intergovernmental relations in Canada: The emergence of collaborative federalism. *Publius: The Journal of Federalism, 32*(2), 49–71.

Canada Department of Finance. (2007). *Federal transfers to provinces and territories*. Retrieved from www.fin.gc.ca/FEDPROV/fmAcce.html

Canada Health Infoway. (2007). *Infoway: Establishing electronic health records for Canadians.* Retrieved from www.infoway-inforoute.ca/en/WhoWeAre/Overview.aspx

Canadian Health Coalition. (2008). *Grading the government.* Ottawa: Canadian Health Coalition.

Facal, J. (2005). *Social policy and intergovernmental relations in Canada: Understanding the failure of SUFA from a Quebec perspective.* Regina: The Saskatchewan Institute of Public Policy.

Fortin, S., Noel, A. & St-Hilaire, F. (Eds.). (2003). *Forging the Canadian Social Union: SUFA and beyond.* Montreal: Institute for Research on Public Policy.

Fuller, C. (2000). *Health accord is welcome, but national standards still in jeopardy.* Ottawa: Canadian Centre for Policy Alternatives.

Gibbins, R. (2003). Shifting sands: Exploring the political foundations of SUFA. In S. Fortin, A. Noel & F. St-Hilaire (Eds.), *Forging the Canadian Social Union: SUFA and beyond,* 31–46. Montreal: Institute for Research on Public Policy.

Health Canada. (2006). *Healthy Canadians: A federal report on comparable health indicators 2006.* Ottawa: Health Canada.

Jackson, A. (2004). The unhealthy Canadian workplace. In D. Raphael (Ed.), *Social determinants of health: Canadian perspectives,* 79–94. Toronto: Canadian Scholars' Press Inc.

Lazar, H. (2000). *The Social Union Framework Agreement: Lost opportunity or new beginning?* Kingston: School of Policy Studies, Queen's University.

Maioni, A. (2000a). Assessing the Social Union Framework Agreement. *Policy Options,* 21(3), 39–41.

McIntosh, T. (2000). Is the Social Union too "healthy"? Re-thinking labour market policy. *Policy Options,* (April), 48–49.

Myles, J. (1998). How to design a "liberal" welfare state: A comparison of Canada and the United States. Social Policy and Administration, 32(4), 341–364.

Noel, A. (2001). Power and purpose in intergovernmental relations. *Policy Matters/Enjeux publics, 2*(6), 1–28.

Noel, A., St-Hilaire, F. & Fortin, S. (2003). Learning from the SUFA experience. In S. Fortin, A. Noel & F. St-Hilaire (Eds.), *Forging the Canadian social union: SUFA and beyond,* 1–29. Montreal: Institute for Public Policy Research.

Prince, M.J. (2003). SUFA: Sea change or mere ripple for Canadian social policy? In S. Fortin, A. Noel & F. St-Hilaire (Eds.), *Forging the Canadian Social Union: SUFA and beyond,* 125–156. Montreal: Institute for Research on Public Policy.

Rachlis, M. (2004). *Prescription for excellence: How innovation is saving Canada's health care system.* Toronto: HarperCollins.

Simeon, R. & Willis, E. (1997). Democracy and performance: Governance in Canada and the United States. In K. Banting, G. Hoberg & R. Simeon (Eds.), *Degrees of freedom: Canada and the Untied States in a changing world,* 150–186. Montreal & Kingston: McGill-Queen's University Press.

Smiley, D.V. (1980). *Canada in question: Federalism in the eighties* (3rd ed.). Toronto: McGraw-Hill Ryerson Limited.

Teeple, G. (2000). *Globalization and the decline of social reform: Into the twenty-first century.* Aurora: Garamond Press.

Tremblay, D.G. (2004). Unemployment and the labour market. In D. Raphael (Ed.), *Social determinants of health: Canadian perspectives,* 53–66 . Toronto: Canadian Scholars' Press Inc.

CRITICAL THINKING QUESTIONS

1. How does Canadian federalism shape the health care reform process?
2. How aware were you of the various health care accords prior to reading this text?
3. Do you think there is a chance these health care accords will save the medicare system? Why?
4. What do you make of the SUFA and the 2000, 2003, and 2004 health accords? How many Canadians do you think are aware of these agreements and their implications for health and social policy in Canada?
5. Considering that very few young Canadians vote, do you think that Canadian governments will be required to respond to their needs in the future?

FURTHER READINGS

Bakvis, H. & Skogstad, G. (Eds.). (2007). *Canadian federalism: Performance, effectiveness, and legitimacy.* Toronto: Oxford University Press.

The 2nd edition of *Canadian Federalism: Performance, Effectiveness, and Legitimacy* is a collection of 18 original essays casting a critical eye on the institutions, processes, and policy outcomes of Canadian federalism. It is divided into three parts: (1) The Institutions and Processes of Canadian Federalism; (2) The Social and Economic Union; and (3) Persistent and New Challenges to the Federation.

Fortin, S., Noel, A. & St-Hilaire, F. (Eds.). (2003). *Forging the Canadian Social Union: SUFA and beyond.* Montreal: Institute for Research on Public Policy.

This volume provides a severe assessment of the 1999 Social Union Framework Agreement. It brings together assessments of various dimensions of the 1999 Social Union Framework Agreement (SUFA) by seven leading experts in social policy and intergovernmental relations.

Health Council of Canada. (2007). *Annual report: Why health care renewal matters: Learning from Canadians with chronic health conditions.* Available online at: http://www.healthcouncilcanada.ca/en/index.php?option=com_content&task=view&id=8&Itemid=10

The Health Council of Canada's first annual report to Canadians focused on access. In its second report, the council focuses on quality. In future reports, the council will examine the collective capacity to measure the performance of health care systems across the country and suggest ways to strengthen transparency and accountability in health care.

RELEVANT WEBSITES

Canadian Federalism and Public Health Care: The Evolution of Federal-Provincial Relations
www.mapleleafweb.com/features/canadian-federalism-and-public-health-care-evolution-federal-provincial-relations
This website has a discussion of the basic division of powers in health care, Canadian federalism and the introduction of public health care, and shifts in this federal-provincial relationship since the 1950s.

Canadian Policy Research Networks
www.cprn.org
CPRN provides timely reports on health care and other federal/provincial issues.

First Ministers' Accord on Health Care Renewal 2003
www.hc-sc.gc.ca/hcs-sss/delivery-prestation/fptcollab/2003accord/index_e.html
First Minister's Meeting on the Future of Health Care 2004
www.hc-sc.gc.ca/hcs-sss/delivery-prestation/fptcollab/2004-fmm-rpm/index_e.html
These websites provide details of the first ministers' health accords of 2003 and 2004.

Institute for Research on Public Policy
www.irpp.org
IRPP seeks to improve public policy in Canada by generating research, providing insight, and sparking debate that will contribute to the public policy decision-making process and strengthen the quality of the public policy decisions made by Canadian governments, citizens, institutions, and organizations.

Social Union Framework Agreement (SUFA)
socialunion.gc.ca/menu_e.html
The "social union" initiative is the umbrella under which governments will concentrate their efforts to renew and modernize Canadian social policy. It focuses on the pan-Canadian dimension of health and social policy systems, the linkages between the social and economic unions, and the recognition that reform is best achieved in partnership among provinces, territories, and the government of Canada.

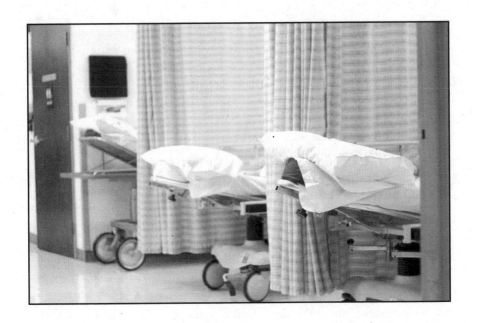

Chapter 11

GLOBALIZATION AND FREE TRADE

■ INTRODUCTION

The late 20th century witnessed radical changes to the world economy related to globalization, the liberalization of trade, and removal of barriers to the flow of investment capital (Banting, Hoberg & Simeon, 1997a; Teeple, 2000). National governments in Canada and other advanced economies have responded to these changes by restructuring their economies. In some nations such as Canada, this has also involved significant reductions in governmental spending on health care and social services. What has been most evident is the decline of the welfare state, which was discussed in Chapter 9. In Canada, beloved social programs such as medicare have been the targets of restructuring and retrenchment. The drastic reduction of the welfare state, however, did not take place in all nations. This is a reflection of national differences in policy priorities (International Labour Organization, 1999; Organisation for Economic Co-operation and Development, 2005).

What is driving these global changes? In a nutshell, the answer is neo-liberal policies that reflect an ongoing commitment to the free movement of goods and services across the globe, as articulated in free trade agreements (Teeple, 2000).

These global changes are also influencing and are influenced by nations' domestic policies. Previous chapters have touched on the implications of neo-liberalism and international trade treaties for the Canadian health care system and also for population health. This chapter further examines how these developments are influencing health policy. The primary focus is the impact of globalization on health care, health-related public policies, and health outcomes. This includes an examination of how these forces may be influencing the democratic process in Canada and other nations.

■ ECONOMIC GLOBALIZATION

Economic globalization refers to the integration of world economies (Banting, Hoberg & Simeon, 1997b). More specifically, economic globalization is "a process of greater integration within the world economy through movement of goods and services, capital, technology and (to a lesser extent) labour, which lead increasingly to economic decisions being influenced by global conditions" (Jenkins, 2004, p. 1). The process of integration can also involve the internationalization of health care services through liberalization or deregulation as directed by provisions found within trade agreements between countries (Bakker, 1996; Teeple, 2000).

The process of economic globalization requires that national governments accept freer markets and global economic integration as the foundation(s) for national macroeconomic policy (Labonte & Schrecker, 2007c). Such changes are frequently presented by governmental and business authorities as inevitable and necessary to ensure economic competitiveness (Bakker, 1996). National governments open up their domestic markets and services to global competition by means of procurement agreements, establishment of dispute-settlement mechanisms, and allowing investment by global financial institutions.

As suggested by its definition, economic globalization is complex and consists of numerous, interrelated policy dynamics (Labonte & Schrecker, 2007a). These dynamics have implications for health care organization and delivery as well as population health outcomes. As suggested earlier, neo-liberal ideology has been applied to justify these changes. In reality, the ideology appears to benefit those whose economic interests lie within the business sector (Langille, 2004).

Capital is more likely to generate larger profits when it can span the globe than when it is limited to one nation. For example, many companies have already experienced increasing profits associated with shifting factories and service industries to lower-wage nations such as India or China. Capital, therefore, seeks freedom from national regulation or other state intervention (Teeple, 2000). Corporate interests are now global or international in scope, although they continue to act

---

Box 11.1: The First Glimpse of Economic Globalization

Karl Marx wrote the following passage in *The Communist Manifesto* more than 160 years ago:

> The need of a constantly expanding market for its products chases the bourgeoisie over the entire surface of the globe. It must nestle everywhere, settle everywhere, establish connections everywhere. [...] The bourgeoisie has, through its exploitation of the world market, given a cosmopolitan character to production and consumption in every country. To the great chagrin of reactionaries, it has drawn from under the feet of industry the national ground on which it stood. All old-established national industries have been destroyed or are daily being destroyed. They are dislodged by new industries, whose introduction becomes a life and death question for all civilized nations, by industries that no longer work up indigenous raw material, but raw material drawn from the remotest zones; industries whose products are consumed, not only at home, but in every quarter of the globe. In place of the old wants, satisfied by the production of the country, we find new wants, requiring for their satisfaction the products of distant lands and climes. In place of the old local and national seclusion and self-sufficiency, we have intercourse in every direction, universal inter-dependence of nations. And as in material, so also in intellectual production. The intellectual creations of individual nations become common property. National one-sidedness and narrow-mindedness become more and more impossible, and from the numerous national and local literatures, there arises a world literature.

Source: Marx, Karl. (1848). *The communist manifesto*, 223–224. New York: Penguin Classics.

---

upon national jurisdictions and local domestic policies. These corporations pressure governments to open up more and more goods and services to the market sector.

As a result of these economic and political pressures achieved through a variety of lobbying and other processes, national governments manage and adjust domestic policies to meet the pressures of these transnational, or multinational, market forces (Leys, 2001). Some have suggested that economic globalization, in fact, marks the political demise of the nation-state (Cerny, 1993; Teeple, 2000) because it appears that multinational corporations, not elected governments, can now determine public policy. The ability of national governments to set domestic policy and manage their economies is effectively undermined in the face of commitments to meet international business interests (see Box 11.2).

Box 11.2: The Development of the Global Economy

The development of globalization must be examined in historical context. Its history can be traced to the Second World War when the foundations for a world economy were established. The shift to a globalized economy occurred alongside the development of the welfare state in Canada, the UK, the US, and in the countries of western Europe. The formation of the global economy began toward the end of the Second World War at the United Nations Monetary and Financial Conference held in Bretton Woods, New Hampshire, in 1944 (Leys, 2001; Teeple, 2000). At the conference, the delegates established an international trading regime and the foundation of an international monetary system to enable the development of global trade with a view also to avoid global depressions like the Depression of the 1930s.

The focus of Bretton Woods was the formation of a global economy. The principal components of a framework for a supranational regime of capital accumulation and trade liberalization were formed (Teeple, 2000). These components comprised the principles of liberal democracy that were entrenched in the United Nations, Marshall Aid for reconstruction, the International Monetary Fund (IMF), the World Bank, and the General Agreement on Tariffs and Trade (GATT) to control and liberalize trade around the world. All of these dimensions for a postwar world order were achieved and were up and running by the end of the 1960s.

Observers describe the Bretton Woods conference as a US-led process that culminated in the formation of political and economic structures and policies under the control of the US (Teeple, 2000). There were many reasons why the US was seen as the logical world leader at the end of the war. The US was the only nation-state and the only viable world leader toward the end of the war. It had not suffered the devastation endured by European powers during the war. The US therefore emerged as the only power that could assume a dominant role in global politics and economics. Indeed, Teeple (2000) describes the US as the "pre-eminent capitalist power at the end of the war," (Teeple, 2000, 53) and therefore well placed to restructure and redefine the postwar world economy in its interests. In addition, of all the countries, the US had the largest economy and was eager to identify new markets for trade and investment. Thus, the delegates established an exchange-rate mechanism by setting equivalences of national currencies to be compared with the US dollar.

From this process, the IMF and the World Bank emerged. Among its purposes, the IMF was established to regulate international trade balances, promote international monetary co-operation, exchange stability, and orderly exchange arrangements; to foster economic growth and high levels of employment; and to provide temporary financial assistance to countries to help ease balance of payments adjustments (Articles of Agreement of the International Monetary Fund, adopted at the United Nations Monetary and Financial Conference, Bretton Woods, New Hampshire, July 22, 1944). The purpose of the World Bank was to provide and manage an international fund for economic development.

The General Agreement on Tariffs and Trade (GATT) was formulated in 1947). It was to serve as the institutional means for a negotiated removal of all national barriers to world trade and to develop universal regulations to enable freer commerce (Leys, 2001; Teeple, 2000). At this time, the United Nations (UN) was also created as a supranational, quasi-government and political foundation for the new internationalism. The UN assumed responsibility for peacekeeping operations. It also has been characterized as a vehicle to control the expansion of socialism in Korea, the Congo, Greece, and Indonesia; propagate the principles of liberal democracy and the rights of private property as a political system supporting and consistent with the promotion of capitalism; and develop international laws based on private rights for the "world community" (Teeple, 2000, p. 55).

Teeple and others argue that the intention of the US was to establish the framework for a single world economy of competing capitals (Leys, 2001; Teeple, 2000). The precursors of globalization were set in the Second World War (Teeple, 2000). Before that war, capital was essentially national in character and corporate interests were national interests, protected at home and abroad by means of armed forces, tariff barriers, currency controls, and nationalism and citizenship, and with other national laws and policies. The Bretton Woods agreement facilitated the expansion of global trade. Ultimately, the GATT provided an institutional vehicle for a negotiated lifting of all national barriers to world trade. It also paved the way for the development of global regulations for freer trade.

Indeed, the creation of the welfare state was constructed in tandem with the new era of global capitalism. The welfare state was intended to ameliorate the effects of the market economy, such as unemployment, by providing income and other support programs during periods of unemployment. The aim was unimpeded capital accumulation and mobility. The welfare state appeased the working class while still enabling the capitalist economy to continue to function. All was well until the oil crisis of 1973.

Indeed, national governments become unable to initiate certain economic and social strategies because they are forced to adopt policies consistent with trade treaty requirements. These policy directions may weaken the welfare state. Cerny notes: "The interaction of changing financial market structures on the one hand and states on the other has done more than production, trade or international cooperative regimes to undermine the structures of the Keynesian welfare state and to impose the norms of the competition state ..." (Cerny, 1993, pp. 79–80) (see Box 11.3). In other words, governmental programs associated with the welfare state become incompatible with the requirements of the global market economy. These changes, as one can imagine, may have profound implications for democratic processes. Some critics predict the demise of the nation-state since the requirements of economic globalization have impeded the capacity of national governments to set domestic policy.

Box 11.3: Case Study: The Marketization of the National Health Service

In 1982, Thatcher's cabinet examined several options for privatizing health care (Leys, 2001). The cabinet then pursued three policies to privatize or contract out some hospital services: First, ancillary hospital services such as cleaning, catering, laundry, and pathology tests were contracted out. Second, beginning in 1984, new structures of general managers were set up in hospitals. The general managers replaced senior physicians who had hitherto run hospital boards by consensus or among themselves. Businessmen were appointed to the hospital boards to support the new general managers. Finally, spending was reduced below the growth of needs. Reduced resources forced the NHS to deliver the same level of care for less or cut services.

The result was deteriorating working conditions for staff. Physicians, or consultants, found their view increasingly undermined by general managers on short-term contracts whose chief interest was reducing costs and often lacked any understanding of health care issues. Nurses were no longer able to provide patients the level of care they needed. Cleaning staff and cooks were often transferred to private firms outside hospitals, working for lower wages and inferior terms of employment. In terms of receiving care, increased wait times and cases of acutely ill patients waiting on gurneys for a bed bolstered support for private health care (Leys, 2001). The aim of the reforms was to make the NHS more cost-efficient and, by privatizing aspects of health care, the government thought it had created an "internal market" (p. 171) in 1991 without any public debate or electoral mandate.

Source: Leys, C. (2001). *Market-driven politics*. London: Verso.

As noted elsewhere in this volume, the nation-state was essential in the creation of the welfare state in developed Western political economies. It set national standards to ensure equal access to and quality of services for all citizens regardless of where they lived. This was the basis of the welfare state. Such services were provided on the basis of need, not income or ability to pay. The welfare state was intended to protect workers from the negative effects of market forces. Its creation signified the recognition that the market could not deliver necessary goods such as health care or income support.

The requirements of the global economy for free market conditions and lack of governmental "interference" seem to clash with the collectivist orientation of the welfare state. As noted above, one of the critical tasks of a national government was to mitigate the adverse effects of the market through social provision via the welfare state (Leys, 2001). But these governmental processes have become increasingly market-driven in response to global pressures for deregulation, freer trade, and capital mobility.

National governments, however, have not been deemed totally obsolete. Rather, the process of economic globalization constrains and redefines the powers of national governments to further the process of commodification (Leys, 2001). Commodification refers to the transformation of relationships, formerly untainted by commerce, into commercial relationships of exchange, of buying and selling. The process has also facilitated the growth and mobility of international capital such that national economies become open to foreign investment. Economic globalization effectively comes to increase the power of transnational corporations.

■ ECONOMIC GLOBALIZATION AND NEO-LIBERALISM

Neo-liberalism has become an influential, if not dominant, political ideology that both justifies and drives economic globalization. As an ideology, it is committed to the market economy as the best allocator of resources and wealth in a society (Coburn, 2000). It perceives individuals as motivated chiefly by material and economic considerations, and competition as the primary market instrument for innovations.

Broadly speaking, neo-liberalism seeks to transfer control of the economy from the public to the private sector. This has tremendous policy implications. Williamson has created a short list of policy implications under neo-liberalism (Williamson, 1990):

- trade liberalization—that is, liberalization of imports, with particular emphasis on the elimination of quantitative restrictions (licensing, etc.), and any trade protection to be provided by tariffs

- liberalization of inward foreign direct investment
- privatization of state enterprises
- deregulation—abolition of regulations that impede market entry or restrict competition, except for those justified on safety, environmental, and consumer protection grounds, and prudent oversight of financial institutions
- redirection of public spending away from subsidies
- tax reform—broadening the tax base and adopting moderate marginal tax rates
- interest rates that are market-determined

Economic globalization therefore requires that politics and policymaking be market-driven (Labonte & Schrecker, 2007a, 2007b, 2007c; Leys, 2001; Teeple, 2000). And neo-liberalism justifies the marketization of politics and public policy decisions. It also effectively justifies the marketization of everyday life. As Coburn argues: "the essence of neo-liberalism, in its pure form, is a more or less thoroughgoing adherence, in rhetoric if not in practice, to the virtues of a market economy, and, by extension, a market-oriented society" (Coburn, 2000, p. 138).

The impact of economic globalization and neo-liberal policies on health care organization and delivery and on health-related public policy has been gradual but consistent. From the late 1960s and into the early 1970s, world trade grew at an unprecedented rate as evidenced in increased commodity exchange by over 800 percent (Cypher, 1979). The world market in commodities surpassed national markets, thereby enabling global commodity production. Between 1950 and 1975, foreign direct investment by the United States alone increased substantially, and the returns from abroad grew from 7 percent to more than 25 percent over the same period (Cypher, 1979). As a result of this economic activity, multinational corporations gradually became the primary forces in economic relations between nations (Teeple, 2000), yet there was still interest in human development issues as evidenced by both the creation and general maintenance of the welfare state in most of the advanced economies in the postwar era.

The 1980s changed that. Teeple identifies the 1980s as the critical decade during which welfare state began to decline (Teeple, 2000). This decline coincides with the rise of the global economy and the adoption of neo-liberal policies in countries around the world (Teeple, 2000). For Teeple, the principle behind these policies is unrestricted economic power of private property and capital accumulation. These policies "harmonize" national capitals, accumulated national wealth, and nation-states in order to build a global system of internationalized capital and "supranational" institutions. These policies provide a solid foundation for market forces to play out and, conversely, reduce the role the state plays in the regulation of the market economy. These policies may come to influence the organization and delivery of health care services in Canada.

■ GLOBALIZATION AND CANADIAN HEALTH POLICY

Specific policy areas within the jurisdiction of national governments, such as health care, are particularly vulnerable to global forces. The modern form of the global economy that began after the end of the Second World War saw its resurgence during the 1970s and has some formidable strengths: (1) a wide selection of locations for capital investment; (2) the weight and ubiquity of global financial markets; and (3) the importance to national economies and societal functioning of transnational manufacturing and service corporations.

In his case study on the impact of market forces on British politics and society, Leys argues that, "Capital mobility has not just removed the 'Keynesian capacity' of national governments—their ability to influence the general level of demand. It has made all policy-making sensitive to 'market sentiment' and the regulatory demands of TNCs [Transnational Corporations]" (Leys, 2001, 2).

Impact of Globalization on Health Care

Leys's groundbreaking UK case study of the impact of economic globalization on politics and government policy of the UK can provide insights into the potential transformation of medicare in Canada (Leys, 2001). In his study, Leys describes the increasing privatization of the National Health Service (NHS).

Background

The NHS was the sole provider of medication, equipment, and other medical supplies. It negotiated prices with suppliers. Most Britons received good-quality care at NHS hospitals and, as a result, the NHS was an extremely popular social program. Yet, with demographic changes, medical advances, and other developments, the NHS required constant budget increases—so much so that by late 1970s, the NHS represented 11 percent of total government expenditures and these costs seemed destined to rise. Prime Minister Margaret Thatcher saw the NHS as a drain on the economy and she sought to privatize many of its components. The results were disheartening (Leys, 2001, p. 168) (see Box 11.3).

Armstrong and Armstrong have documented similar changes occurring in Canadian hospitals (Armstrong & Armstrong, 2003; Armstrong et al., 2002). For example, many hospitals contracted out ancillary hospital services such as cleaning and food services. They also reduced the number of nurses on wards. All of these changes can have serious implications for the quality of patient care. Of particular concern is the burden of care that falls to individual households with increased privatization as a result of the failure of hospitals and other health care facilities to provide essential care. The changes that occurred in Ontario in the mid-1990s provide good examples of this.

In a development similar to what happened in the UK during the Thatcher years, Mike Harris's Conservative provincial government (elected in 1995) embarked on an extensive program to reduce public spending in several public policy areas in health, finance, social services, and other ministries. While the Conservatives' attempts to introduce significant private sector involvement in mainline delivery of professional health care services were resisted and eventually dropped for fear of electoral reprisals from voters, the government centralized control of the health budget and privatized some ancillary health care services in the province (Bryant, 2003). The Tory government established community care access centres and required all home care service providers to compete for service contracts. For the first time in history, long-time community health care providers, such as the Victorian Order of Nurses, saw themselves competing with for-profit agencies for service contracts.

In terms of quality of care, these market-oriented reforms can result in reduced access to long-term care for groups with low income and who are therefore unable to pay for care. Another effect of the privatization of home care was that this change placed more responsibility on individual households—usually women—to provide essential care for family members. By taking the responsibility away from state-provided hospital support mechanisms, it shifted the burden to ill-equipped and ill-prepared family members (see Box 11.4).

■ GLOBALIZATION AND HEALTH EQUITY

Privatizing health care services can reduce access for vulnerable populations. Research has shown that user fees and other market-based strategies usually mean that people with low income may do without care (Evans, 1997; Rachlis, 2004).

In addition, health-related public policies that draw upon neo-liberal concepts also can contribute to increased social and health inequalities (Coburn, 2000, 2001, 2004; Hertzman, 2000; Raphael et al., 2001). A substantial research literature now documents exactly how governmental responses to economic globalization have been influencing the social determinants of health, leading to both increasing social inequalities as well as inequalities in health outcomes (Raphael & Bryant, 2006a). This has especially been the case in nations with liberal political economies such as Canada and the United States (Raphael & Bryant, 2006b).

Box 11.4: Gender and Globalization

Much of the globalization literature focuses on the impact on developing and developed nations, but fails to consider globalization's toll on women (Labonte & Schrecker, 2007c). Women, who tend to be the caretakers of both the old and the young of the family, are often consigned to labour that is low-paying and without health benefits. Women's health is jeopardized as a result of working in environments with poor conditions and low pay. Women in developing countries, which experience high levels of absolute and relative poverty, are particularly vulnerable to such conditions (Alarcon-Gonzalez & McKinley, 1999; Sparr, 2000).

Sources: Alarcon-Gonzalez, D. & McKinley, T. (1999). The adverse effects of structural adjustment on working women in Mexico. *Latin American Perspectives, 26,* 103–117; Labonte, R. & Schrecker, T. (2007). Globalization and social determinants of health: The role of the global marketplace. *Globalization and Health, 3*(6), pp. 1–17; Sparr, P. (2000). *Mortgaging women's lives: Feminist critiques of structural adjustment.* London: Zed Books.

Trade Liberalization, Economic Growth, and Poverty Reduction

Some proponents of globalization claim that economic globalization is not necessarily bad for population health. World Bank studies suggest that economies of "globalizers" expanded faster than "non-globalizers." (The so-called high "globalizers"—China, India, Malaysia, Thailand, and Vietnam—were defined as nations whose trade/GDP ratio had increased since 1977; "non-globalizers"— primarily in Africa and Latin America—were those whose ratios decline.) The studies linked globalization with trade liberalization. The World Bank associated this growth with increased resources for delivering health services and access to other social determinants as evidenced by the reduction of extreme poverty. This argument, however, is somewhat flawed. As Labonte and Schrecker note, the World Bank studies measured change and not absolute levels of globalization or trade (Labonte & Schrecker, 2007b). Moreover, the nations identified as "globalizers" were less global than those nations considered to be "non-globalizers." Labonte and Schrecker add that the economic difficulties of non-globalizers can be partly linked to global issues beyond the control of national economic policy decision makers (see Box 11.5).

Labonte and Schrecker argue that while reduction of absolute poverty is an admirable goal, there are several issues to consider before contending that

Box 11.5: Absolute and Relative Poverty

Absolute poverty is defined as living without the most basic resources for survival such as food, shelter, and clothing. Starvation is the basic measure in this definition. For families living in absolute poverty, the sole daily preoccupation is the struggle to find enough food and water to survive another day. The tendency has been to maintain that absolute poverty is exceedingly rare in a country like Canada. Yet, the number of people living on the streets is growing and while it is known that people are dying from starvation and inadequate shelter, especially during Canadian winters, the number of these casualties remains unknown.

Relative poverty is defined as families and individuals whose income and other resource levels are scant in comparison to the majority of people in Canadian society. The number of people living in relative poverty fluctuates with economic conditions. The measure of relative poverty is the number of people living below a certain percentage of the average income level of the rest of the country. This arbitrary measure can mask the real circumstances in which many "poor" people are living because income is not an accurate indicator of quality of life. While low income may not result in starvation, it can negatively affect development and future opportunities, barring impoverished people from full participation in society (Ryerse, 1990).

Source: Ryerse, C. (1990). *Thursday's child. Child poverty in Canada: A review of the effects of poverty on children 3.* Ottawa: National Youth in Care Network.

globalization leads to poverty reduction (Labonte & Schrecker, 2007c). To the extent that globalization is related to growth, it seems to enhance population health only *if* growth reliably reduces poverty without triggering other negative outcomes (Deaton, 2004; Labonte & Schrecker, 2007c). In actuality, the presumed relationship between globalization and poverty reduction is weak, with more evidence indicating that growth without equitable distribution is generally ineffective in reducing poverty (Woodward & Simms, 2006). This is so because the increases in national wealth associated with globalizing may not be distributed equitably among the population. This has clearly been the case in Canada where the economic growth over the past two decades—supposedly an outcome of increased trade associated with NAFTA—has primarily accrued to the most well-off (Statistics Canada, 2004).

Conversely, trade liberalization has been shown to weaken many people's economic circumstances (Labonte & Schrecker, 2007c). In a nutshell, globalization has been found to benefit the wealthy and failing to assist the poor. A wide range of measures show inequality between regions and ratios, and comparisons of incomes of rich and poor groups in nations consistently show that inequality continues to increase (Sutcliffe, 2004). It may very well be that the gap between the rich and the poor in Canada will continue to increase as well unless Canadian governments initiate efforts to protect the population from the negative effects of economic globalization.

■ LABOUR MARKETS AND GLOBAL RESTRUCTURING OF PRODUCTION

Labour markets and global restructuring constitutes another way in which economic globalization may influence the social determinants of health (Labonte & Schrecker, 2007c). An important aspect of economic globalization is the restructuring of production and service provision across numerous national borders by transnational corporations (TNCs) (Dicken, 2003; Millen & Holtz, 2000; Millen, Lyon & Irwin, 2000).

Research on globalization and markets identifies several trends that appear to be related. For example, the most important trend with respect to health care and health equity is this: Competition for foreign direct investment and outsourced production leads governments to lean favourably toward private corporations. These corporations then attempt to influence public policy to favour business interests. Policy changes that favour business include lowering labour practice standards, reducing health and safety regulations, and weakening policies that redistribute income and wealth (Cornia, 2005). Cerny argues that globalization forces the convergence of national social and economic policies toward the ideal of the competition state, directed to "promotion of economic activities, whether at home or abroad, which will make firms and sectors located within the territory of the state competitive in international markets" (Cerny, 1993, p. 136). Because these changes are economically driven—that is, for the benefit of businesses, not necessarily people's health—they can, in effect, increase health inequities.

The related restructuring of labour markets affects men and women in different ways (Elson, 2002; Elson & Cagatay, 2000; Petchesky, 2003). In addition to increasing the insecurity of work for both men and women, restructured work can have particularly negative health effects for women. For example, work in the garment industry (where women are the majority of garment workers) can be dangerous. Poor working conditions and long hours of work are acceptable due to the lack of alternatives for many women in developing countries with few economic opportunities. Similarly, changes in working conditions in the health care sector can affect women who constitute the majority of health workers (Armstrong, 2006; Armstrong et al., 2002; Armstrong & Armstrong, 2002). In conclusion, globalization may lead to new economic opportunities, but these opportunities may be available only at "the price of exposure to hazardous working conditions" (Labonte & Schrecker, 2007c, p. 11).

Debt Crises: The Market under Pressure

Via the International Monetary Fund (IMF), the World Bank has lent funds to many developing nations. These loans have helped countries to restructure their economies with a view to enabling them to pay external creditors (Labonte & Schrecker, 2007c). With these loans, Labonte and Schrecker argue that the World Bank and the IMF "promoted multiple, more or less coordinated domestic policies of integrating national economies into the global marketplace" (p. 14). Debt crises, however, have severely limited the capacity of developing countries to address basic needs in public health, education, water, sanitation, and nutrition.

Studies on health impacts of debt crises are unable to isolate the effects of structural adjustment (namely, debt) from the effects of globalization-related economic difficulties (Labonte & Schrecker, 2007c). In over 76 studies, the Commission on Macroeconomics and Health noted predominantly negative effects, particularly in Africa. However, this commission de-emphasized the case against structural adjustment (or debt), which was attributable to incomplete sampling of the literature. Labonte and Schrecker argue that the authors of this commission carried out a limited review of country cases, and excluded ethnographic studies and country-level participatory evaluations that can explicate the negative impact of adjustment policies (or debt) on population health. They thus conclude that debt affects social determinants "both directly and indirectly" (p. 15). For example, reductions in food subsidies, government wages, and employment have direct negative effects on access to nutrition and household income. Labonte and Schrecker further suggest that the major impacts on social structure are related to poverty, income inequality, and changing gender relations such as the unequal impact on women's incomes and their household responsibilities. Poverty and economic insecurity have significant impacts on exposure and vulnerability offset by housing, working conditions, among other considerations. Health systems were also affected via decreased health spending and use of cost-recovery measures.

Summary: Globalization and the Social Determinants of Health

All of these issues linked to neo-liberalism can adversely affect the social determinants of health—namely, employment, access to nutritious food, education, and housing (Labonte & Schrecker, 2007c). They can also impede access to health services. This means that the working poor and unemployed may lack the financial resources to pay for care.

■ GLOBALIZATION, TRADE AGREEMENTS, AND THE CANADIAN HEALTH CARE SYSTEM

In Canada, the federal government has tried to protect health care from the free market. Successive Canadian federal governments have promised to protect health care in trade treaty negotiations and have assured that the health care system cannot be touched by free trade treaties, in particular the North American Free Trade Agreement (NAFTA) and the General Agreement on Trade in Services (Grieshaber-Otto & Sinclair, 2004). In virtually all recent trade negotiations, Canada has tried to ensure its ability to preserve existing health measures and to enact new health ones (Grieshaber-Otto & Sinclair, 2004).

The 2001 Mazankowski Report on Health Care outlined a broad range of themes and recommendations to reform health care in Alberta. The Kirby Report, a federal report of the next year, also stressed the need for co-operation among all stakeholders to reduce problems of maldistribution, undersupply, and jurisdictional competition (Kirby, 2002; Mazankowski, 2001). Both reports recommended market-based reforms. There is particular concern that these recommendations, if implemented, could lead to challenges relating to potential profit: Health care presents a huge and tempting commercial opportunity for the private sector (Kirby, 2002; Mazankowski, 2001).

Concern about the lure of profit is indeed justified. Both Mazankowski and Kirby espouse market values and discipline as necessary to improve health care. Mazankowski advocates a larger role for private financing and for-profit delivery of health care. Kirby supports public financing and enlarging the medicare monopoly to include new services, but calls for incorporating market-based methods and a larger private sector role in health care delivery.

Current federal and provincial government policies are contributing to the erosion of the public health care system through under-resourcing and increasing privatization of elements of the system (Grieshaber-Otto & Sinclair, 2004). Importantly, there is no going back: Once an area is privatized, international trade treaties—to which governments are bound—can potentially lock in these market-based health care reforms (see Box 11.6).

Grieshaber-Otto and Sinclair have carried out an extensive analysis of the potential implications of the North America Free Trade Agreement (NAFTA) and the General Agreement on Trade in Services (GATS) for health care in Canada. Specifically, these researchers examined how some of Mazankowski's and Kirby's recommendations for market-based reforms could interact with Canada's trade obligations under these treaties. The following discussion provides an overview of these issues.

Box 11.6: Impact of Expanding Private Sector Involvement in Health Care

1. Cutbacks in health insurance will be difficult and costly to reverse. Canada listed health insurance as one of its specific commitments in GATS. This means that the GATS National Treatment and Market Access rules will pertain to this sector. Trying to bring delisted services back into the realm of publicly insured services could limit foreign service providers' commercial opportunities. They, in turn, could urge their own governments to launch trade challenges against Canada.
2. Delisting health care services from publicly insured services would impede efforts to regulate aspects of privately insured services within Canada.

Source: Grieshaber-Otto, J. & Sinclair, S. (2004). *Bad medicine: Trade treaties, privatization, and health care reform in Canada.* Ottawa: Canadian Centre for Policy Alternatives.

■ NAFTA, GATS, AND THE CANADIAN HEALTH CARE SYSTEM

Canada is a participant in both NAFTA and GATS, even though it may very well be that medicare, a cherished social program in Canada, will come to be incompatible with the terms of these treaties (Grieshaber-Otto & Sinclair, 2004). Like other nations, Canada has declared that it is committed to upholding its existing health care system and reserves the right to implement new health care measures. However, there are a number of exemptions, exceptions, and reservations being created to allow health care issues to fall outside trade treaty rules. Some of these procedures pertain to all nations, and others only to Canada (see Box 11.7).

The scope of NAFTA is far-reaching. Its services and investment chapters cover all measures in all sectors with the exception of those for which national governments have negotiated specific exclusions or exemptions. The GATS is equally broad, and pertains to all provisions by governments that can have an impact on services, including the ways in which these services are delivered. The only area outside of GATS regulation is that provided "in the exercise of governmental authority" (Grieshaber-Otto & Sinclair, 2004, p. 23) This means that those services provided are within the jurisdiction of government and may continue.

NAFTA contains two reservations—that is, country-specific exceptions that shelter government policies in health care. Annex I is a general reservation against

Box 11.7: Implications of the North America Free Trade Agreement for Medicare

Under the NAFTA, foreign health care insurers and companies can invoke the treaty's expropriation-compensation rules (Grieshaber-Otto & Sinclair, 2004). These rules affect medicare and are more inclusive than related Canadian domestic law. Moreover, NAFTA's investor-to-state dispute settlement process supports these rules. In particular they could make for-profit health care difficult to reverse. NAFTA articles cover all aspects in all sectors except those for which governments negotiated explicit exclusion.

Among these is Annex I, which is a general reservation against some of NAFTA's provisions that allow each of the three NAFTA signatories to retain all nonconforming provincial and state government measures that were in place when NAFTA came into force January 1, 1994.

Annex I reservation applies against the NAFTA national treatment, most favoured nation treatment, local presence, performance requirements, and senior management and board of directors articles. And this provision is bound, which means that any current nonconforming measures can only be amended to be consistent with the terms of NAFTA. There is no possibility of restoring a measure once it has been eliminated or amended. Any protection provided by Annex I will disappear over time.

The most favoured nation (MFN) treatment rule contends that governments must extend the best treatment given to any foreign goods, investments, or services to all like foreign goods, investments, or services, or "favour one, favour all." Measures that are formally non-discriminatory can breach these non-discrimination rules if they adversely affect the "equality of competitive opportunities" of foreign investors or service providers. Canada negotiated a second reservation that excludes the Canadian health care sector from a few NAFTA provisions in the agreement's investment and services chapters.

Under NAFTA's Annex II-C-9, Canada has the right to implement or retain health care measures that may contravene national treatment provisions if they pertain to health services that are deemed to be social services or are provided for a "public purpose" (Grieshaber-Otto & Sinclair, 2004, p. 26) This annex is unbound. In other words it protects existing nonconforming policies or statutes, and permits Canadian governments to adopt new policies that would be considered to run counter to the intent of NAFTA. It contains a reservation that specifies that any such measures should pertain to health to the extent that it is "a social service established or maintained for a public purpose" (p. 26). Grieshaber-Otto and Sinclair argue that these terms are undefined, and US and Canadian governments have applied different interpretations, thereby contributing to uncertainty about the true scope of the Annex II reservation (Grieshaber-Otto & Sinclair, 2004).

The General Agreement on Trade in Services (GATS) has a similarly broad scope and covers all services, except those provided "in the exercise of governmental authority." Specific GATS provisions such as the most favoured nation rule are top-down and cover all sectors. The most serious provisions are "bottom-up," which means they apply to sectors that governments specifically decide to include. According to Grieshaber-Otto and Sinclair, the federal government has made no commitments to cover direct "health services" as classified in GATS.

The GATS excludes services that are provided in the "exercise of governmental authority." Such services are defined as services that are not provided on a commercial or competitive basis.

Grieshaber-Otto and Sinclair note that because Canadian health care comprises considerable private financing and delivery of services, governmental authority exclusion cannot be considered sufficient to protect the Canadian health care system from GATS rules, but apparently Canada's decision not to list direct health services under the GATS will provide much more protection. Canada has covered specific health-related services, such as health insurance. Not good. Under GATS, Canadian negotiators decided to include private health insurance under the World Trade Organization's trade-in-services agreement. According to Grieshaber-Otto and Sinclair, the provision enables American and European governments to challenge Canadian initiatives to expand public health insurance into new areas, such as pharmacare or home care, on the grounds that it denies their private insurers access to these health care markets. Under GATS rules, such a dispute could lead to trade sanctions against Canadian exports to Europe or the US. The threat of litigation may be enough to deter the federal government from initiating such reforms.

Source: Grieshaber-Otto, J. & Sinclair, S. (2004). *Bad medicine: Trade treaties, privatization, and health care reform in Canada.* Ottawa: Canadian Centre for Policy Alternatives.

some of NAFTA's terms that allows each of the three NAFTA countries to retain all nonconforming provincial and state government programs and policies that were in place when NAFTA came into effect on January 1, 1994. The Annex I reservation is *bound,* which means that existing public policy programs and policies can only be adjusted to make them more consistent with NAFTA provisions. If a program or policy is abolished, it cannot be later reinstated and remain outside NAFTA regulations. Understandably, a major concern about the protection provided by the Annex I reservation is that once it ceases, it cannot be reinstated.

Canada negotiated a second reservation in NAFTA. Annex II, also referred to as the NAFTA social services reservation, is unbound. It protects existing policies and programs that are not consistent with NAFTA and also allows the Canadian government to implement new policies and programs that are also not NAFTA consistent. These programs are protected if they are health related and are established as a social service for a public purpose. According to Grieshaber-Otto and Sinclair, these terms are somewhat ambiguous, and the US and Canadian governments have interpreted them differently. This lack of clarity contributes to uncertainty about the range of the Annex II reservation.

The concerns raised by these trade agreements are enough to cause Grieshaber-Otto and Sinclair and others to argue that the safeguards do not fully protect the Canadian health care system. NAFTA's very broad provisions against "expropriation"—that is, usurping an established enterprise without compensation—cover all sectors, including health. Grieshaber-Otto and Sinclair suggest that even where safeguards protect health services, they may at the same time enhance the commercial element in financing or delivery.

Similarly, the GATS does not apply to services provided by governments. It applies only if the services are provided as not-for-profit. One difficulty with this is that the Canadian health care system comprises both public and private financing and delivery. This means that the governmental authority exclusion may not provide sufficient protection of the Canadian health care system from GATS rules that "do not fully exclude the Canadian health care system" (Grieshaber-Otto & Sinclair, 2004, p. 25). Of particular concern is that trade treaties have the potential to lock in privatization and market-oriented strategies that have been proposed to reform medicare.

■ TRADE AGREEMENTS AND PUBLIC-PRIVATE PARTNERSHIPS

Many argue that protecting the health care system can be ensured only by a traditional approach where governments purchase and pay for the services directly (Grieshaber-Otto & Sinclair, 2004). This is the "single-payer" model, which is the current Canadian model, albeit with some private finance and delivery.

In contrast to this traditional and established Canadian model, public-private partnerships (P3s) are a particular form of health care commercialization. Some consider P3s to be particularly risky since they cover a substantial range of health care services (National Union of Public and General Employees, 2006). Of particular concern is that fact that P3s have a strong potential to enable foreign corporations to use trade policy rules to misrepresent key aspects of Canadian health care policy (Grieshaber-Otto & Sinclair, 2004). Further, trade treaty rules favour the rights of the foreign investor, which requires host governments to financially compensate foreign corporations.

■ EFFECTS OF GLOBALIZATION: IMPACT ON THE LABOUR MARKET

In Canada, since the NAFTA came into being, the country has lost numerous jobs in the manufacturing sector and now 25 percent of the jobs in the Canadian labour market are low-paying (Innocenti Research Centre, 2005). This is one of the highest percentages of low-paying jobs among advanced economies. Such changes have contributed to a widening gap between high-income groups and low-income groups; these changes have effectively increased health inequalities (Coburn, 2001; Yalnizyan, 1998, 2007). Other countries involved in neo-liberalist trade agreements, particularly the United States and the United Kingdom, have similarly experienced a growth in inequalities, in the distribution of income, and in health outcomes (see Box 11.8).

Box 11.8: Proposed MRI Project Renews Privatization Debate
By Angela Hall
Leader Post

No ground has been broken for the proposed project, no pricey equipment is in place, and no stamps of government approval have been made.

But even before details are clear about the latest proposal to put the first privately-owned magnetic resonance imaging (MRI) machine in Saskatchewan, it has renewed general debate about the private sector's role in the province's health-care system.

The recently elected Saskatchewan Party government says the idea of private facilities delivering some publicly funded health services isn't new, but any proposals to expand what's currently done would need to be closely examined.

"I think the debate is 'Do we want to pragmatically look at ways that can reduce wait times for diagnostics?'" Premier Brad Wall said to reporters this week.

"That might include (the provincial government) not owning every single MRI. Right now they don't in terms of X-ray technology, in terms of other diagnostics, the government doesn't have to own it all."

However, the premier said offering medical services such as an MRI for a fee "seems to be outside the Canada Health Act," and is [an] area where the government doesn't want to tread.

Wall said he will look at what proposal comes forward from Kawactoose First Nation, which this week along with Siemens Canada announced plans for a health centre in east Regina that would include MRI services. Officials at a news conference Monday said patients would not be able to jump to the front of the queue by paying out-of-pocket, but rather that the proposed centre would work with the existing system.

However, the provincial NDP says that even if the province pays for MRI scans that take place in a facility it doesn't own in the same way it does for those in a public hospital, there are questions about the effectiveness of such a system.

Health critic Judy Junor said private facilities could hurt publicly funded hospitals by luring away trained health professionals, citing that as one problem in Ontario before private MRI clinics were ultimately purchased back into the public fold.

"You can buy the machine, that's the easy part. It's whose [sic] going to work it on a day to day basis," Junor said.

Meanwhile, University of Saskatchewan health economist Allen Backman doubts that a private MRI service could stay afloat without offering both insured and non-insured services.

"What it means is that they would take public patients paid for by the government ... but they would also have to take private patients who pay in order to get in ahead of line or who pay for services that aren't ordinarily funded by government insurance, things like preventative full body scans," Backman said.

Such a move in Saskatchewan would "really mean a new direction in health care," he said.

A few provinces have already headed in the direction of offering MRIs for a fee. In Alberta, patients have long had the option of purchasing such a scan outside of the public system at one of six private clinics, according to Alberta Health. A Vancouver-based company, meanwhile, refers patients willing to pay for certain services, including MRIs, to a private facilities that can do the job fast.

Clients from Saskatchewan that contact the company seeking MRIs typically end up in Alberta for the scan, said Richard Baker, the businessman who founded Timely Medical Alternatives.

The last time a Saskatchewan group proposed a private MRI machine was in 2004 when Muskeg Lake First Nation said it wanted to own and operate an MRI unit on its Saskatoon reserve—either through an agreement with the then-NDP government or possibly by charging patients. Plans for a wellness and diabetes centre there were announced last year but without an MRI component. Muskeg Lake officials this week declined comment.

Source: Leader Post (February 15, 2008), p. A3.

In contrast, Sweden and other countries with a social democratic tradition seem to be less vulnerable to the negative effects of globalization. Figure 11.1 shows that Sweden and the other Nordic countries have higher expenditures on health and social programs and better population health as a result. All of these countries have a social democratic tradition that seems to have provided resistance to the market-driven policies of neo-liberalism. This and other evidence on social spending suggests that some political traditions appear to be more susceptible to the negative affects of globalization. Esping-Andersen identified examples of liberal welfare states or liberal political economies which are susceptible to globalization.

The political system can, in part, protect its citizens from the negative effects of globalization *if* the political system intrinsically values the social welfare net. Some researchers found that democratic countries with developed welfare states experienced lower poverty rates and better health in general (Alesina & Glaeser, 2004; Navarro & Shi, 2002).

■ CONCLUSIONS

Economic globalization and neo-liberalism are prominent forces that have effectively changed the role of governments in advanced Western economies and, as a result, they have restructured society. Economic globalization, associated with the ongoing expansion of the market economy, has been linked to a decline in the depth and quality of the welfare state (Banting et al., 1997a; Leys, 2001; Teeple, 2000). Indeed, the rise of neo-liberalism and economic globalization has led to concerns about the maintenance of a public health care system and health-related policies that promote health.

Labonte and Schrecker have identified pathways by which economic globalization influence population health outcomes and the social determinants of health. Their work, and that of others, strongly suggests that collective responses that focus on the redistribution of wealth in order to improve the health and living conditions of Canadians in general, and vulnerable populations in particular, definitely need to be developed.

■ REFERENCES

Alesina, A. & Glaeser, E.L. (2004). *Fighting poverty in the US and Europe: A world of difference.* Toronto: Oxford University Press.

Armstrong, H. & Armstrong, P. (2003). *Wasting away: The undermining of Canadian health care.* Toronto: Oxford University Press.

Armstrong, P. (2006). Gender, health, and care. In D. Raphael, T. Bryant & M. Rioux (Eds.), *Staying alive: Critical perspectives on health, illness, and health care,* 287–303. Toronto: Canadian Scholars' Press Inc.

Armstrong, P., Amaratunga, C., Bernier, J., Grant, K., Pederson, A. & Wilson, K. (2002). *Exposing privatization: Women and health care reform in Canada*. Toronto: Garamond.

Armstrong, P. & Armstrong, H. (2002). *Thinking it through: Women, work, and caring in the new millennium*. Halifax: Canadian Institutes of Health Research (CIHR), Nova Scotia Advisory Council on the Status of Women, and Atlantic Centre of Excellence for Women's Health (ACEWH).

Bakker, I. (1996). Introduction: The gendered foundations of restructuring in Canada. In I. Bakker (Ed.), *Rethinking restructuring: Gender and change in Canada*, 3–25. Toronto: University of Toronto Press.

Banting, K., Hoberg, G. & Simeon, R. (1997a). Introduction. In K. Banting, G. Hoberg & R. Simeon (Eds.), *Degrees of freedom: Canada and the United States in a changing world*, 3–19. Montreal & Kingston: McGill-Queen's University Press.

Banting, K., Hoberg, G. & Simeon, R. (Eds.). (1997b). *Degrees of freedom: Canada and the United States in a changing world*. Montreal & Kingston: McGill-Queen's University Press.

Bryant, T. (2003). A critical examination of the hospital restructuring process in Ontario, Canada. *Health Policy, 64*, 193–205.

Cerny, P. (1993). The deregulation and re-regulation of financial markets in a more open world. In P. Cerny (Ed.), *Finance and world politics: Markets, regimes, and states in the post-hegemonic era*, 51–85. Aldershot: Edward Elgar.

Coburn, D. (2000). Income inequality, social cohesion, and the health status of populations: The role of neo-liberalism. *Social Science & Medicine, 51*(1), 135–146.

Coburn, D. (2001). Health, health care, and neo-liberalism. In P. Armstrong, H. Armstrong & D. Coburn (Eds.), *Unhealthy times: The political economy of health and care in Canada*, 45–65. Toronto: Oxford University Press.

Coburn, D. (2004). Beyond the income inequality hypothesis: Globalization, neo-liberalism, and health inequalities. *Social Science & Medicine, 58*, 41–56.

Cornia, G.A. (2005). *Policy reform and income distribution, ST/ESA/2005/DWP/3*. New York: United Nations Department of Economic and Social Affairs.

Cypher, J.M. (1979). The transnational challenge to the corporate state. *Journal of Economic Issues, 13*(2), 513–542.

Deaton, A. (2004). *Health in an age of globalization*. Washington: Brookings Institution.

Dicken, P. (2003). *Global shift: Reshaping the global economic map in the 21st century* (4th ed.). New York: Guilford Press.

Elson, D. (2002). Gender justice, human rights, and neo-liberal economic policies. In M. Molyneux & S. Razavi (Eds.), *Gender justice, development, and rights*, 78–114. Oxford: Oxford University Press.

Elson, D. & Cagatay, N. (2000). The social content of macroeconomic policies. *World Development, 28*, 1347–1364.

Evans, R.G. (1997). Going for the gold: The redistributive agenda behind market-based health care reform. *Journal of Health Politics, Policy, and Law, 22*(2), 427–465.

Grieshaber-Otto, J. & Sinclair, S. (2004). *Bad medicine: Trade treaties, privatization, and health care reform in Canada*. Ottawa: Canadian Centre for Policy Alternatives.

Hertzman, C. (2000). Social change, market forces, and health. *Social Science & Medicine, 51*(7), 1007–1008.

Innocenti Research Centre. (2005). *Child poverty in rich nations, 2005*. Report Card No. 6. Florence: Innocenti Research Centre.

International Labour Organization. (1999). *Country studies on the social impact of globalization: Final report.* Geneva: International Labour Organization.

Jenkins, R. (2004). Globalization, production, employment, and poverty: Debates and evidence. *Journal of International Development, 16,* 1–12.

Kirby, M.J. (2002). *The health of Canadians: The federal role.* Ottawa: Standing Senate Committee on Social Affairs, Science, and Technology.

Labonte, R. & Schrecker, T. (2007a). Globalization and social determinants of health: Introduction and methodological background. Part 1 of 3. *Globalization and Health, 3*(5), 1–10.

Labonte, R. & Schrecker, T. (2007b). Globalization and social determinants of health: Promoting health equity in global governance. Part 3 of 3. *Globalization and Health, 3*(7), 1–15.

Labonte, R. & Schrecker, T. (2007c). Globalization and social determinants of health: The role of the global marketplace. *Globalization and Health, 3*(6), 1–17.

Langille, D. (2004). The political determinants of health. In D. Raphael (Ed.), *Social determinants of health: Canadian perspectives,* 283–296. Toronto: Canadian Scholars' Press Inc.

Leys, C. (2001). *Market-driven politics.* London: Verso.

Mazankowski, D. (2001). *A framework for reform: Report of the Premier's Advisory Council on Health.* Edmonton: Government of Alberta.

Millen, J.V. & Holtz, T.H. (2000). Dying for growth, Part I: Transnational corporations and the health of the poor. In J.Y. Kim, J.V. Millen, A. Irwin & J. Gershman (Eds.), *Dying for growth: Global inequality and the health of the poor,* 177–223. Monroe: Common Courage Press.

Millen, J.V., Lyon, E. & Irwin, A. (2000). Dying for growth, Part II: The political influence of national and transnational corporations. In J.Y. Kim, J.V. Millen, A. Irwin & J. Gershman (Eds.), *Dying for growth: Global inequality and the health of the poor,* 225–244. Monroe: Common Courage Press.

National Union of Public and General Employees. (2006). *Public-private partnerships: What they are, why they're a bad idea.* Retrieved from www.nupge.ca

Navarro, V. & Shi, L. (2002). The political context of social inequalities and health. In V. Navarro (Ed.), *The political economy of social inequalities: Consequences for health and quality of life,* 403–418. Amityville: Baywood.

Organisation for Economic Co-operation and Development. (2005). *Society at a glance: OECD social indicators 2005 Edition.* Paris: Organisation for Economic Cooperation and Development.

Petchesky, R.P. (2003). *Global prescriptions: Gendering health and human rights.* London: Zed Books.

Rachlis, M. (2004). *Prescription for excellence: How innovation is saving Canada's health care system.* Toronto: HarperCollins.

Raphael, D. & Bryant, T. (2006a). Maintaining population health in a period of welfare state decline: Political economy as the missing dimension in health promotion theory and practice. *Promotion and Education, 13,* 236–242.

Raphael, D. & Bryant, T. (2006b). The state's role in promoting population health: Public health concerns in Canada, USA, UK, and Sweden. *Health Policy, 78,* 39–55.

Raphael, D., Renwick, R., Brown, I., Steinmetz, B., Sehdev, H. & Phillips, S. (2001). Making the links between community structure and individual well-being. Community quality of life in Riverdale, Toronto, Canada. *Health and Place, 7*(3), 17–34.

Statistics Canada. (2004). *Income of Canadian families: 2000 census.* Ottawa: Statistics Canada.

Sutcliffe, B. (2004). World inequality and globalization. *Oxford Review of Economic Policy, 20*(1), 15–37.

Teeple, G. (2000). *Globalization and the decline of social reform: Into the twenty-first century.* Aurora: Garamond Press.

Williamson, J. (1990). *Latin American adjustment: How much has happened?* Washington: Institute for International Economics.

Woodward, D. & Simms, A. (2006). *Growth isn't working: The unbalanced distribution of benefits and costs from economic growth.* London: New Economics Foundation.

Yalnizyan, A. (1998). *The growing gap: A report on growing inequality between the rich and poor in Canada.* Toronto: Centre for Social Justice Foundation for Research and Education (CSJ).

Yalnizyan, A. (2007). *The rich and the rest of us.* Ottawa: Canadian Centre for Policy Alternatives.

CRITICAL THINKING QUESTIONS

1. What is economic globalization? What does it mean for the social determinants of health and health policy?

2. How can national governments, such as the Canadian federal government, resist global pressures?

3. What role can citizens play in challenging neo-liberal policies?

4. What are the supposed benefits of free trade agreements for Canadians? What are some of the threats to the health care system and the health of Canadians inherent within these treaties?

5. What are some of the reasons why governments agree to these trade agreements?

FURTHER READINGS

Grieshaber-Otto, J. & Sinclair, S. (2004). *Bad medicine: Trade treaties, privatization, and health care reform in Canada.* Ottawa: Canadian Centre for Policy Alternatives.

Jim Grieshaber-Otto and Scott Sinclair examine a recurring theme in Canada's health care debate: the role of private financing and for-profit delivery of health care. They explore Canada's international trade-treaty obligations and how these interact with this important issue. Available online at: http://www.policyalternatives.ca/documents/National_Office_Pubs/bad_medicine.pdf

Labonte, R. & Schrecker, T. (2007). Globalization and social determinants of health: Introduction and methodological background (Part 1 of 3). *Globalization and Health, 3*(5), pp. 1–10.

Labonte, R. & Schrecker, T. (2007). Globalization and social determinants of health: The role of the global marketplace (Part 2 of 3). *Globalization and Health, 3*(6), 1–17.

Labonte, R. & Schrecker, T. (2007). Globalization and social determinants of health: Promoting health equity in global governance (Part 3 of 3). *Globalization and Health, 3*(7), 1–15.

These three articles sketch out the implications of economic globalization for the social determinants of health. By doing so they bring to light the processes by which larger economic forces shape the form that health and health inequalities take in different nations.

Labonte, R. & Schrecker, T. et al. (2007). *Towards health-equitable globalization.* Geneva: WHO Commission on the Social Determinants of Health.

This is the final report of the Globalization and Health Knowledge Network of the Commission on the Social Determinants of Health. Available online at: www.who.int/social_determinants/resources/globlalization_kn_07_2007.pdf

Leys, C. (2001). *Market-driven politics.* London: Verso.

Market-Driven Politics is an analysis of global economic forces and national politics in two fields of public life that are both fundamentally important and familiar to everyone—television broadcasting and health care. Public services like these play an important role because they both affect the legitimacy of the government and are targets for global capital.

Navarro, V. (Ed.). (2007). *Neo-liberalism, globalization, and inequalities: Consequences for health and quality of life.* Amityville: Baywood Press.

This book assembles a series of articles that challenges neo-liberal ideology. Written by well-known scholars, these articles question each of the tenets of neo-liberal doctrine, showing how the policies guided by this ideology have adversely affected human development in the countries where they have been implemented.

RELEVANT WEBSITES

Globalization and Health
www.globalizationandhealth.com/articles/browse.asp
   The journal *Globalization and Health* publishes manuscripts that consider the positive and negative influences of globalization on health. *Globalization and Health* is affiliated with the London School of Economics.

Globalization and Health Equity
www.globalhealthequity.ca/welcome/index.shtml
   The Globalization and Health Equity Research Unit is established within the Institute of Population Health at the University of Ottawa. The research group examines how contemporary globalization (post-1980) is affecting social determinants of health and the health status of different population groups within and among nations.

Globalization Knowledge Network
www.who.int/social_determinants/knowledge_networks/globalization/en/index.html
   The network examines how globalization's dynamics and processes affect health outcomes. These include trade liberalization, integration of production of goods, consumption and lifestyle patterns, and household level income. The uneven distribution of globalization's gains and losses and the impact it has on inequities will be analyzed to inform policies aimed at mitigating the actual and potential harmful effects of globalization on health.

Progressive Economic Forum (PEF) Globalization Section
www.progressive-economics.ca/category/globalization
   The PEF aims to promote the development of a progressive economics community in Canada. The PEF brings together over 125 progressive economists working in universities, the labour movement, and activist research organizations. This site provides information about PEF, and its research and education products, and ways to contribute to its growth and success through membership, meetings and conferences, and their annual student essay contest.

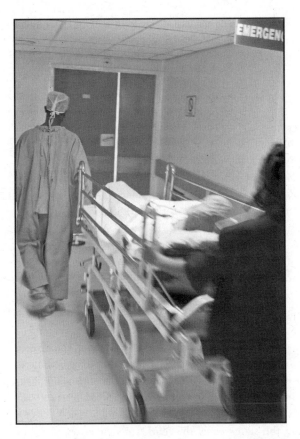

Chapter 12

THE FUTURE OF HEALTH POLICY IN CANADA

■ INTRODUCTION

This book has discussed several themes and issues for understanding current directions in health care and health policy in Canada and in other countries. These themes have identified various shifts in health policy since the development of the federal health care program—or medicare—in Canada from 1961 through to the present.

This chapter highlights the key issues and concepts discussed in the volume and their relevance for understanding health policy in Canada. As discussed, numerous forces have shaped health policy, including the health professions, pharmaceutical industry, and social movements. This chapter emphasizes the links between health and social policies and the efforts by Canadian governments to resist challenges to progressive health and social policies. It proposes future directions in health policy for consideration.

■ POLIS VERSUS THE MARKET

The polis versus the market has been an important theme throughout this volume. Chapter 1 distinguished between the polis or collectivist approaches and market-oriented approaches to public policy. The polis refers to an ideal political society in which citizens are engaged in the political process (Stone, 1988). They participate in decisions to ensure the social and economic security of citizens, and the well-being of the population as a whole. The market refers to a society in which individuals engage in exchanges to satisfy their welfare (Stone, 1988). People are in competition with one another to obtain basic goods and services. They try to obtain goods at the lowest cost to themselves.

Stone (1988) discusses how the market distorts the polis. The polis represents the ultimate political society in which the collective decides on issues that affect the society as a whole and shares risk across the population. In contrast, the market represents individualist approaches toward social and health policy issues. Market-oriented policies lead to an emphasis on individual responsibility for health, and hence a minimal state role in health provision as reflected in the biomedical and lifestyle approaches to health presented in Chapter 2.

The dichotomy between the state versus the market characterizes many of the current health care debates in Canada and elsewhere. The market focus seems to preclude consideration of broader health considerations and recognition that health policy is more than management of the health care system. The welfare state reflects a collectivist orientation in which society as a whole pays for provision of health care and other social programs to ensure all citizens have access.

■ THE KEYNESIAN WELFARE STATE

The welfare state—and the creation of a public health care system in Canada and other developed economies—represents a collectivist approach to health and social policy that characterizes the approach to public policy following the Second World War. The state is actively involved in health and social provision. The state intervened in housing, social services, and health care. In Canada, the first public health care program was established in Saskatchewan in 1947. The federal health care program, medicare, was established in 1966. Canadian medicare is a much-valued social program among citizens. It shares risk for health care costs across the population. Health care is paid for through general revenues, and thus is provided on the basis of need, not on ability to pay. Medicare and the other program components of the welfare state are redistributive measures in a society. They help redistribute wealth and other resources from high-income to low-income populations in Canada. As redistributive policy, it runs counter to the market and market-based policies.

Esping-Andersen (1990) devised one of the most used welfare state typologies to differentiate between social democratic, liberal, and conservative welfare regimes. Of the three regimes, social democratic regimes have the most generous health and social benefits as they have a commitment to reduce poverty and inequality. The Nordic countries are considered social democratic regimes. Conservative, also termed "corporatist," regimes (e.g., Beligum, France, Austria) emphasize the role of the family in social provision, but provide more generous benefits than liberal welfare states. The liberal welfare states are Canada, the United States, the United Kingdom, Australia, and New Zealand.

Of the all the liberal regimes, the United States is the only country without a public health care system. Some American employers provide health insurance benefits to employees, but employment no longer assures health insurance. As of 2005, almost 47 million Americans had no health insurance (National Coalition on Health Care, 2007). It would seem that the liberal regimes are more susceptible to neo-liberalism, which has seen a resurgence in recent years, and economic globalization, which requires minimal state involvement in health and social provision. Economic globalization and neo-liberal policies have been associated by many observers with the decline of the welfare state (Teeple, 2000). Esping-Andersen identified political ideology as an important determinant of the extent of the welfare state in a country.

In Canada, municipal governments usually have responsibility for public health. Provincial legislation specifies the mandatory services and programs that local public health units must provide. Mandatory programs comprise anti-tobacco, infant and maternal health, dental, school-based programs, infection control, and sanitation. In recent years, however, provincial governments have emphasized conservative approaches to public health, forcing a shift from community-based health promotion programs to biomedical foci on disease and infection control. These foci contribute to an emphasis on individual risk behaviours and individualized approaches to health intervention. Such approaches emphasize individual risk factors and individual lifestyle behaviour change to improve health.

■ INDIVIDUAL RESPONSIBILITY FOR HEALTH

The shift to market-oriented health care has driven the emphasis on individual responsibility for health as reflected in the biomedical and lifestyle perspectives on health presented in Chapter 2. The lifestyle perspective emphasizes personal behavioural changes as contributing to health. Governments frequently invoke the lifestyle and individual responsibility message to justify governments' reduced role in social provision. Governments admonish citizens to adopt healthy lifestyles that include exercise, nutritious diet, moderate alcohol consumption, and smoking cessation. Sarah Nettleton refers to these elements as the "holy trinity of risks" (Nettleton, 1997).

The lifestyle message is pervasive and is a top-down approach to health, emphasizing the expertise of the health professions and others to advise on a healthy lifestyle to reduce risk factors for chronic diseases such as cardiovascular disease and type 2 diabetes. When such is the case, the emphasis on lifestyle and individual responsibility excludes the social determinants of health such as income and employment security, housing, and education, among others. The lifestyle and biomedical approaches individualize health and justify the state's reduced role in health and social provision.

The dominant health message masks a larger issue that needs to be addressed if governments want to reduce health expenditures. The emphasis on individual risk factors and market-oriented health highlight the influence of neo-liberalism and economic globalization.

■ BARRIERS TO THE DEVELOPED WELFARE STATE: NEO-LIBERALISM AND ECONOMIC GLOBALIZATION

Neo-liberalism, as the dominant political ideology in Canada and other countries, has provided the rationale for economic globalization. Coburn and others define neo-liberalism as a market ideology that advocates an unfettered market as the source of all innovation and social provision (Coburn, 2000; Teeple, 2000). Neo-liberalism and economic globalization are not new ideas. Capitalism has always been global in character (McNally, 2006). What makes the current phase of neo-liberalism and globalization distinctive is the development of corporate monopolies and the concentration of vast wealth. It has led to increased commodification of health care. Health care is seen as an investment opportunity for foreign, private, for-profit health care providers.

Thus, the market has redefined public services and the role of government. It requires deregulation and hence a minimal government role and extols the virtues of an unregulated market in health care provision. Yet there is little evidence to support market proponents' claims that private care is better and more efficient. These developments have contributed to widening income gaps within so-called globalized economies and concomitant inequalities in health outcomes within the populations of these economies.

■ IMPACT OF TRADE AGREEMENTS ON HEALTH CARE AND HEALTH POLICY

The origins of the current emphasis on market strategies in health care have been attributed to the rise of neo-liberal policies, the dominant political ideology, and economic globalization (Teeple, 2000). In Canada, the United Kingdom, and other Western countries, market-oriented strategies have been adopted to reduce government expenditures on health, and ostensibly to preserve the public health care system. Market-based strategies include public-private partnerships (P3s); user fees for assorted health services; and allowing private, for-profit health care providers to deliver health care services. These changes are driven by the belief that allowing a parallel private health care system to develop will relieve some of the pressure on the public system. P3s represent a particular type of health care commercialization. Because they can cover a considerable range of health care services, they represent a risk that foreign corporations will bend important elements of Canadian health care policy by using trade policy rules to claim that Canada is depriving these foreign entities of a profit (Grieshaber-Otto & Sinclair, 2004). As noted, trade treaty rules, particularly NAFTA investment clauses, favour the rights of foreign investors.

There is much evidence, cited in this volume and elsewhere, that shows such measures reduce vulnerable, low-income populations' access to health care. For example, these populations will do without health care that they may need if they are required to pay user fees. Evans and others have shown that user fees and private health care in general are not cost-efficient and are inferior in quality compared to public health care services. Indeed, as discussed in Chapter 6, the single-payer system that is synonymous with Canada is cost-efficient and delivers higher quality care than private, for-profit care.

If medicare is fraying at the edges—with reports of long wait times for care or people being sent to the United States at provincial governments' expense for care that is not available in Canada—many have argued that its problems can be attributed to reduced federal transfers for health care to the provincial and territorial governments. It may also be an issue of resource allocation within the system. Canada ranks as one of the highest health spenders, so perhaps what is needed is better management of resources and rational approaches to treatment, professional responsibilities, and means of controlling costs such as those associated with pharmaceuticals (Lexchin, 2007).

■ GROWING INEQUALITIES IN HEALTH

Another important theme related to the theme of markets and the growth of health care markets in Canada and other countries is growing inequalities in health

Figure 12.1: Child Poverty in Wealthy Nations, Late 1990s

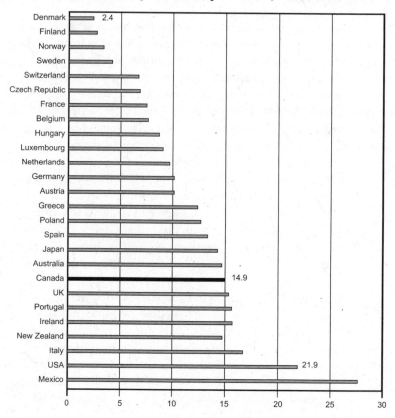

Percentage of Children Living in Relative Poverty Defined as Households with <50% of the
National Median Household Income

Source: Adapted from Innocenti Research Centre. (1999). *A league table of child poverty in rich nations* (p. 4). Florence: Innocenti Research Centre.

outcomes. Inequalities in health grow out of the shift from redistributive policies to market-based policies described above (Leys, 2001; Teeple, 2000). Indeed, health policy observers have attributed growing inequalities between the developed and developing world, and between rich and poor within developed economies such as Canada, the US, and the UK to economic globalization. Figure 12.1 shows the child poverty rates in different countries.

■ NEW INSTITUTIONALIST PERSPECTIVE ON THE PROSPECTS FOR HEALTH CARE REFORM IN CANADA: THE IMPACT OF CANADIAN FEDERALISM

From a new institutionalist perspective, institutions structure political debate and the range of solutions that policy-makers will consider to address public problems (Hall, 1993; Hall & Taylor, 1996). In health care, for example, Canadian federalism has sometimes led to innovations, as in the creation of medicare, but it has also resisted change (Hutchison, Abelson & Lavis, 2001).

Federal and provincial institutions can impede meaningful reforms of the health care system, particularly in relation to resourcing and managing medicare. The ongoing wrangling between the federal and provincial governments over financing of health care has led to little productive debate on how to change the system to improve and sustain Canadian medicare. The two levels of government, therefore, structure health care debate and can limit the range of solutions that will be considered to reform the system and improve service and health outcomes (see Box 12.1).

Box 12.1: Health Care's Cure Has Failed: Five Years on, Most of Roy Romanow's Plans to Fix Medicare Remain Unfulfilled
By Thomas Walkom
Toronto Star

Five-and-a-half years ago, Roy Romanow's far-reaching recommendations for medicare were heralded as a blueprint for the 21st century.

"The Romanow report will not gather dust on a shelf," then-prime minister Jean Chrétien vowed in late 2002, after the royal commissioner released his final report on the future of health care. "We will move quickly."

Indeed, the timing seemed right for quick, decisive action. The Canadian Medical Association, the country's main lobby group for physicians, was on side with most of Romanow's 47 recommendations. So were nurses, health-care unions and most premiers.

True, there were important dissenters. The governments of Alberta, Ontario and Quebec were hostile. Stephen Harper, then head of the opposition Canadian Alliance, dismissed Romanow's report as "pie-in-the-sky."

But polls showed that among the general public, the health-care commission report—with its description of medicare as an expression of Canadian values—struck a chord. For a while, the former Saskatchewan premier was treated as a kind of folk hero.

By 2004, Ottawa had pledged an additional $68 billion for health care over 10 years. The aim, the then-Liberal government said, was to finance the kinds of reforms Romanow was calling for.

Today, however, most of those bold reforms remain unfulfilled. Even Romanow is not sure how much his 18-month, $15 million commission accomplished. At times he seems darkly pessimistic.

On the one hand, he says, by resonating with the vast majority of Canadians who want medicare to continue, his 356-page report slowed down those who want to privatize the country's national health-insurance system.

But he is also clearly frustrated—at times almost bitter—about the failure of federal and provincial governments to capitalize on that popular sentiment.

During an hour-long interview with the *Toronto Star*, these warring sentiments keep bubbling to the surface. When he speaks of the "heartbreak and hopeful stories" he heard during months of public hearings, his eyes light up.

But when he turns to governments, his mood shifts. Searching for the right words, Romanow talks of how Ottawa and the provinces demonstrated "areas of inconsistency," how they cherry-picked some of his recommendations while ignoring others and how, in the end, the politicians emphasized "form over substance."

Even the most concrete reform to come from his report—the decision of governments to focus on reducing wait times in five specific medical areas—has been a mixed blessing, he says. Those who need help in those five areas, which range from cancer care to cataract surgery, may be better off. But the downside, Romanow says, is that wait-time reduction has become a surrogate for real reform.

"This five-guarantees concept was a kind of snazzy way of saying we're really moving on wait time, but it ignores the more substantive issues where heavy lifting is required," he says.

During months of hearings, Romanow heard countless pleas to protect the Canada Health Act, the federal statute that lets Ottawa financially penalize provinces that don't follow medicare standards.

Yet Ottawa still refuses to enforce the rules. In British Columbia, for instance, private clinics that allow wealthier patients to jump the queue operate with impunity.

"The Canada Health Act," says Romanow, "is almost becoming a dead letter of the law."

His mood darkening, Romanow ticks off the reforms that have not occurred. He recommended that Ottawa amend the Canada Health Act to specifically include limited home care and diagnostic tests as so-called medically necessary services. It didn't.

He recommended a limited national pharmacare program, as well as reforms to curb the accelerating cost of drugs. Nothing. He called on governments to tell voters how they spend health dollars. They still don't. He recommended that Ottawa give the provinces significantly more money for health care (which it did), but also that it insist this money be used for essential structural reforms (which it did not).

He is particularly irked by the failure of governments to deal with the massive health problems of aboriginal communities. "This is a blight on the nation," he says angrily.

"We are one of the richest nations in the world. Heartbreaking! There has been nothing."

It would be easy to dismiss his critique as the angry words of a commissioner peeved by governments' failure to heed his every word. Romanow is aware of this danger and keeps checking himself, qualifying his criticisms and offering rationales for what he clearly suggests was—and is—a fundamental political failure.

But his grim judgment is supported by the very body Ottawa set up to measure its progress on health reforms, the Health Council of Canada. It looked, for instance, at:

- *Primary care:* Romanow had recommended that provincial governments reorganize family medicine into teams so that doctors, aided by nurse practitioners and others, could provide seamless care for all, 24 hours of every day.

   In 2003, Ottawa and the provinces watered that down, promising instead that, within eight years, half of Canadians would have access to an "appropriate health-care provider." Yet in 2005, the Health Council reported Canada is unlikely to meet even this "modest" goal.

- *Record-keeping:* Romanow had recommended that governments computerize health records to make medicare more efficient and limit faulty prescribing. In 2004, governments promised to ensure that half the population had electronic health records within six years. Yet by 2007, only 5 per cent of such records were computerized.

- *Home care:* Currently, medicare covers only payments to physicians and hospitals. But increasingly, patients are being released early from hospital to recover at home. Romanow recommended that home care for the mentally ill, those recently released from hospital and those near death be covered by medicare, arguing this would be both fairer and—ultimately—cheaper.

Governments took this relatively modest proposal and whittled it down even further. "Home care is not the integral part of health care that Canadians deserve and expect," concluded the Health Council, in a report released this week.

Drugs: Romanow recommended that Ottawa cover half the cost for those who have to spend more than $1,500 a year on pharmaceuticals. Equally important, he made a series of recommendations aimed at curbing escalating drug costs—including changes to the Patent Act and the establishment of a national agency to negotiate prices with the big pharmaceutical firms.

Governments responded by promising to "take action" by 2006 and "develop a national pharmaceutical strategy." Yet, as the Health Council points out, even these limited goals haven't been achieved.

"We have not yet seen the nation-wide action to establish catastrophic drug protection that the accord promised," it says in this week's report. "The current patchwork of government drug plans leaves millions of Canadians with little or no protection."

To the Health Council, the major success story of the past five years involves government attempts to reduce wait times for heart and cancer patients, as well as those needing hip and joint surgery, cataract operations or diagnostic tests. Here, it says, there has been "real progress in some cases."

It also points out that Ottawa did keep its promise to give employment insurance benefits to those caring for sick relatives.

But in other areas, the council echoes Romanow's frustrations. It notes that while Ottawa announced a $200 million aboriginal health fund in 2004, three years later it had not spent any of this money.

And it says that, in spite of government pledges, there has been no progress made on another key Romanow recommendation, one that would have required provincial governments to explain to voters what exactly they get for their health-care dollars.

Even so, some analysts argue that the health-care commission was more successful than Romanow thinks. Most of his specific recommendations may not have been implemented. But, by badgering Ottawa to pay its historical share of health-care funding, he forced the national government back into the medicare game as a real player.

Moreover, at a crucial point in the political battle over health care, his report set the terms of debate.

"He helped to clarify the issues," says University of Toronto health policy analyst Raisa Deber.

Before Romanow, it was fashionable to decry medicare as both unfair and unaffordable. His commission reminded the country that national public health insurance exists in Canada because Canadians want it and because it works.

He quite properly dismissed those who fret about the so-called sustainability of government-financed health care by pointing out the obvious: We have to pay for our health care one way or another; if, as all the evidence indicates, we can get better results at a lower cost by pooling our money through government, then medicare is not a problem but a bargain.

There are few who think the Romanow exercise was an unalloyed success. Michael Rachlis, a Toronto physician and health-policy consultant who did some work for the royal commission, argues Romanow missed an opportunity to promote a comprehensive vision of medicare embracing both quality and prevention. "I don't think it accomplished a lot," says Rachlis.

But at the same time, Romanow's report and others effectively derailed those who would have completely dismantled Canada's public health-insurance system.

As University of Toronto law professor and health policy analyst Colleen Flood noted in an email, Romanow can take credit for "the fact that we have medicare as we know it (mostly)."

Now the debate has moved to a different level. The critics no longer take direct aim at what some used to call socialized medicine. Instead, they raise different questions: Should Canada's medicare system be more like that of, say, Germany? What is the role of the private sector in delivering medicare?

Even Harper, now the country's prime minister, says that medicare is here to stay.

Still, it is understandable that Romanow is weary of it all. A successful politician (he was premier of Saskatchewan for 10 years and one of the key architects of Canada's 1982 constitutional patriation), he has been ground down. After spending 18 months on the report and an additional three years proselytizing, he says he is deeply frustrated by the half-hearted response of his fellow politicians.

"I can't do any more," he says. "I'm tired. I'm beat."

Now, he focuses on the Canadian Index of Wellbeing, an effort to measure broad-based social progress. He's also a director of two Canadian corporations, including Torstar Corp., the company that owns this newspaper.

Five years ago, Canada was ready to reform medicare, he says. All that was missing was political drive at the top, the kind of drive exhibited by former prime minister Lester Pearson when he introduced national medicare 42 years ago.

"If you have a combination of political leadership and proper timing and a proper report, you have made a huge step in Pearson-like nation building," says Romanow. "A reformed health-care system would be a nation-building exercise for the 21st century."

That combination did not happen. During the Liberal years, the feud between Chrétien and his successor, Paul Martin, drained the government's energy. Today, Harper favours a strict-constructionist theory of federalism that gives his government little incentive to involve itself in social policies like health.

To Romanow this is all grim news. He is asked if the country missed its chance to fix medicare.

"Our chances have been drastically reduced, not missed entirely," he answers carefully. "But the window is closing ... I hope the inability of governments to do it doesn't stand as an example of Canada's diminishing will."

Source: Toronto Star (June 07, 2008), A1,A10.

This volume has lamented the continuous wrangling over health care between the two levels of government in spite of recent infusions of federal funds toward health care. Maioni describes health care as a "political football" (Maioni, 2003, p.52). The federal government has used health care to control how the provinces and territories use federal transfers, while at the same time paring back its contributions, which are so essential to maintain the health care system. While not the most important determinant of health and well-being, the lack of a public health care system denies access to quality health care for low-income populations and contributes to growing inequalities in health outcomes within a population.

The first ministers meet frequently to discuss health and social spending issues. As discussed in Chapter 10, they signed the Social Union Framework Agreement (SUFA) and the 2000, 2003, and 2004 health accords ostensibly to renew their commitment to social and health provision (Noel, St-Hilaire & Fortin, 2003). The purpose of these agreements was to restore the spirit of co-operation that characterized the relationship between the federal and provincial governments in the 1950s and 1960s when they cost-shared health care and other social programs.

On the heels of SUFA, the first ministers signed the 2003 Health Accord to target funding in key health care areas as recommended by Romanow in his report on health care reform (Romanow, 2002). Following Romanow's recommendation, the 2003 Accord created the Health Council of Canada to monitor the performance of the health care system.

The accord, however lacked accountability mechanisms and contained no restrictions on public funding that some provinces had allocated to for-profit health care operators. The 2004 Health Accord was a 10-year plan (Health Canada, 2006). In the accord, the federal government promised $41.3 billion in new federal transfers to the provinces and territories over 10 years (2004–2013) (Department of Finance Canada, 2007). The federal government will use the funding to enhance its ongoing financial contributions through the Canada Health Transfer. The 2004 Health Accord is also intended to tackle wait times and other outstanding health care issues.

In its report card on the performance of the Harper government, the Canadian Health Coalition assigns the Harper Conservatives in Ottawa a grade of D in its ability to resolve the issue (Canadian Health Coalition, 2008). It may very well be that the federal and provincial governments sign these accords with little consideration of the key issues that need to be addressed. As a result, these agreements may sometimes not lead to tangible results. This leads us to question the commitment of the two levels of government to address health care issues.

While not perfect, the health accords provide some direction on health policy. Most importantly, they recognize the government's important role in health care provision. The two levels of government must uphold the promises made in the accords if medicare is to survive the current debate. The SUFA and the Health Accords may provide a rallying point for civil society actors such as the labour movement, the health advocacy organizations, and others to lobby the federal and provincial governments to protect health care. Governments' recent inaction suggests that these accords need to be supported by concrete action by both levels of government (see Box 12.2).

Box 12.2: Health Care Renewal in Canada: Measuring up? What Governments Promised: A Summary

2003 First Ministers' Accord on Health Care Renewal

In February 2003, the prime minister and premiers signed an accord on health care renewal, worth $36 billion over five years. They pledged to increase access to health care providers, diagnostic procedures and treatments, home and community care services, and necessary drugs. They also agreed to establish the Health Council of Canada.

The 2004 10-Year Plan to Strengthen Health Care

In September 2004, the prime minister and premiers signed a second health care agreement which committed an additional $41 billion in federal funds over the next 10 years. In it, they reconfirmed their commitment to the principles of the Canada Health Act and also promised to collaborate, share best practices, and be accountable to the public with respect to the progress of renewal. The Health Council was given additional responsibilities to report on the health status of Canadians and on health outcomes.

Aboriginal Health Transition Fund

In September 2004, a special meeting of First Ministers and national Aboriginal leaders announced a $200 million Aboriginal health transition fund, to be created over five years. The fund was designed to improve the integration of federal and provincial health services, improve access to health services, make available health programs and services that are better suited to Aboriginal peoples, and increase the participation of Aboriginal peoples in the design, delivery, and evaluation of health programs and services.

2005 Annual Conference of Ministers of Health

At this conference, the ministers of health made a number of important commitments regarding drug coverage and pharmaceuticals management, including accelerating work on options for catastrophic drug coverage, developing a common drug review, and working toward a national formulary. As well, they agreed on a set of goals for improving the health of Canadians.

2005 Kelowna Accord and Blueprint on Aboriginal Health

In November 2005, a two-day summit of first ministers was held in Kelowna, British Columbia. At this meeting the federal government pledged $5 billion over five years to improve the lives of Aboriginal peoples in the areas of health care, housing, and education. The leaders from 19 jurisdictions, including the government of Canada, every province and territory, and five national Aboriginal groups (the Assembly of First Nations, the Inuit of Canada, the Métis National Council, the Congress of Aboriginal Peoples, and the Native Women's Association of Canada) agreed to the tenets of this commitment, subject to further discussion on the funding and how it was to be spent.

The Blueprint on Aboriginal Health, a 10-year transformative plan to help close the gap in health outcomes between Aboriginal peoples and the general Canadian population, was tabled at this meeting. The federal government committed to use the blueprint in creating Aboriginal health programs; since then, no funding has been committed to the blueprint by the federal government. As a collective, the provinces and territories have not indicated their commitment to the blueprint as their framework for the development or implementation of such programs.

2006 First Ministers' Conference

In the 2004 10-Year Plan to Strengthen Health Care, governments committed to establish a ministerial task force to develop and implement a national pharmaceuticals strategy (NPS), including coverage for catastrophic drug costs, and to report on progress by June 30, 2006. At the conclusion of the Council of the Federation meeting in St. John's on July 28, 2006, the premiers accepted a task force report on the NPS and directed provincial and territorial health ministers to release a report by September 2006 on the status of NPS and to "continue to work on key elements ... with a special focus on the Catastrophic Drug Program."

On September 21, 2006, the provincial and territorial ministers of health released a progress report. The federal minister did not participate in the release. The report recommended, among other things, that the task force focus further on policy, design, and costing analysis for options for catastrophic drug coverage.

Source: Health Council of Canada. (2007). *Health care renewal in Canada: Measuring up?*, p. 6. Toronto: Health Council of Canada.

■ FUTURE DIRECTIONS: HEALTH CARE REFORM

Reforming health care and health policy provide some avenues for altering government approaches to health and changing health policies to promote better health outcomes for the population as a whole. Many provincial efforts to reform the health care system have tended to focus on market-based strategies to the exclusion of public-based solutions.

Of the three main health reform reports, only Romanow recognizes public support for medicare. Romanow also argues that the public health care system is sustainable and urged moving forward to "transforming it into a truly national, more comprehensive, responsive and accountable health care system" (Romanow, 2002, p. xv). Romanow cites the considerable body of evidence that shows private care is frequently of poorer quality than public health care and less cost-efficient. Moreover, Romanow reiterates the need for a publicly funded and administered system while also recognizing the need to reform and improve the health care system. Further, Romanow notes that most Canadians are satisfied with the care they receive and see little need to privatize. He affirms the role of the state in health care provision.

As noted in Chapter 7, the health reform reports of Mazankowski and Kirby endorsed a larger role for local authorities in health (Kirby, 2002; Mazankowski, 2001). Governments have justified the adoption of commercial strategies that fundamentally restructure health care and their implications for accessing health care are presented, not only as necessary to reduce public spending, but as inevitable (Bakker, 1996). Governments in Canada, the United Kingdom, and other countries with public health care systems have deregulated or privatized elements of health care in order to save money. They also deregulate health care and other public services to attract investment and facilitate the process of commodification and maintain their competitiveness in the global economy (Leys, 2001). These changes may lead governments to reduce health expenditures to deal with moribund civil services. These actions, together with reduced senior government financing, appear to be elements of a larger agenda to meet the requirements of economic globalization.

Also discussed in Chapter 7, both Mazankowski and Kirby recommend privatization measures such as user fees for services in order to sustain the system and expanding the role of the private sector in health care delivery. Opting for private measures or an expanded role for the private sector is an ideological position. It prescribes roles and relationships for private institutions and government within a society. The private institutions identified to improve health care represent the market and market-oriented strategies such as user fees, medical savings accounts

(MSAs), and public-private partnerships (P3s). This orientation is consistent with Stone's (1988) market model. P3 arrangements involve transferring a public service to a private provider to design, build, and deliver. In the end, the new service will belong to a private corporation. Critics argue that once these arrangements are in place, it will be almost impossible to reverse these arrangements to bring these goods or services back into the public realm.

All three reports are concerned with sustaining medicare, but present very different solutions to ensure its sustainability. Mazankowski (2001) recommends user fees and medical savings accounts (MSAs) to reduce inappropriate use. Kirby (2002) recommends public over private funding, but also recommends MSAs for similar reasons to Mazankowski and devolution of health to regional authorities. Romanow unequivocally states that public funding makes the most sense and notes the lack of evidence that privatization will improve the quality of care. These and other aspects of the reports reflect different conceptions of society and how best to deliver health care.

Drawing on Stone's (1988) distinction between the polis and the market, it is clear that the market underlies Mazankowski's and Kirby's approaches to health care reform. Both imply that making the health care system run more like a private business will ensure its sustainability. They recommend market solutions such as medical savings accounts as necessary to ensure the sustainability of the system and make consumers more aware of the cost of health care.

In contrast, the Romanow Report reflects the polis in articulating the collective responsibility of Canadians to decide how to reform and sustain the health care system. Romanow does not consider health care a commodity to be bought and sold in the market, but rather as a public good. He cites evidence that shows that public health care provides better quality care compared to private health facilities and is less costly than private care. Romanow's perspective is also more consistent with the views of the Canadian public in the desire to preserve the system.

Maioni (2003) argues that unless the federal, provincial, and territorial governments understand their shared responsibility for medicare, Romanow's solutions may not be workable. She specifically describes federal-provincial relations as toxic, and therefore not conducive—and potentially detrimental—to addressing the problems of medicare and preserving it. She also makes an interesting argument about three reforms with respect to money: "more money, money better spent, and accountability for the money" spent on health care (Maioni, 2003, p. 51) (see Box 12.3).

There is also institutional resistance to expand the system not only to provide sufficient resources to support core functions of medicare, but also to expand the system's scope to include dental care, home care, and pharmacare, as recommended as early as 1964 by Emmett Hall's first report to the federal government. Mazankowski and Kirby only recommend catastrophic drug coverage and were opposed to expanding the scope of medicare to include home care and dental services (see Box 12.4).

Box 12.3: Health Coverage Still Falls Short, Report Finds

By Gloria Galloway
Globe and Mail

OTTAWA—Canadians still lack uniform access to medical essentials such as catastrophic drug coverage and primary care five years after the signing of a federal-provincial health-care accord to address those types of problems.

A report to be released today by the Health Council of Canada, the body created to track the progress of the accord, finds that key pledges in the document the first ministers signed on Feb. 5, 2003, have not been honoured.

"We characterize this as being a glass half full, half empty," Don Juzwishin, the Health Council's executive director, said yesterday in a telephone interview. "There are successes that are remarkable across the country—but they are pockets of success."

Five years ago, then-prime minister Jean Chrétien and the provincial and territorial premiers hammered out a plan to shorten waiting times for medical care and increase the number of family doctors. There was also consensus that there should be universal access to prescription drugs and home care. The deal came with an injection of $36-billion in federal funds over five years—and a second accord in 2004 offered an additional $41-billion over 10 years.

The Health Council report finds that some of the promises of those deals have been realized, including major purchases of medical equipment and improvements in the management of waiting lists.

But progress has been much slower in other areas and less collaborative than the accord envisioned, says the report. One problem area "is the catastrophic drug coverage and safe appropriate prescribing," Mr. Juzwishin said.

"The (2003) accord has promised that all Canadians, by the end of 2006, would have reasonable access to protection from financial hardship from the cost of pharmaceuticals. That hasn't happened. The National Pharmaceutical Strategy is very, very silent and so those issues that surround the prescription-drugs issue continue in limbo."

The accord also promised that all Canadians would have access to short-term, publicly financed home care. Many jurisdictions now offer two weeks of coverage, "but this is not adequate for what many people need," says the Council.

The report found progress in aboriginal health care is far from what the first ministers envisioned, the nationwide progress on the provision of primary care has been uneven, and the health-care work force has "serious mismatches" between the supply and demand.

In addition, the goal of having electronic health records for half of all Canadians by 2010 is going to be difficult, if not impossible, to reach. The records would make patients' health histories easily accessible by different doctors in different jurisdictions, promoting safety and more efficient care.

Federal Health Minister Tony Clement said yesterday that his government has made some systemic changes since the 2004 accord to address these problems. For instance, another $400-million has been invested in the electronic health record "and we attached those to some improvements we wanted to see in wait times," Mr. Clement said.

Source: Globe and Mail (June 4, 2008), p. A9.

Box 12.4: Health Accord Promises Not Being Met

The agency charged with monitoring and reporting on the quality of Canadian health care says provincial and territorial governments have not lived up to the promises they made in the health accords of 2003–04.

The Health Council of Canada, created in Dec. 2003 following the recommendations of Roy Romanow's Royal Commission on Health Care, says the jurisdictions have failed to create a system that allows health care access to be compared from province to province.

Under the 2004 health care accord, all provinces and territories except Quebec and Alberta agreed to create such measurable standards by the end of 2005.

The lack of compliance raises questions about whether the agreements should be regarded as binding contracts or merely agreements in principle.

In the 26-member council's second annual report, it says only four jurisdictions made public their plans to increase the supply of health care professionals by the end of last year. These were to include targets for recruitment and training.

The 2003 accord committed $36 billion in federal funds over five years, and the 2004 deal increased that amount by $41 billion over 10 years.

Council chair Michael Decter said the focus on wait times has led politicians to forget about quality, citing "adverse patient events" and regional disparities in care in the report, titled "Health Care Renewal in Canada: Clearing the Road to Quality."

It said Canadians spend an estimated 1.1 million unnecessary extra days in hospital due to such "adverse events," suggesting doing things right the first time would drastically improve wait times.

The Council also believes electronic health records should be available for all Canadians by 2010.

"I believe that many Canadians think that when they are in a hospital bed, or they're in an emergency or they're in a doctor's office, that that provider does have access to a great deal of information that they don't actually have access to," Decter said.

"There is a very fragmented paper system at the moment.

"If we're going to deliver quality care in the country, those people providing care have to know all the medications you are on, have to be able to know all the conditions you have, or it's a little too much of a hunt in the dark."

Council members were appointed by the participating provinces, territories and the Government of Canada. They come with a broad spectrum of health care experience including community care, Aboriginal health, nursing, health education and administration, finance, medicine and pharmacy.

Some of the Council's key recommendations include:

- To improve patient safety, make accreditation for health care facilities mandatory, a condition of public funding.
- Speed up the development of electronic health records.
- Strengthen legislation to ban all forms of direct-to-consumer advertising of prescription drugs in Canada.
- Create information systems that identify patients whose waits are becoming unusually long, triggering an audit.
- Increase the number of inter-professional teams providing primary health care beyond the goal set out in the 2003 and 2004 agreements, which currently call for 50 per cent of residents to have 24/7 access to health care teams by 2011.
- Address the needs of people without any drug coverage or without coverage that protects them from catastrophic drug costs.

Source: CTV News, updated February 7 2006, http://www.ctv.ca/servlet/ArticleNews/story/CTVNews/20060207/health_care_060207?s_name=&no_ads=

■ DEFICIT-REDUCTION DRIVEN HEALTH CARE REFORM

Of key dynamics that influence health care and health policy in Canada, chief among these is an emphasis on deficit reduction among Canadian governments since the 1980s (Maioni, 2003). The focus on deficit reduction and health care seems to have precluded consideration of alternative approaches to health care reform, in particular strategies that consider how to improve the health of the population in addition to concerns about health care.

Some concerns and perceptions of the public have shaped the debate about health care (Mendelsohn, 2002a). First, the Canadian public hears that the health care system as it is currently organized, i.e., public financing and private provision, is unsustainable. Second, the media and politicians propagate the view that the system is in crisis. Finally, the first two perceptions promote the argument that some form of privatization is the only solution to address the problems of the health care system.

In addition, Canadians support the five principles of the Canada Health Act and its core elements. While they perceive that the system has deteriorated since its inception and may need to change to reflect changing needs and technology in the health care field, they are concerned about losing medicare. They are willing to accept some modifications to ensure its sustainability into the future. Canadians, however, also have some contradictory views concerning two-tiered medicine (Mendelsohn, 2002a).

For example, as noted earlier in this volume, a public opinion poll that showed 33 percent of Canadians were prepared to accept two-tiered medicine, while 73 percent support the option of private facilities if they are unable to receive timely access in the public system (Mendelsohn, 2002b). What is driving these attitudes and perceptions about medicare and health care reform? It would seem that the media and politicians drive public perceptions about key health issues to achieve particular objectives. For example, they argue that long wait times in the public health care system is proof that medicare is not working (Sanmartin, 2004). This, in turn, justifies allowing a parallel private health care system to develop to meet health care needs.

■ NEW DIRECTIONS FOR HEALTH POLICY: SOCIAL DETERMINANTS OF HEALTH

As emphasized throughout this volume, public health refers both to healthy public policy, health care services, building strong communities, protecting citizens from environmental threats, and promoting healthy behaviours (Raphael & Bryant,

2006). Much of the emphasis since the Second World War has been on health care provision. Until the 1970s and 1980s, there had been little attention to social determinants such as housing, income, and education and their impact on population health and well-being. Yet the Canadian and other national governments developed housing and other programs to ensure that families and individuals were able to meet their basic needs (Myles, 1998). To reflect the interest in the welfare of the population, the federal government established the federal department Health and Welfare Canada. The department name recognized the close relationship between health and social policies in improving and maintaining the health of the population.

For several decades, Canadian governments and professional associations such as the Canadian Public Health Association emphasized the importance of the social determinants of health—that is, living conditions—and the importance of healthy public policies in promoting and maintaining the health and well-being of a population. The social determinants emphasize a model of health that is consistent with the political economy approach to health as defined in Chapter 2. The social determinants are the material conditions of living (or simply living conditions), such as income security, employment security, education, food security, housing security, and access to health care services, among others. The model conceptualizes health as related to social structures such as public policies that strongly influence health and well-being. The social determinants reinforce a belief in collective well-being and state or government provision of services such as health care, as in the Keynesian welfare state.

Moreover, an emphasis on social determinants requires public policies that will enhance population health. In short, the social determinants of health approach requires government intervention to ensure quality health and social programs and to maintain the health of a population. In addition, much research evidence supports a state role in improving the health of a population (Coburn, 2000; Deaton, 2004). Many lists of social determinants have been devised by such organizations as the World Health Organization and the Canadian Institute for Advanced Research. However, those lists that emphasize public policy as strong influences on the social determinants of health are most helpful in explicating the importance of a state role in health and social provision.

During the 1980s and early 1990s, Canada was a world leader in health promotion and innovative approaches to public health (Restrepo, 1996). Canadian researchers made significant contributions to health promotion principles of equity and participation, and the focus in the population health field on the determinants of health. The decade of the 1990s marked a departure from progressive approaches to public health. Canada now lags behind other countries in applying its own concepts for promoting health and well-being (Canadian Population Health Initiative, 2002). Behavioural and lifestyle approaches, as defined in Chapter 2, have become the new mantra.

Addressing the social determinants requires redistributive social policy changes. That is, policies that would redistribute wealth from higher-income groups to the poorest income groups. Health policy as defined in the social determinants of health approach is broader than merely being concerned with the health care system and the delivery of quality health care services across a population as is the focus in Canada. Health policy is also concerned with the determinants or influences on population health. The countries of northern Europe, such as Sweden and Denmark, recognize these important connections, have implemented policies that maintain high public spending on health and social services, and have been able to improve population health status. Canada has yet to learn this lesson about the importance of implementing redistributive policies to improve the overall health of the Canadian population. What are some of the barriers?

■ STATE ROLE IN HEALTH CARE PROVISION

The research cited in the previous sections underscores the important role of the state in managing and financing the system to ensure all citizens have access to health care services, but also in ensuring national standards. Such standards ensure that all citizens, regardless of where they live in a country, have access to high-quality health care services. When the national health care program in Canada was first established in 1961, governments were committed to cost-sharing the program to ensure universal access and a high quality of care. The reluctance to act highlights the political and economic forces that influence health policy in Canada. There is a need for guidance on the key issues affecting health policy and health care. It is important to consider public alternatives, which have been shown to be cost-efficient health care provision.

Moreover, intergovernmental relations must be more co-operative as they were at the creation of the Canadian welfare state. The federal and provincial governments must move beyond concerns of deficit reduction, and devise measures to strengthen medicare. Consistent with a social determinants of health approach, they must pursue prevention, a component that Tommy Douglas, the founder of Canadian medicare, stressed was key to its sustainability.

■ HEALTH COUNCIL OF CANADA

In his health reform report, Romanow recommended the creation of a health council to promote collaborative relations between the territorial, provincial, and federal governments (Romanow, 2002). The council would monitor the performance of the health care system and produce regular reports on its findings. Romanow considered the council to provide direction for preserving and improving the health care system (see Box 12.3). The council is independent of the federal and provincial governments and provides evidence on key indicators on the performance of the health care system.

In the 2003 Accord on Health Care Renewal, the first ministers created the Health Council of Canada and expanded its role in the 2004 Health Accord. It was part of the 10-year plan devised to support health care. The council provides regular reports on the development of health care renewal, the health status of the Canadian population, and the outcomes produced by the health care system. The council membership consists both of governmental and non-governmental representatives with experience in health, education, and finance. Its mandate is to report directly to the Canadian public on the process of implementing the 2003 and 2004 health care agreements.

The Health Council is unique in providing a national, comprehensive perspective on health care reform and reports annually to the Canadian public on the state of the Canadian health care system. Its mandate is to provide advice on how to enhance access to health care, the quality of health care services, and population health outcomes. As such, the council provides much-needed information on the performance of the health care system and the important role of the state in health and social provision for advocacy organizations to demand transparency and government action on health care.

■ THE ROLE OF CIVIL SOCIETY IN HEALTH POLICY AND DEMOCRATIC PROCESS

Many different forces and groups in civil society—such as the pharmaceutical industry, the health professions (particularly doctors), and others—act on the political system to influence health policy outcomes. Canadian social movements—such as the Canadian Health Coalition, the Ontario Health Coalition, the Canadian Centre for Policy Alternatives, and other civil society organizations—have played a critical role in health care and health policy by drawing attention to efforts to privatize health care services. They have provided public education on key policy issues that affect health care and health policy in general. Such groups advocate community-based health care to ensure accessibility for marginalized populations in Canadian society. They have also played a role in bringing health inequalities and the social determinants of health, and the impact of income distribution on health outcomes into health policy discourse in Canada.

Social movements and public policy organizations, such as the Canadian Centre for Policy Alternatives and the Canadian Policy Research Networks, play a critical role as well in ensuring government accountability to the population in protecting medicare. Social movements also play an important part in ensuring the democratic process and government accountability. These organizations need to be strengthened to ensure their continued vigilance of social and health issues that affect all Canadians and future generations of Canadians.

■ CONCLUSIONS

The volume has drawn attention to many key issues and tried to expand the understanding of health policy. Health policy is not simply about managing the health care system. It is also concerned with the government's role in improving and maintaining the health of the population.

Health policy is about power, politics, and process. It is driven by values and conflict among different groups in society about how government dollars should be spent on health issues. Health policy is as ideological as other public policy areas, if not more so. It is about intergovernmental relations and the capacity of the two levels of government to move beyond deficit-reduction health reform to resolve long-standing health policy issues through transparent deliberations that enable civil society actors to have input into how these issues should be addressed.

■ REFERENCES

Bakker, I. (1996). Introduction: The gendered foundations of restructuring in Canada. In I. Bakker (Ed.), *Rethinking restructuring: Gender and change in Canada*, 3–25. Toronto: University of Toronto Press.

Canadian Health Coalition. (2008). *Grading the government*. Ottawa: Canadian Health Coalition.

Canadian Population Health Initiative. (2002). *Canadian Population Health Initiative brief to the Commission on the Future of Health Care in Canada*. Retrieved from http://secure. cihi.ca/cihiweb/en/downloads/cphi_policy_romanowbrief_e.pdf

Coburn, D. (2000). Income inequality, social cohesion, and the health status of populations: The role of neo-liberalism. *Social Science & Medicine, 51*(1), 135–146.

Coburn, D. (2001). Health, health care and neo-liberalism. In P. Armstrong, H. Armstrong & D. Coburn (Eds.) *Unhealthy Times: The political economy of health and care in Canada*, 45–65. Toronto: Oxford University Press.

Deaton, A. (2004). *Health in an age of globalization*. Washington: Brookings Institution.

Department of Finance Canada. (2007). *Federal investments in support of the 10-Year Plan to Strengthen Health Care*. Retrieved from www.fin.gc.ca/FEDPROV/typhc_e.html

Esping-Andersen, G. (1990). *The three worlds of welfare capitalism*. Princeton: Princeton University Press.

Grieshaber-Otto, J. & Sinclair, S. (2004). *Bad medicine: Trade treaties, privatization, and health care reform in Canada*. Ottawa: Canadian Centre for Policy Alternatives.

Hall, P. (1993). Policy paradigms, social learning, and the state: The case of economic policymaking in Britain. *Comparative Politics, 25*, 275–296.

Hall, P.A. & Taylor, R.C.R. (1996). Political science and the three institutionalisms. *Political Studies, 44*, 936–957.

Health Canada. (2006). *Healthy Canadians: A federal report on comparable health indicators 2006*. Ottawa: Health Canada.

Hutchison, B., Abelson, J. & Lavis, J. (2001). Primary care in Canada: So much innovation, so little change. *Health Affairs, 20*(3), 116–131.

Kirby, M.J. (2002). *The health of Canadians: The federal role*. Ottawa: Standing Senate Committee on Social Affairs, Science, and Technology.

Langille, D. (2004). The political determinants of health. In D. Raphael (Ed.), *Social determinants of health: Canadian perspectives*, 283–296. Toronto: Canadian Scholars' Press Inc.

Lexchin, J. (2007). No excuse for denying drug coverage: It's time to end Canadians' long wait for pharmacare. *The CCPA Monitor 14*(7 Dec.), 1,6. Ottawa: The Canadian Centre for Policy Alternatives, National Office.

Leys, C. (2001). *Market-driven politics*. London: Verso.

Maioni, A. (2003). Romanow—A defence of public health care, but is there a map for the road ahead? *Policy Options, 24*(2), 50–53.

Mazankowski, D. (2001). *A framework for reform: Report of the Premier's Advisory Council on Health*. Edmonton: Government of Alberta.

McNally, D. (2006). *Another world is possible: Globalization and anti-capitalism*. Winnipeg: Arbeiter Ring Publishing.

Mendelsohn, M. (2002a). Canadians prepared to accept medicare reform in primary care, poll shows. *Policy Options* (November), 27–29.

Mendelsohn, M. (2002b). *Canadians' thoughts on their health care system: Preserving the Canadian model through innovation*. Saskatoon: Commission on the Future of Health Care in Canada.

Myles, J. (1998). How to design a "liberal" welfare state: A comparison of Canada and the United States. *Social Policy and Administration 32*(4), 341–364.

National Coalition on Health Care. (2007). *Facts on health care insurance coverage*. Washington: National Coalition on Health Care. www. nchc.org/facts/coverage.shtml

Nettleton, S. (1997). Surveillance, health promotion, and the formation of a risk identity. In M. Sidell, L. Jones, J. Katz & A. Peberdy (Eds.), *Debates and dilemmas in promoting health*, 314–324. London: Open University Press.

Noel, A., St-Hilaire, F. & Fortin, S. (2003). Learning from the SUFA experience. In S. Fortin, A. Noel & F. St-Hilaire (Eds.), *Forging the Canadian social union: SUFA and beyond*, 1–29. Montreal: Institute for Public Policy Research.

Raphael, D. & Bryant, T. (2006). Public health concerns in Canada, USA, UK, and Sweden: Exploring the gaps between knowledge and action in promoting population health. In D. Raphael, T. Bryant & M. Rioux (Eds.), *Staying alive: Critical perspectives on health, illness, and health care*, 347–372. Toronto: Canadian Scholars' Press Inc.

Restrepo, H.E. (1996). Introduction. In Pan American Health Organization (Ed.), *Health promotion: An anthology* (pp. ix–xi). Washington: Pan American Health Organization.

Romanow, R.J. (2002). *Building on values: The future of health care in Canada*. Saskatoon: Commission on the Future of Health Care in Canada.

Sanmartin, C. & Ng, E. (2004). Joint Canada/United States survey of health, 2002–03. Ottawa: Statistics Canada.

Savas, E.S. (2005). Privatization and public-private partnerships. Adapted from Privatization in the city: Successes failures, lessons. Washington: CQ Press. Online at: www. cesmadrid.es/documentos/Sem200601_MD02_IN.pdf

Stone, D. (1988). *Policy paradox and political reason.* Glenview: Scott, Foresman.

Teeple, G. (2000). *Globalization and the decline of social reform: Into the twenty-first century.* Aurora: Garamond Press.

COPYRIGHT ACKNOWLEDGEMENTS

Box 2.1 (part 2): "The Social Determinants 10 Tips for Better Health" adapted from Dr. David Gordon, "Alternative Tips for Better Health," Townsend Centre for International Poverty Research, London. Copyright © 1999. Reprinted by permission of the author.

Figure 2.1: From Grabb, *Theories of Social Inequality 4/E.* © 2002 Nelson Education Ltd. Reproduced by permission. www.cengage.com/permissions.

Figure 2.2: "Social Determinants of Health" by E. Brunner and M.G. Marmot in "Social Organization, Stress, and Health" from *Social Determinants of Health* edited by M.G. Marmot and R.G. Wilkinson. Copyright © 2006 Oxford University Press. Reprinted by permission of Oxford University Press.

Box 2.5: Reprinted from *The Lancet,* 11 May 2002, W. Kondro, "Poverty and Heart Disease," p. 1679. Copyright © 2002 with permission from Elsevier.

Figure 3.1: "Easton's Model of the Political System" from *A Framework for Political Analysis* by D. Easton. Copyright © 1965. Reprinted with permission of Professor David Easton.

Figure 3.2: "Introduction: The Contours of Social Exclusion," by J. Percy-Smith, in *Policy Responses to Social Exclusion: Toward Inclusion* (p.5), by J. Percy-Smith (Ed.), 2000, Buckingham, UK: McGraw-Hill

Box 3.3: D. Coburn, "Income Inequality, Social Cohesion and the Health Status of Populations: The Role of Neo-Liberalism" was published in *Social Science and Medicine* 51 (2000): 135–146. Copyright Elsevier 2003. Reprinted with permission.

Box 4.1: Hall, P.A. (1993). "Policy Paradigms, Social Learning and the State: The Case of Economic Policy Making in Britain." *Journal of Comparative Politics* 25(3), 175–196. Copyright © Journal of Comparative Politics. Reprinted by permission of the Journal of Comparative Politics.

Figure 4.1: From D. Raphael, *Social Determinants of Health.* Copyright © 2004 Canadian Scholars' Press. Reprinted by permission of Canadian Scholars' Press.

Box 4.3: "Editorial: Flawed Premise on Health-Care," *Toronto Star,* August 24, 2007.

Box 4.4: Adapted from P. Park, "What Is Participatory Research? A Theoretical and Methodological Perspective," in P. Park, M. Brydon-Miller, B. Hall, and T. Jackson (Eds.), *Voices of Change: Participatory Research in the United States and Canada.* Toronto: Ontario Institute for Studies in Education. 1993.

Figure 5.1: From "Convergence or Resilience? A Hierarchical Cluster Analysis of the Welfare Regimes in Advanced Countries" by S. Saint-Arnaud and P. Bernard, *Current Sociology* 51(5) (2003): 503. Reprinted by permission of Sage Publications.

Box 5.1: "Shocks and Public Policymaking" by Lenora Todaro from *The Best of 2007, Village Voice,* November 27, 2007, www.villagevoice.com/books/0749.asdf.78504.10.html/3. Copyright © Lenora Todaro. Reprinted by permission of the author.

Box 5.2: "Structural Change and Health Policy in Venezuela"

Muntaner, C., Salazar, R.M., Guerra, Benach, J. and Armada, F. (2006). "Venezuela's Barrio Adentro: An Alternative to Neoliberalism in Health Care." *International Journal of Health Services* 36:4, 803-811. Reprinted with permission of the Baywood Publishing Company.

Box 5.4: "Private Health Care in Quebec" by Josée Legault from *The Edmonton Journal,* February 24, 2008, A18. Originally appeared in *The Gazette.* Copyright © Josée Legault. Reprinted by permission of the author.

Box 5.6: An excerpt from "How Politics Pushed the HPV Vaccine" by Andre Picard originally published in the *Globe and Mail,* Saturday, August 11, 2007, A1, A11. Copyright

"Canadians Prepared to Accept Medicare Reform in Primary Care, Poll Shows," *Policy Options* 24(2) (2002): 27–29. Reprinted with permission of the Institute for Research on Public Policy. www.irpp.org.

Table 8.1: Excerpted from Figure5.2.1 *Health at a Glance 2007: OECD Indicators*, OECD 2007, www.oecd.org/health/healthataglance. Reprinted by permission of the OECD.

Box 8.1: "Private Health Care Legal but Unprofitable in Canada" by Sue Toye from *University of Toronto Bulletin*, March 22, 2001.www.news.utoronto.ca/bin1/010322d. asp. Copyright © 2001 University of Toronto Bulletin. Reprinted with permission.

Box 8.4: "Public-Private Partnerships" by H. MacKenzie from *Financing Canada's Hospitals: Public Alternatives to P3s*, www.healthcoalition.ca/3p.pdf. Copyright © 2004 Canadian Health Coalition. Reprinted by permission of the Canadian Health Coalition.

Box 8.5: Extracted from *Experts Tell Romanow Commission that Public Private Partnerships Are Not the Answer*. Copyright © 2002 Canadian Union of Public Employees. Reprinted by permission of the Canadian Union of Public Employees.

Box 8.6: Woolhandler, S., Campbell, T., and Himmelstein, D. U. (2003). "Costs of Health Care Administration in the United States and Canada." *New England Journal of Medicine* 349(8): 768.

Box 8.7: Excerpted from "No Easy Cure for Health Tax" by Thomas Walkom, *Toronto Star,* September 9, 2007. Reprinted with permission – Torstar Syndication Services.

Table 9.1: Gosta Esping-Andersen, *The Three Worlds of Welfare Capitalism.* ©1990 Gosta Esping-Andersen. Reprinted by permission of Princeton University Press.

Table 9.2: "Public Expenditurs on Health 1960–1990, percent of GDP" from V. Navarro and L. Shi (2001), "The Political Context of Social Inequalities and Health." *International Journal of Health Services* 31(1), 11–21. Reprinted by permission of Baywood Publishing Company.

Figure 9.1A: "Public Expenditure on Health as % of GDP, 2001"from *Social Expenditure Database* www.oecd.org/els/social/expenditure. Copyright © 2004 OECD. Reprinted by permission of the OECD.

Figure 9.1B: "Public Expenditure on Old Age as % of GDP, 2001   "from   *Social Expenditure Database* www.oecd.org/els/social/expenditure. Copyright © 2004 OECD. Reprinted by permission of the OECD.

Figure 9.1C: "Public Expenditure on Incapacity-Related Benefits as % of GDP, 2001" from *Social Expenditure Database* www.oecd.org/els/social/expenditure. Copyright © 2004 OECD. Reprinted by permission of the OECD.

Figure 9.1D: "Public Expenditure on Family as % of GDP, 2001"from *Social Expenditure Database* www.oecd.org/els/social/expenditure. Copyright © 2004 OECD. Reprinted by permission of the OECD.

Figure 9.2: "Average Percentage of Net Replacement Rates over 60 Months of Unemployment, for Four Family Types and Two Earnings Levels without and with Social Assistance, 2002" from *Society at a Glance: OECD Social Indicators 2005 Edition* (p.43) by Organisation for Economic Co-operation and Development (Paris, France). Copyright © 2005 OECD. Reprinted by permission of the OECD.

Figure 9.3: "Average Net Incomes of Social Assistance Recipients as Percentage of Median Equivalent Household Income, Married Couple with Two Children, 2001" from *Society at a Glance: OECD Social Indicators 2005 Edition* (p.45) by Organisation for Economic Co-operation and Development (Paris, France). Copyright © 2005 OECD. Reprinted by permission of the OECD.

Figure 9.4: "Net Incomes at Statutory Minimum Wages, Married Couple with Two Children as Percentage of Median Household Income, 2001" from from *Society at a*

INDEX